Hematologic and Oncologic Emergencies

HEMATOLOGIC AND ONCOLOGIC EMERGENCIES

Edited by

William R. Bell, M.D.

Edythe Harris Lucas-Clara Lucas Lynn Professor
Division of Hematology
Department of Medicine
The John Hopkins University School of Medicine
Director
Special Coagulation Laboratory
The Johns Hopkins Hospital
Baltimore, Maryland

Churchill Livingstone
New York, Edinburgh, London, Madrid, Melbourne, Tokyo

Library of Congress Cataloging-in-Publication Data

Hematologic and oncologic emergencies / edited by William R. Bell.
p. cm.
Includes bibliographical references and index.
ISBN 0-443-08871-3
1. Hematologic emergencies. 2. Oncologic emergencies. I. Bell, William Robert, date.
[DNLM: 1. Hematologic Diseases—complications. 2. Neoplasms—complications. 3. Emergencies. WH 100 H4833 1993]
RC636.H3845 1993
616.1'5025—dc20
DNLM/DLC
for Library of Congress 93-12498
CIP

Distributed in the United Kingdom by Churchill Livingstone, Robert Stevenson House, 1–3 Baxter's Place, Leith Walk, Edinburgh EH1 3AF, and by associated companies, branches, and representatives throughout the world.

Accurate indications, adverse reactions, and dosage schedules for drugs are provided in this book, but it is possible that they may change. The reader is urged to review the package information data of the manufacturers of the medications mentioned.

The Publishers have made every effort to trace the copyright holders for borrowed material. If they have inadvertently overlooked any, they will be pleased to make the necessary arrangements at the first opportunity.

Acquisitions Editor: *Robert A. Hurley*
Copy Editor: *Paul Bernstein*
Production Supervisor: *Jeanine Furino*
Cover Design: *Susan Fung*

Printed in the United States of America

First published in 1993 7 6 5 4 3 2 1

CONTRIBUTORS

William R. Bell, M.D.
Edythe Harris Lucas-Clara Lucas Lynn Professor, Division of Hematology, Department of Medicine, The Johns Hopkins University School of Medicine; Director, Special Coagulation Laboratory, The Johns Hopkins Hospital, Baltimore, Maryland

Hayden G. Braine, M.D.
Associate Professor, Departments of Medicine and Oncology, The Johns Hopkins University School of Medicine; Director, Hemapheresis Treatment Center, Department of Oncology, The Johns Hopkins Hospital, Baltimore, Maryland

Samuel Charache, M.D.
Professor, Departments of Medicine and Pathology, The Johns Hopkins University School of Medicine; Director, Hematology Laboratory, The Johns Hopkins Hospital, Baltimore, Maryland

R. Ben Dawson, M.D.
Professor, Department of Pathology, Associate Professor, Department of Medicine, Director, Blood Research Laboratory, University of Maryland School of Medicine; Director, Therapeutic Apheresis Center, Baltimore RH Typing Laboratory, Baltimore, Maryland

Thomas S. Kickler, M.D.
Associate Professor, Departments of Pathology and Medicine, The Johns Hopkins University School of Medicine; Associate Director, The Johns Hopkins Hospital Blood Bank, The Johns Hopkins Hospital, Baltimore, Maryland

Harvey G. Klein, M.D.
Chief, Department of Transfusion Medicine, National Institutes of Health, Bethesda, Maryland

Mabel Koshy, M.D.
Professor, Department of Medicine, University of Illinois College of Medicine; Director, Sickle Cell Clinic, Department of Hematology, University of Illinois Hospital, Chicago, Illinois

Michael W. Lankiewicz, M.D.
Fellow, Division of Hematology, Department of Medicine, The Johns Hopkins University School of Medicine, Baltimore, Maryland

Kathleen A. Leonard, M.D.
Senior Staff Fellow, Department of Transfusion Medicine, National Institutes of Health, Bethesda, Maryland

Maurie Markman, M.D.
Director, Cleveland Clinic Cancer Center and Chairman, Department of Hematology and Medical Oncology, The Cleveland Clinic Foundation, Cleveland, Ohio

Paul F. Milner, M.D.
Professor, Departments of Pathology and Medicine, Medical College of Georgia School of Medicine, Augusta, Georgia

Paul M. Ness, M.D.
Associate Professor, Departments of Pathology and Medicine, The Johns Hopkins University School of Medicine; Director, The Johns Hopkins Hospital Blood Bank, The Johns Hopkins Hospital, Baltimore, Maryland

Diane J. Nugent, M.D.
Director of Coagulation Research and Hemostasis-Thrombosis Program, Pediatric Subspecialty Faculty, Department of Hematology/Oncology, Children's Hospital of Orange County and Pediatric Oncology Research Center, Orange, California

Oscar D. Ratnoff, M.D.
Professor Emeritus, Department of Medicine, Case Western Reserve University School of Medicine; Physician, Department of Medicine, University Hospitals of Cleveland, Cleveland, Ohio

Alexander P. Reiner, M.D.
Senior Fellow, Division of Hematology, Department of Medicine, University of Washington School of Medicine, Seattle, Washington

PREFACE

Blood, the complex non-Newtonian fluid, the nutritional support system for the survival of all organs and associated tissues in the human body, is truly the essence of life. It is the biochemical communication network that facilitates the function of all cells. Primary defects in the blood are instantaneously sensed by all organs in the human body. The obvious possibility exists that any aberration in the blood could be promptly and systemically transmitted with the potential of extensive multiorgan damage.

The overwhelming majority of diseases of the blood require emergency attention. Alteration in the blood must be quickly reversed or the consequences of extensive cellular damage and death may result. For these reasons the authors of this text have made considerable effort to identify the most practical methods that should be employed to quickly and correctly identify various hematologic and oncologic emergencies and to enable their optimal expedient management. Thoughtful consideration has been given to maintaining a balance between the most recent scientific knowledge applicable to the situation and the most practical clinical approach.

The advances presented in this text have been derived from insights into the pathophysiology and pathogenesis of hematologic and oncologic disease processes. All contributors have tried to enable the reader to remain current in those areas where new discoveries have induced an explosively expanding mass of information and knowledge. We are not pretending that the information herein is complete and final. Controversy still exists and new discoveries will be forthcoming. However, the reader will recognize a consensus, not disagreement, among the contributors to this text. A reasonably extensive bibliography that is current and, where possible, restricted to available journals, follows each chapter. This will provide for the interested reader more detailed supportive information that in some instances is abstruse and accompanied by considerable controversy.

All contributors to the text dedicate their efforts to their wives, children, and loved ones. Special thanks to Jean Propf, who typed and retyped several of the manuscripts and who coordinated this effort.

William R. Bell, M.D.

CONTENTS

1

THE MANAGEMENT OF ACUTE EPISODES OF BLEEDING

OSCAR D. RATNOFF

The treatment of acute episodes of bleeding in patients with hemostatic defects is as diverse as the underlying disorders themselves. A bleeding tendency may reflect inborn or acquired disease or a combination thereof. This chapter concerns the care of patients with relatively commonplace complications of a bleeding tendency.

Although patients with hemostatic defects may bleed so severely that they die of exsanguination, this is, in fact, distinctly rare. Much more often they sustain localized bleeding that creates temporary or permanent tissue damage. Joint damage from recurrent bleeding may be so extensive in severe hemophilia that the patient may be permanently crippled; this is so prominent a feature of hemophilia that in the mid-nineteenth century this disorder was classified as a rheumatic disease.

The logical treatment of patients with hemostatic defects may then include measures to control potentially dangerous bleeding, correct deficiencies of clotting factors, and prevent or ameliorate tissue damage. Repair of the deficiency of a clotting factor requires some concept of the concentration in plasma of this factor that will provide hemostasis and of the rate at which an infused clotting factor disappears from plasma (i.e., the rate of its catabolism) (Table 1-1).

Repair of the deficiency of a clotting factor requires knowledge of the concentration in plasma that will provide hemostasis and of the rate at which an infused clotting factor disappears from the plasma (i.e., the rate of catabolism of a given procoagulant factor).

To be administered effectively in the treatment of patients with hemostatic defects, plasma or its fractions must be deficient in isohemagglutinins that might be expected to induce hemolytic reactions or must be given in a type-specific manner. Needless to say, precautions must be taken in the preparation of plasma or its fractions to minimize transmission of bloodborne infectious agents. And, in preparation for surgery or dental extraction, the patient's plasma must be tested for circulating anticoagulants (i.e., autoantibodies) against the patient's deficient factor.

TABLE 1-1. Plasma Concentration and Biologic Half-Life of Some Plasma Hemostatic Factors

Factor	Concentration (mg/dL)	Hemostatic Level	Biologic Half-Life
Fibrinogen (factor I)	200–400	100 mg/dl	3–4 days
Prothrombin	12–15	40–50%	3 days
Factor VII	0.05–0.06	20%	4–5 h
Proaccelerin (factor V)	0.4–1.4	25%	15–30 days
Stuart factor (factor X)	0.7–1.2	10%	24–36 h
Antihemophilic factor (factor VIII)	0.005–0.015	30%	10–12 h
von Willebrand factor	0.5–1.0	?	10–24 h
Christmas factor (factor IX)	0.3–0.5	10–25%	18–24 h
Plasma thromboplastin antecedent (factor XI)	0.4–0.6	< 20%	2–3 days
Hageman factor (factor XII)	1.5–4.5	0%	2 days
Plasma prekallikrein	3.5–4.5	0%	35 h
High-molecular-kininogen	8–9	0%	6 days
Fibrin-stabilizing factor (factor XIII)	1–2	10%	11–12 days

The titer of clotting factors in a patient's plasma and in the plasma or plasma fractions used in the treatment is standardized in comparison with pooled normal plasma (1 ml of which contains 1 U of each clotting factor). The only exception is plasma fibrinogen, which is measured on a weight basis.

The titer of clotting factors in the patients' plasma and in the plasma or plasma fractions used in treatment is standardized in comparison with pooled normal plasma, 1 ml of which is said to contain one unit (U) of each clotting factor except for fibrinogen, which is measured gravimetrically, and calcium ions, which cannot be measured in plasma samples because of the presence of citrate ions.

SOME HEMOSTATIC AGENTS DERIVED FROM BLOOD

Early in the nineteenth century the British surgeon Lane reported that transfusion of blood controlled the abnormal bleeding of a boy who, in retrospect, may have had hemophilia.[1] No substantial progress in the treatment of hemorrhagic disorders ensued until 1925, when Feissly[2] reported that transfusion of normal plasma shortened the clotting time of patients with hemophilia. Plasma transfusions, however, did not come into common use until the 1940s and 1950s with the development of blood banking and the capacity to store plasma in the frozen condition.[3] Fresh-frozen, pooled normal plasma contains all the plasma clotting factors and inhibitors, but its titers of coagulant antihemophilic factor (factor VIII) and proaccelerin (factor V) are usually significantly less than those of freshly prepared unfrozen plasma. Plasma is still useful when no safe and reliable plasma fraction is available or, as in hepatic disease, when the patient may have multiple defects. Plasma is also helpful in controlling bleeding complicating oral anticoagulant therapy. In all these situations a commonly used dose in adults is 1,000 ml, administered intravenously, followed by 500 ml every 12 hours; exceptionally in the case of a deficiency of fibrin-stabilizing factor (factor XIII), 500 ml every 48 hours should provide adequate hemostasis.

In the mid-1930s Patek and Stetson[4] and Patek and Taylor[5] corrected the clotting defect of a patient who, in modern terms, had classic hemophilia (hemophilia A, factor VIII deficiency) by transfusion of a crude fraction of normal plasma. Their reports marked the beginnings of modern replacement therapy, whereby patients with deficiencies of clotting factors are infused with appropriate fractions of plasma or with purified clotting factors synthesized by recombinant DNA technology.

Patek's crude antihemophilic factor (factor VIII) was not a practical solution to the problem of bleeding in hemostatic disorders. The first practical agent for treatment of classic hemophilia was so-called Cohn fraction I, a fraction precipitated from plasma by addition of ethanol to a concentration of 8 percent.[6] Cohn fraction I proved to be unsatisfactory in the treatment of hemophilia because its content of antihemophilic factor varied widely from lot to lot and because, being made from pools of the plasmas of many donors, it often transmitted hepatitis to its recipients. Moreover, Cohn fraction I was ineffective in patients with the clinically identical disorder Christmas disease (hemophilia B, factor IX deficiency), which was not distinguished from classic hemophilia until 1952.

The spur provided by the use of Cohn fraction I led to the development of techniques that made possible treatment of hemostatic disorders with appropriate fractions of plasma. By the mid-1960s two techniques were devised that radically changed the care of patients with classic hemophilia. Pool and her associates[7] found that a crude, insoluble precipitate remaining after frozen plasma was allowed to thaw at refrigerator temperatures was rich in antihemophilic factor and that such cryoprecipitates could be used therapeutically. Cryoprecipitates are also rich in fibrinogen and are currently the only practical source of this protein; each bag contains 200 to 250 mg of fibrinogen on the average.[8] At about the same time that Pool et al.'s studies were made, Wagner et al.[9] and Webster et al.[10] initiated studies that evolved into methods for the preparation of lyophilized purified antihemophilic factor (factor VIII). These preparations made possible self-treatment of minor hemorrhages by patients with classic hemophilia.

Both cryoprecipitates and these early lyophilized concentrates of antihemophilic factor (factor VIII) were relatively crude. Further purification was difficult because coagulant antihemophilic factor, the agent deficient in classic hemophilia, circulates in noncovalent combination with another protein, von Willebrand factor, the agent deficient in von Willebrand disease. Zimmerman[11] put this noncovalent complex to good use to purify factor VIII. He prepared murine monoclonal antibody against von Willebrand factor and attached it to an insoluble matrix. He then prepared a column of the insolubilized antibody and trickled through the column a source of the antihemophilic factor–von Willebrand factor complex, for example, Pool et al.'s cryoprecipitate. The complex adsorbed on the insolubilized antibody was freed of contaminating proteins by washing the column, and factor VIII was then separated from the immobilized, adsorbed von Willebrand factor. The highly purified antihemophilic factor (factor VIII) prepared in this way could be lyophilized and then used therapeutically. Variations of this technique have been used by different manufacturers. Most recently, highly purified factor VIII has been prepared by recombinant DNA technology.[12,13] Notably, the earliest preparations of factor VIII contained both the coagulant (factor VIII) and von Willebrand factor portions of the factor VIII–von Willebrand factor complex, allowing treatment of both classic hemophilia and von Willebrand disease. This advantage has been lost in most but not all of the more recent purified products; Humate-P (Armour Pharmaceutical Co.), Profilate HP (Alpha Therapeutic Corp.), and Koate-HS (Miles-Cutter) are products available in the United States that are said to contain therapeutic amounts of von Willebrand factor, but thee products may not be able to correct the prolonged bleeding time of patients with von Willebrand disease in a sustained fashion.[14]

After infusion of factor VIII, the patient should be watched closely for evidence of a hypersensitivity reaction; should this occur, diphenhydramine hydrochloride (Benadryl), in a dosage in adults of 50 mg by mouth, may be helpful. Administration of Benadryl in advance of treatment may be a useful prophylactic measure in patients who have had hypersensitivity reactions.

The development of other plasma fractions followed a

parallel course. Deficiencies of the vitamin K-dependent clotting factors [prothrombin, factor VII, Christmas factor (factor IX), and Stuart factor (factor X)] were first treated solely by transfusion of plasma. Later, the vitamin K-dependent factors were partially purified (without separating one from another) by adsorbing them to insoluble salts of certain cations or on diethylaminoethyl cellulose or Sephadex.[15,16] These prothrombin complex preparations in lyophilized form have been used to repair acquired or hereditary deficiencies of each of these factors[17,18]; however, their efficacy as agents for replacement therapy varies. For example, Proplex T (Baxter-Hyland) is reportedly more effective than other preparations in correcting severe factor VII deficiency. Unfortunately, use of the prothrombin complex preparations has been accompanied by thrombotic events or myocardial necrosis,[19,20] which may be due to the presence of activated clotting factors in the preparations. Two deliberately activated preparations, Autoplex T and factor VIII inhibitor bypassing activity (FEIBA), have been made available for the sole purpose of treating patients with antibodies against clotting factors (i.e., circulating anticoagulants). More recently, monoclonal antibody–purified and nonimmunologic affinity–purified Christmas factor (factor IX) have been introduced for the care of patients with Christmas disease,[21,22] as well as plasma-derived or recombinant activated factor VII (factor VIIa) for treatment of patients with circulating anticoagulants against factor VIII.[23,24]

A major problem in the use of blood products has been the transmission of viruses pathogenic for humans, including the viruses responsible for hepatitis, the acquired immunodeficiency syndrome (AIDS), and parovirus infection.[25] More careful donor selection, testing of blood or plasma products for possible viral contamination, and virucidal treatment of plasma fractions with heat, organic solvents, or both have greatly reduced but not totally eliminated the risk of transmission of these agents. Ideally, the effectiveness of infusions of the various clotting factors can be monitored by measuring the titer of the appropriate agent in the patient's plasma. When the patient is being prepared for elective surgery, this may be a practical measure, but in the stress of an emergency, quantitative assays may not be immediately available. A satisfactory way to monitor therapy in many patients with classic hemophilia, von Willebrand disease, or Christmas disease is to measure its effect upon the patient's abnormally long partial thromboplastin time with use of a published nomogram[26] (Table 1-2). The values obtained by interpolation into this nomogram have been remarkably accurate when compared with quantitative assays.

A technique to monitor therapy in patients with classic hemophilia, von Willebrand disease, or Christmas disease is to measure its effect upon the patient's abnormally prolonged activated partial thromboplastin time.

TABLE 1-2. Partial Thromboplastin Time of Normal Plasma Serially Diluted With Plasma of Patients with Hereditary Deficiencies of Individual Clotting Factors[a]

	Partial Thromboplastin Time (s) (% increase in aPTT)								
Percent Normal Plasma	100%	90%	80%	60%	50%	40%	20%	10%	0%
Hageman factor (factor XII)	44.5	48.6 (9%)	49.5 (11%)	53.7 (21%)	54.8 (23%)	55.9 (26%)	69.0 (56%)	85.0 (91%)	>300 (>500%)
Prekallikrein	45.4	45.1 (0%)	46.5 (2%)	48.8 (7%)	48.8 (7%)	51.8 (14%)	53.2 (17%)	60.1 (32%)	>300 (>500%)
HMW-kininogen	45.1	46.3 (2%)	45.4 (0%)	45.9 (1%)	46.1 (2%)	48.1 (6%)	49.6 (10%)	57.0 (26%)	>300 (>500%)
PTA (factor XI)	46.3	46.6 (0.6%)	48.1 (4%)	49.2 (6%)	51.0 (10%)	53.1 (15%)	59.0 (27%)	64.4 (39%)	119.5 (158%)
Christmas factor (factor IX)	45.1	49.9 (11%)	51.2 (14%)	52.4 (16%)	54.1 (20%)	54.1 (20%)	60.2 (33%)	69.2 (53%)	122.2 (170%)
Antihemophilic factor (factor VIII)	43.4	45.2 (4%)	45.9 (5%)	49.2 (13%)	49.8 (15%)	53.0 (22%)	62.6 (44%)	79.2 (82%)	141.6 (226%)
Stuart factor (factor X)	46.6	50.6 (8%)	50.7 (8%)	54.1 (16%)	55.3 (19%)	64.8 (39%)	71.4 (53%)	88.2 (89%)	154.7 (232%)
Proaccelerin (factor V)	47.5	47.5 (0%)	49.7 (4%)	50.5 (6%)	52.9 (11%)	52.9 (11%)	58.7 (23%)	62.0 (30%)	186.9 (293%)
Prothrombin	47.5	48.8 (2%)	49.6 (4%)	50.2 (5%)	50.2 (5%)	52.2 (9%)	53.9 (13%)	59.6 (25%)	84.2 (77%)
Fibrinogen	46.7	47.5 (1%)	49.5 (5%)	51.1 (9%)	51.8 (10%)	52.8 (13%)	55.2 (18%)	63.9 (36%)	>300 (>500%)

Abbreviations: aPTT, activated partial thromboplastin time; HMW, high molecular weight; PTA, plasma thromboplastin antecedent.

[a] aPTT of mixtures of normal plasma and plasmas deficient in single clotting factors. The values in parentheses represent the percent increase in the aPTT brought about by the indicated reduction in the concentration of each factor.

(From Gordon et al.,[26] with permission.)

SOME OTHER HEMOSTATIC AGENTS

DDAVP

The vasopressin analog, 1-desamino-8-D-arginine vasopressin (DDAVP, Stimate), increases the plasma concentration of the factor VIII–von Willebrand factor complex in normal subjects whether administered intravenously, subcutaneously, or by nasal spray.[27–31] A common assumption is that DDAVP directly or indirectly releases the factor VIII–von Willebrand factor complex from its bodily stores, particularly vascular endothelium. This property suggested the use of DDAVP as a hemostatic agent in patients with mild classic hemophilia (factor VIII deficiency) or von Willebrand disease.[32,33] Although DDAVP is indeed effective in these disorders, its use has been complicated by disturbing side effects, perhaps as a result of hyponatremia, which include convulsions in infants and thrombotic events in adults.

DDAVP is not helpful in patients with Christmas disease (factor IX deficiency) or with deficiencies of other clotting factors.

Ascorbic Acid (Vitamin C)

Although scurvy is now rare in developed countries, the unremitting plagues of starvation that persists in some of the world's areas reminds us that this disorder has undoubtedly been responsible more than any other for severe acute and chronic bleeding. Although gastrointestinal or intracranial bleeding may be fatal, much more to be feared is unexpected sudden death. Scurvy is therefore a true medical emergency, and if this diagnosis is entertained, the patient should be treated with 250 mg of ascorbic acid daily without waiting until the results of assays for vitamin C are available.[34]

Antifibrinolytic Agents

ε-Aminocaproic acid (EACA, Amicar) and tranexamic acid (AMCA, Cyclokapron) are antifibrinolytic agents, which act primarily by inhibiting the conversion of plasminogen to plasmin, a potent plasma fibrinolytic enzyme. As will be described, they are useful in preventing bleeding after dental extraction in patients with hereditary hemorrhagic disorders. These agents have also been used to decrease blood loss after prostatectomy.[35] Oral antifibrinolytic agents have also been recommended to control bleeding in patients with amegakaryocytic or immune thrombocytopenic purpura.[36–38]

ACUTE BLOOD LOSS IN PATIENTS WITH HEREDITARY BLEEDING DISORDERS

As noted earlier, severe blood loss is a relatively infrequent problem in patients with hereditary hemostatic disorders, particularly classic hemophilia or Christmas disease, although fear of this complication compounds the anxieties of patients and their families. Blood loss can be external, from trauma (occasionally self-inflicted), or into the soft tissues or body cavities, in which case the trauma may not be recognized or recalled by the patient. Massive bleeding may also occur from peptic ulcer or from esophageal varices, sometimes the result of the hepatic complications of therapy. Blood loss should be treated as in other patients by local control by pressure over open blood vessels and by maintenance of blood volume through transfusion of packed red blood cells and if necessary solutions of electrolytes. At the same time, the specific hemostatic defect should be corrected to the extent possible (e.g., by infusion of lyophilized monoclonal antibody-purified factor VIII or IX). In severe classic hemophilia, an infusion of 50 units of factor VIII per kilogram of body weight (U/kg) will raise the plasma titer of factor VIII by 100 U/dl (i.e., enough to bring the coagulant titer of factor VIII to that of the average normal individual). The same regimen is appropriate for patients with severe Christmas disease, using infusions of Christmas factor (factor IX) rather than antihemophilic factor (factor VIII). If the patient is actively bleeding, supplementing the initial infusion with half the dosage after each half-disappearance time may not be sufficient to maintain a normal titer; if possible, the original dose should be repeated.

In the treatment of a patient who is actively bleeding, supplementation of the initial infusion with half the initial dose after each half-disappearance time may not be sufficient to maintain a normal titer; if possible, the original full dose should be repeated.

Severe blood loss that threatens exsanguination is distinctly uncommon in patients with other hereditary disorders of clotting. When it occurs, in addition to transfusion of red blood cells to sustain the peripheral circulation, intravenous infusions of plasma may help to correct the hemostatic defect; these may have to be repeated if blood loss continues to be a problem. An initial dosage of 1 L of plasma followed by 500 ml every 6 to 12 hours may control a hemostatic defect, but of course this does not raise the titer of the deficient factor to normal levels. If hemostasis does not ensue and the presence of a circulating anticoagulant can be excluded, there are two other approaches, namely, to use larger volumes of plasma while administering a diuretic to shrink the plasma volume and to perform exchange transfusion with normal plasma. Clearly, neither of these expedients is a happy choice.

In the exceedingly rare instance of congenital afibrinogenemia, transfusion of cryoprecipitates may promote hemostasis. Each bag of cryoprecipitate contains, on the average, 200 to 250 mg of fibrinogen.[8] Transfusion of one bag of cryoprecipitate for every 2 kg of body weight will raise the plasma fibrinogen level by about 200 to 250 mg/dl, safely above the level required for hemostasis. Fibrinogen is catabolized relatively slowly, but if continued blood loss occurs, the infusions may have to be repeated. Although means for determining fibrinogen levels are readily available at some hospitals, in others one may take advantage of the fact that the prothrombin time and partial thromboplastin time may be elevated by severe hypofibrinogenemia, giving a crude guide to therapy.

Transfusion of one bag of cryoprecipitate for every 2 kg of body weight will raise the plasma fibrinogen level by about 200 to 250 mg/dl, which is more than adequate to maintain hemostasis.

OTHER FORMS OF ACUTE BLEEDING IN DISORDERS OF HEMOSTASIS

Intracranial Bleeding

By all odds the most frightening problem in patients with hemostatic defects is intracranial bleeding, which in only about half the cases is attributable to overt head trauma.[39–41] A contrary view, that in about half of cases there is no evidence of trauma, has been expressed.[40] Relatively speaking, the rare disorders, deficiencies of congenital factor VII and factor XIII (fibrin-stabilizing factor), are probably those most likely to be complicated by lethal intracranial hemorrhage.[42] Patents or their families should be warned about the dangers of head trauma and the need to be alert to such symptoms as visual changes, severe headache, or coma.[43] In my experience automobile accidents have been the most frequent cause of intracranial bleeding. One severely disturbed patient with a circulating anticoagulant deficiency complicating severe classic hemophilia repeatedly banged his head against a wall, presumably to induce lethal bleeding or to call attention to himself. To minimize automobile injuries the use of over-the-shoulder seat belts should be repeatedly stressed; I do not know whether air bags will add safety in this specific situation, but their use seems sensible.

Patients with known hemostatic defects should be taught to treat even the slightest head injury as potentially dangerous, and they should immediately go to their physician, hemophilia clinic, or emergency room for care. If they are in a home therapy program and the injury seems minor, before they come to the hospital they should as soon as possible self-administer the appropriate clotting factor at a level that will bring the titer of the deficient factor to 100 percent of normal (e.g., 50 U/kg of factor VIII or factor IX). The same dosage should be used if the patient presents with head injury at a treatment site. Treatment should be

Patients with known hemostatic defects should be taught to treat even the slightest head injury as potentially dangerous, and they should immediately obtain the services of their physician, the hemophilia clinic, or the emergency room for care.

continued for at least 1 week.[40] Because the increased plasma volume produced by infusions is dangerous in individuals with intracranial hemorrhage, appropriate measures should be taken to minimize this risk, including the use of diuretic agents. As already noted, this problem is particularly difficult when plasma is either the only agent available for treatment, as in deficiencies of proaccelerin (factor V), PTA (factor XI), or fibrin-stabilizing factor (factor XIII) or when it is prudent to minimize the risk of thrombosis, as in factor VII deficiency. The patient (if an adult) should receive a transfusion of 1 L of plasma, followed by at least 500 ml every 6 hours, administered slowly and with the caution just noted about overloading the circulation.

Patients with known hemostatic defects who suffer any type of head trauma or symptomatology should receive neurologic and/or neurosurgical consultation, and even if they have severe headache, use of aspirin must be avoided.

Needless to say, neurologic or neurosurgical consultation should be sought promptly, and despite the occurrence of headache, the use of aspirin should be avoided. Furthermore, it is imperative to determine whether a circulating anticoagulant is present, as surgical intervention may be needed. Spinal tap should be performed only after the patient's defect is corrected and therefore must be avoided when it is not possible to neutralize or circumvent the action of circulating anticoagulants (antibodies). Intracranial bleeding is particularly difficult to control in patients with circulating anticoagulants, whether these represent a complication of a hereditary hemostatic defect or are "acquired." Under these circumstances treatment is often most unsatisfactory.[43]

Examination of the cerebrospinal fluid via lumbar puncture must be avoided when it is not possible to neutralize or circumvent the action of circulating anticoagulants.

The prognosis of intracranial bleeding in patients with hereditary hemorrhagic disorders is grave. Death occurs in 30 to 40 percent of cases, and of those patients who survive, almost half have permanent neurologic damage.[40,44] Intracranial bleeding may be a recurrent event without overt trauma in patients with hereditary clotting defects. In one such patient, an infant with a severe deficiency of Stuart factor (factor X), prophylaxis with infusions of prothrombin complex through a central venous catheter at a rate of 40 U/kg twice weekly seemed to be effective.[45] Intracranial bleeding may also complicate acquired hemostatic disorders, particularly those induced by oral anticoagulant therapy and by severe thrombocytopenia of whatever cause.

Hemorrhage into the Spinal Cord

Fortunately bleeding into the spinal cord is rare in patients with hereditary clotting diseases. In one 17-year-old boy with Stuart factor (factor X) deficiency, treatment of incomplete transverse paralysis at the 6th thoracic level by administration of prednisolone, 30 mg/day, and prothrombin complex for 8 days resulted in remission of symptoms.[46]

Peripheral Nerve Damage

Damage to peripheral nerves, relatively uncommon, is usually brought about by pressure from hematomas. Although the femoral, ulnar, and median nerves seem particularly prone to damage, other nerves may also be involved.[41,47,48] Replacement therapy is imperative. Silverstein[47] recommends that this be continued "for some time" after signs of active bleeding have subsided. Surgical relief of pressure on nerves should be attempted only after correction of the hemostatic defect.

Surgical relief of pressure on nerves or any other body structure should be attempted only after the hemostatic defect has been adequately corrected.

Bleeding into the Anterior Neck

Another truly frightening site of bleeding is the anterior neck. Bleeding may appear to start in the pharynx or beneath the tongue, dissecting down into the neck and compressing the trachea so as to compromise breathing, or the first evidence of bleeding may be in the soft tissues of the neck. Among 24 episodes observed over the last 28 years at University Hospitals of Cleveland, 3 occurred in association with circulating anticoagulants, 2 were complications of classic hemophilia, and 1 was of spontaneous origin. There were no fatalities.

In confronting this dangerous complication, otolaryngologic consultation should be sought early. It is best to refer all patients to the same physician to take advantage of that specialist's experience with this problem. Preparations for emergency tracheotomy should also be made; this procedure was more frequently performed before the advent of modern replacement therapy. In those patients without circulating anticoagulants, specific correction of the hemostatic defect should be made as quickly as possible, whereas in those who do have circulating anticoagulants, more heroic attempts to control hemostasis should be instituted, including transfusion of porcine factor VIII or recombinant factor VIIa if these agents are available.

Hemarthrosis

In severely affected patients with classic hemophilia or Christmas disease (i.e., those in whom the titer of the deficient factor is less than 1 percent) commonplace sites of bleeding are the joints, particularly those of the knees, hips, ankles, shoulders, and elbows; curiously, hemarthrosis is unusual in the joints of the hands, feet (below the ankle), and the vertebral column. Hemarthrosis has also been described in severely affected patients with other hereditary clotting deficiencies, including those of prothrombin, factor VII, and Stuart factor (factor X).

Hemarthrosis may follow an overt stress to the joint, or it may appear out of the blue. Although hemarthrosis is seldom a critical event, the severe pain that may accompany it demands rapid therapy to provide relief. Moreover, prompt therapy may minimize permanent joint damage in patients with severe classic hemophilia, although this is more difficult to establish. The joint should be encased in icebags to minimize pain, the patient should be given analgesics or narcotics (but neither subcutaneously nor intramuscularly), and the hemostatic defect should be corrected by intravenous infusion of plasma or the appropriate plasma fraction. For example, in classic hemophilia an intravenous infusion of 40 U of antihemophilic factor (factor VIII) per kilogram of body weight, given in the form of a virus-inactivated concentrate or as cryoprecipitate, suffices to control pain and swelling and presumably also to minimize joint damage, although this is more speculative. Gill et al.[49] suggest somewhat higher doses for bleeding into the hip. Before the current AIDS epidemic, we routinely added prednisone therapy to this regimen, as suggested by Kisker and Burke,[50] but this now seems an added stress to the patient's possibly compromised immune system. Only seldom is a second infusion of antihemophilic factor needed. A similar course of therapy is recommended for patients with Christmas disease (factor IX deficiency, hemophilia B) who appear to have acute hemarthrosis, using infusions of plasma or of concentrates containing Christmas factor rather than concentrates of factor VIII. Hemarthrosis in patients with severe deficiencies of Stuart factor (factor X), prothrombin, or factor VII should be treated by intravenous infusions of plasma or concentrates of the vitamin K-dependent factors, while keeping in mind the possible thrombogenicity of such concentrates.[51,52]

Bleeding into Soft Tissues

Hematomas, usually the result of obvious trauma, are rarely immediately life-threatening but may be a source of considerable discomfort. They can occur anywhere, and the chief concern is that pressure from the extravasated blood may damage adjacent structures, including bone, where they cause the formation of pseudocysts, and peripheral nerves. However, hematomas may present other problems for the patient. In one 41-year-old man with severe classic hemophilia treated at University Hospitals of Cleveland, a football-sized subcutaneous hematoma appeared on the left lateral abdominal wall after a coughing spell; bleeding dissected into the scrotal sac, and the patient's hematocrit dropped acutely from 41 to 21 percent.

Although the patient was treated by transfusions of cryoprecipitates, it was unclear whether these contributed to the cessation of bleeding.

Hematomas may be a source of diagnostic difficulty when they are located in areas not easily accessible to the examiner. For example, in one 25-year-old patient with severe classic hemophilia, bleeding occurred in the mesocolon or omentum, as demonstrated by both computed tomography (CT) scan and ultrasound. The lesions resolved on treatment with large doses of lyophilized concentrates of antihemophilic factor (factor VIII).

The treatment of bleeding into soft tissues is similar to that recommended for hemarthrosis, namely analgesia, immobilization of the affected part, cooling with an ice pack, and transfusion of appropriate clotting factors.[40] Other forms of soft tissue bleeding in patients with hereditary hemostatic disorders should be treated in much the same way; hematomas in subcutaneous or intramuscular areas may be sufficiently large or may impinge on nerves or other structures so as to require treatment.

In patients with mild classic hemophilia or von Willebrand disease, transfusion of fractions of plasma may be avoided by intravenous infusion of DDAVP at a dosage of 0.3 μg per kilogram of bodyweight in a volume of 50 ml of saline solution, repeated after 12 or more hours. In our local experience this is not always appropriate; if the hemorrhage is such as to require treatment, a transfusion of the deficient clotting factor or plasma should be given.

Probably the most important rule in the care of patients with hematomas is to avoid surgical procedures if at all possible because of the risk of infection.[40] Of course, pressure on peripheral nerves may make surgery unavoidable.

Urinary Tract Bleeding

Gross hematuria is a common symptom in severe classic hemophilia or Christmas disease, and once this occurs, it is not unusual for the patient to experience repeated episodes.[53] This symptom is unusual in childhood, appearing most often in adolescence. Bleeding is thought to be responsible for some of the many abnormalities of the renal tract seen in hereditary bleeders.[54] When a patient presents with gross hematuria, a diligent search should be made for an underlying lesion, with use of both intravenous and retrograde cystoscopy as appropriate and always with correction of the hemorrhagic defect as the first step. Usually no underlying lesion is found, but in one unfortunate Cleveland patient, investigation of the cause of his gross hematuria demonstrated both a staghorn calculus and a primary renal tumor. Similarly, in a patient of Greer et al.[55]

von Willebrand disease, gross hematuria proved to be due to renal carcinoma.

Treatment of gross hematuria includes bed rest, not necessarily a logical step, and correction of the hemostatic defect. The temptation to use antifibrinolytic agents such as EACA and AMCA is great because these agents inhibit lysis of clots that might be induced by urinary urokinase. However, severe renal damage from obstruction by undissolved clots has been recorded repeatedly, and antifibrinolytic agents should be avoided.

Bleeding after Dental Extraction

Prophylaxis by infusion of a sufficient quantity of the appropriate clotting factor to raise its titer to 50 percent of normal, followed by a 10-day course of oral EACA or AMCA nearly always prevents significant bleeding after any dental extraction or dental surgery.

At one time protracted bleeding after dental extraction could be anticipated in patients with severe hemostatic de fects. Prophylaxis by infusion of enough of the appropriate clotting factor to raise its titer to 50 percent of normal, fol lowed by a 10-day course of oral EACA (Amicar) or AMCA (Cyklokapron), nearly always prevents significant bleeding.[56] EACA and AMCA inhibit the conversion of a plasminogen to plasmin and thereby reduce the chance that clotted blood in the dental socket will dissolve before the wound has healed. Our practice in adults is to administer 4 g of EACA by mouth every 4 hours, day and night, for 10 days, and proportionately less in children. The corresponding dose of AMCA is 0.5 g every 8 hours. Other practitioners use lesser amounts. EACA has also been used to reduce bleeding from the inevitable wounds to the oral mucosa, particularly in children. Patients should be cautioned not to drive a car while taking oral antifibrinolytic agents, as faintness is among the many side effects of these potent substances.

Gastrointestinal Bleeding

The principal cause of gastrointestinal bleeding in patients with hereditary hemostatic defects is peptic ulcer disease, although in about half of cases there are no earlier symptoms pointing to this diagnosis.[57,58] The emergency treatment is no different than in nonbleeders except that one must additionally infuse the appropriate fraction of plasma itself. Peptic ulcer disease may not be more frequent in bleeders than in nonbleeders, but bleeding is more life-threatening.

In patients with hereditary disorders of blood clotting, particularly classic hemophilia, Christmas disease, and von Willebrand disease, bleeding from the gastrointestinal tract is usually from a discrete lesion such as a peptic ulcer, an intestinal polyp, or hemorrhoids. Peptic ulcer occurs in at least 13 percent of patients with hemophilia or Christmas disease, and often this disorder is responsible for gross or microscopic hemorrhage.[40] The diagnostic and therapeutic procedures appropriate for the underlying gastrointestinal problem should be carried out whenever possible, but only after administration of full therapeutic doses of the patients' missing factor.

Bleeding from the gastrointestinal tract is particularly to be feared in patients with von Willebrand disease, in whom this complication may be lethal despite an otherwise benign course. Identification of the site of bleeding, despite exploratory surgery, may be difficult. In a few cases bleeding has been attributed to angiodysplasia. Treatment of gastrointestinal bleeding in von Willebrand disease is also difficult. In these patients repeated infusion of cryoprecipitates at a dosage of two to four bags per kilogram of body weight every 12 hours is not necessarily helpful; cryoprecipitate infusions supplemented by infusions of DDAVP may possibly provide hemostasis in some cases.

Bleeding from hemorrhoidal disease can also be difficult to treat. In one moderately affected Cleveland patient with classic hemophilia, despite rather massive efforts to control his hemostatic abnormality by infusions of cryoprecipitate and lyophilized preparations of factor VIII, repeated surgical procedures were required before bleeding was controlled by local application of sutures.

Gastrointestinal hemorrhage was a prominent symptom in the interesting case of a newborn girl with qualitatively abnormal prothrombin; therapy with infusions of plasma and of prothrombin complex preparations appeared to be beneficial.[59]

Intraperitoneal and Intrapleural Bleeding

Intraperitoneal bleeding is unusual in patients with either hereditary or acquired hemostatic disorders. An instructive case has been described above. I have not yet encountered intrapleural bleeding as a complication of hereditary clotting disease, but I believe that this complication should be treated, as in patients without hemostatic defects, by removing the bloody pleural effusion to avoid compromising respiratory function. Bloody pleural fluid was a manifestation of the bleeding tendency of a patient studied at University Hospitals of Cleveland who had thrombocythemia as an element of polycythemia vera.

BLEEDING IN PATIENTS WITH CIRCULATING ANTICOAGULANTS

Circulating anticoagulants are abnormal endogenous components of blood that inhibit its coagulation.[60] So-called lupus anticoagulants, which interfere with the conversion of prothrombin to thrombin by factor X (Stuart factor), are usually not associated with an abnormal hemorrhagic tendency, but they often occur in patients who have other causes of bleeding such as thrombocytopenia.

Circulating anticoagulants directed against antihemophilic factor (factor VIII) occur in as many as 20 percent of patients with severe classic hemophilia, but only in those patients who at some time have been treated with agents containing factor VIII; rare exceptions to this rule have been described. Similar circulating anticoagulants against factor VIII are seen in nonhemophilic patients, either as a rare complication of pregnancy (or the postparturient state) or apparently arising spontaneously. Among this last group are patients with a variety of cutaneous eruptions or systemic lupus erythematosus and patients who had ingested either penicillin-like compounds or phenytoin shortly before the appearance of their bleeding tendency. Circulating anticoagulants against factor VIII are immunoglobulins that neutralize the clot-promoting properties of this clotting factor. Nonhemophilic patients with such circulating anticoagulants have symptoms resembling those of patients with severe classic hemophilia, compounded by their resistance to ordinary forms of therapy because the antibodies neutralize the clot-promoting effects of factor VIII.

The titer of circulating anticoagulants against antihemophilic factor (factor VIII) is most often quantified by the Bethesda method, which measures the residual functional concentration of the clotting factor after incubation of the patient's plasma with normal plasma.[61] For many years we have used a similar method, which seems simpler to perform, has a low error, and avoids certain methodologic problems.[62,63]

Circulating anticoagulants against other clotting factors have also been described, particularly in patients with Christmas disease (factor IX deficiency) and plasma thromboplastin antecedent (PTA or factor XI deficiency). Inhibitors of Christmas factor, like those inhibiting antihemophilic factor (factor VIII), may arise in patients with Christmas disease or in previously normal individuals.[64,65] As in patients with classic hemophilia, inhibitors arise in patients with Christmas disease who have received transfusions of plasma or factor IX-rich fractions.

In patients with low-titer anticoagulants directed against factor VIII, massive infusion of human factor VIII may provide temporary control of hemostasis, but in some patients this may be followed by an anamnestic rise in antibody titer. Kasper[66] recommends that if a hemorrhage is critical, attempts should be made to raise the patient's factor VIII level to 30 to 50 U/dl or higher—that is, to 30 to 50 percent of the average normal titer. In those in whom the anticoagulant titer is high, this may not be practical, and currently a helpful emergency measure is the transfusion of porcine factor VIII at reported dosages of 20 to 100 U per kilogram of body weight, which is efficacious because porcine factor VIII is relatively resistant to human antibodies against this clotting factor.[67–70] The use of porcine factor VIII has made possible dental and other surgical procedures that would otherwise have been avoided because of the risk of bleeding. Still, although transfusion of porcine factor VIII apparently controlled bleeding in two of our patients with spontaneous inhibitors against factor VIII, a serious complication was transient but severe thrombocytopenia. A major deterrent to therapy with porcine factor VIII is its extraordinarily high cost.

Other measures that have been recommended to control bleeding in patients with circulating anticoagulants include infusion of prothrombin complex preparations, particularly those in which some of the clotting factors have been deliberately activated, such as Autoplex and FEIBA.[71] Although this therapy has been widely used, its effect on hemostasis is erratic and its use is risky, as it appears to induce thrombosis or myocardial necrosis in some patients, complications noted above and reviewed by Lusher[72,73] and Kasper.[66] Recombinant factor VIIa may provide hemostasis without the drawbacks of prothrombin complex preparations, but treatment failures and induction of disseminated intravascular coagulation (DIC) have been reported.[74,75] This agent has not yet been approved except for investigational use. Intensive exchange transfusion, using normal plasma, human albumin, or concentrates of factor VIII as the exchange fluid, may help to reduce the titer of the anticoagulant but not necessarily sufficiently to allow hemostasis.[76–79] In one recent report, a patient with classic hemophilia who had a high titer of circulating anticoagulant and a life-threatening lingual hemorrhage was successfully treated by continuous infusion of monoclonal antibody–purified factor VIII at a rate of 75 U/kg/h for 5 days.[80]

The principles of treatment in patients with circulating anticoagulants against factor IX are the same as in patients with inhibitors of factor VIII. In those patients in whom the titer of the anticoagulant is relatively low, bleeding may be controlled by administration of larger than usual doses of prothrombin complex concentrates or, if available, purified factor IX. In those in whom this procedure is insufficient to stop bleeding or in those with high-titered inhibitors, the various expedients used to provide hemostasis in the presence of a circulating anticoagulant against factor VIII may be tried, including infusions of *activated* prothrombin complex preparations, which contain factor IX.

I have had no experience with emergency reduction of

the titer of anticoagulants against factors VIII or IX by extracorporeal filtration of the patient's blood through columns of staphylococcal protein A bound to an insoluble matrix such as agarose (Sepharose) or silica. In this procedure, IgG immunoglobulins (except those of subclass 3) in the patient's plasma are removed from the circulation by binding through their FC portions to protein A. This maneuver may reduce the titer of antibody to the point that hemostasis can be achieved by transfusion of factor VIII or IX concentrates.[81,82] Alternatively, anticoagulants against Christmas factor (factor IX) have been removed by adsorption to a purified factor IX preparation that has been covalently linked to Sepharose.[83]

Because treatment of acute episodes of bleeding in patients with circulating anticoagulants is so often unsatisfactory, consideration should be given to more definitive therapy. Among proposed methods are administration of immunosuppressive agents and desensitization to the offending antigen, (e.g., antihemophilic factor [factor VIII]).[72,79,84] In some patients, particularly those with spontaneously acquired anticoagulants, treatment with intravenously administered IgG, 0.4 g/kg/day for 5 days, has led to a decreased titer of the anticoagulant or even to its apparent disappearance.[85,86]

DISSEMINATED INTRAVASCULAR COAGULATION AS A CAUSE OF ACUTE BLEEDING

Acquired hypofibrinogenemia as a consequence of DIC may cause life-threatening bleeding. Acute DIC is of particular importance in such complications of pregnancy as amniotic fluid embolism, premature separation of the placenta, and intrauterine retention of a dead fetus, in which life-threatening blood loss, particularly from the uterus, may occur.[87] Regardless of other forms of therapy, every effort should be made to empty the uterus, as this will often suffice to halt the progress of DIC. In patients with amniotic fluid embolism, severe blood loss should be met by transfusion of packed red blood cells, plasma, and platelets to combat shock and correct the hemostatic defect. Transfusion of cryoprecipitates (as a source of fibrinogen) is useful only in those patients with hypofibrinogenemia; the dosage schedule is the same as that described above for congenital afibrinogenemia. Infusions of plasma may also aid hemostasis by correcting deficiencies of plasma clotting inhibitors such as antithrombin III that may result from DIC. Of greater importance is treatment of the respiratory distress that accompanies amniotic fluid embolism by administering oxygen and positive end-expiratory pressure (PEEP) ventilation. Despite these measures, the prognosis is poor; amniotic fluid embolism is the principal cause of death during childbirth. Severe blood loss is also a commonplace result of premature separation of the placenta. Nearly always, the hemostatic defect is readily corrected by emptying the uterus, which avoids the need to transfuse cryoprecipitates.

Although hypofibrinogenemia occurs in perhaps one-fourth of patients who retain a dead fetus in utero, exsanguinating bleeding is unusual. The hypofibrinogenemia can be corrected by interrupting the process of DIC by administration of heparin, as first suggested by Phillips and Sciarra[88] and Lerner et al.[89] Heparin may be infused intravenously at a rate of 1,000 U/h for 24 hours,[90] or alternatively, subcutaneously at a rate of 5,000 to 10,000 U twice daily.[91] This is usually sufficient to bring the patient's fibrinogen to a normal level. Heparin therapy may then be discontinued and the uterus emptied, with resolution of the patient's hemorrhagic problem. Although heparin therapy has been recommended in other forms of DIC, its efficacy is not established, and the risk of compounding an already severe bleeding tendency must be kept in mind.

DIC is also a complication of a host of diseases, including sepsis, shock, neoplasia, and cirrhosis of the liver. As in the case of DIC arising during pregnancy or parturition, a prime effort should be directed at the cause of the syndrome (e.g., vigorous antibiotic treatment when infection seems to be at the root of the problem). As in the pregnancy-related syndromes, heparin therapy is of limited value.

A patient whose bleeding is associated with hypofibrinogenemia and who requires treatment because of impending or overt shock should be infused intravenously with cryoprecipitates, one bag for every 2 kg of body weight followed by one bag for every 15 kg every day until hemostasis is achieved.[92] Moreover, when bleeding is alarming, sufficient platelets should be infused to keep the platelet count above about 50,000/μl with adequate volumes of plasma and packed red blood cells.

DIC is of particular consequence in patients with acute leukemia, particularly promyelocytic leukemia, in which the contents of the abnormal leukocytes are clot-promoting. In this situation heparin therapy may be of some help in promoting hemostasis.[93] Low-dose heparin therapy (50 U/kg every 6 hours) may be sufficient and may help to avoid additional bleeding.[94] Since the therapy of acute leukemia may induce transient hypofibrinogenemia, prophylaxis with intravenously administered heparin has been recommended and, although some doubt its merits, this appears to be a helpful measure.[92] An alternative view of the pathogenesis of the bleeding syndrome in acute leukemia has been revived recently, namely, the hypothesis that the hemostatic defect is due to acute fibrinolysis.[95] If this proves to be correct, antifibrinolytic therapy with, for example, EACA would be a rational choice.

BLEEDING IN DISORDERS OF VITAMIN K METABOLISM AND HEPATIC DISEASE

The synthesis of four clotting factors—prothrombin, factor VII, Stuart factor (factor X), and Christmas factor (factor IX)—takes place in hepatocytes via a process requiring the presence of vitamin K. The hepatocytes synthesize inactive precursor proteins of the vitamin K-dependent clotting factors, and these proteins are then transformed into functionally capable proenzymes by insertion of a third carboxyl group into certain glutamic acid residues. This transformation is brought about in a post-translational step by a hepatic microsomal enzyme that uses vitamin K as a needed cofactor; vitamin K is the generic name for a group of naphthoquinone derivatives that serve this function.

The natural vitamin K compounds are absorbed from the gut in the same way as lipids and like lipids require bile salts for absorption. Anything interfering with absorption of vitamin K (e.g., exclusion of bile salts from the gut by obstruction of the ampulla of Vater or intra- or extrahepatic obstruction of the common duct) results in deficiencies of the vitamin K-dependent clotting factors and as a consequence generalized bleeding tendency. Similarly, disorders such as sprue that impair the absorptive function of the gut may be complicated by bleeding, usually ecchymoses and in women, menorrhagia. In all these cases, intramuscularly injected vitamin K_1 at a dosage of 25 mg will correct the defect within hours, but parenteral treatment must be continued until the basic problem is corrected. If bleeding is alarming, transfusion of 1,000 ml of normal plasma in adults and proportionately less in children will provide immediate but transient correction of the deficiency state. Further transfusions of 500 ml of plasma every 6 hours may be required until synthesis of the vitamin K-dependent factors is adequate. Administration of diuretics may help to prevent circulatory overload.[96]

Patients with hepatic disease also may have a general bleeding tendency, but its genesis is more complex. In those with cirrhosis of the liver, gastrointestinal bleeding leading to major blood loss is usually a consequence of bleeding from esophageal varices, although the possibility that the hemorrhage may be from such other lesions as peptic ulcer, gastritis, or mucosal tears should not be overlooked. Bleeding problems in patients with hepatic disease are usually compounded by impairment of hemostatic mechanisms, including deficiencies of the vitamin K-dependent clotting factors, proaccelerin (factor V) and, unusually, fibrinogen, as well as by significant thrombocytopenia and (at least as measured in the test tube) enhanced fibrinolytic activity. In contrast to patients in whom deficiencies of the vitamin K-dependent factors reflect deficiency of vitamin K, in patients with liver disease these deficiencies are due to impaired synthesis of the precursor proteins by hepatocytes. Such patients respond poorly if at all to parenteral injection of vitamin K, but, exceptionally, patients in whom intrahepatic obstruction of the bile ducts is prominent may respond to parenteral vitamin K_1. The deficiency of proaccelerin (factor V) is not improved by vitamin K.

In most cases therapy directed against variceal bleeding is of prime importance; replacement of blood volume with packed red blood cells and plasma is usually necessary. To correct the clotting abnormality, Burns[97] recommends infusion of 1,200 ml or more of fresh-frozen plasma, the dosage depending on the degree of prolongation of the prothrombin time. Additionally, he recommends that transfusions of platelets, at an initial dosage of 8 U, be given to patients with platelet counts below 70,000/μl.

HEMORRHAGIC DISEASE OF THE NEWBORN

The continual occurrence of hemorrhagic disease of the newborn is discouraging, particularly that subset of cases that occur 3 to 6 weeks after birth. Hemorrhagic disease of the newborn may bring about bleeding into the gastrointestinal tract or elsewhere; especially to be feared is intracranial hemorrhage.[98] This disorder, which is more likely to occur in babies fed human rather than cow's milk, is clearly related to deficiency of vitamin K and can be prevented by a single parenteral injection of 0.5 to 1.0 mg of vitamin K_1 or an oral dose of 1.0 to 2.0 mg.[99] Occasionally, therapy must be repeated.

BLEEDING AS A COMPLICATION OF ANTICOAGULANT THERAPY

A major complication of treatment with *oral* anticoagulants is hemorrhage, and as in the case of the hereditary disorders of hemostasis, intracranial bleeding is particularly dangerous. Frequently but not always, the prothrombin time is higher than the usual therapeutic range. If hemorrhage does not appear to be life-threatening, treatment by intramuscular injection of vitamin K_1 (25 to 50 mg Aquamephyton, Merck) will usually correct the hemostatic defect within a few hours; the effect of this therapy can be judged by repeated measurements of the prothrombin time. If the prothrombin time remains long and the diagnosis seems secure, a second injection of vitamin K_1 may be given 6 to 8 hours after the first. When bleeding is more alarming, either in volume or because of its site, immediate correction of the clotting defect can be provided by intravenous transfusion of 1 L of plasma; this will bring the concentration of the vitamin K-dependent factors to a temporarily safe level. This treatment, however, is not a substitute for treatment with vitamin K_1, which must also be carried out to overcome the effects of the oral anticoagulant. Oral anticoagulant therapy should not be reinstituted until the patient's bleeding appears to be controlled. Therapy should be reinstituted cautiously, as the response to oral anticoagulants will be blunted by any residual effect of the vitamin K administered until this agent has been metabolized.

A more subtle problem is recognition of self-induced administration of oral anticoagulants. The patient nearly always has ready access to the drugs, either as a nurse, technician, or a member of a physician's family. The sudden onset of a generalized bleeding tendency in the absent of an overt cause should arouse suspicion; the diagnosis is supported by a prolonged prothrombin time and is ultimately confirmed by obtaining assays for warfarin in the patient's plasma. Treatment is the same as for hemorrhagic complications of oral anticoagulant therapy, but additionally, psychiatric help should be sought as soon as the diagnosis is evident. I have avoided confronting the patient with our suspicions in an attempt to avert a more dramatic attempt at self-destruction.

Bleeding as the result of heparin therapy is unfortunately also frequent. Depending upon the perceived urgency of the problem, one may attempt empiric neutralization of heparin by intravenous infusion of protamine sulfate at a dosage of 1 mg per 100 U of heparin, administered over a 10-minute period; the half-disappearance time of heparin from plasma is 1 to 2 hours. Or one can try to estimate the needed dosage by measuring the thrombin time of the patient's plasma to which varying amounts of protamine sulfate have been added.

BLEEDING AS A COMPLICATION OF UREMIA

Major hemorrhagic events are now much less frequent in uremic patients than in former years, not only because of the use of dialysis but also because of attention to other contributing factors.[100] Among the laboratory features that may be found are thrombocytopenia; qualitative changes in platelet function that are principally responsible for the characteristic prolongation of the bleeding time (perhaps enhanced by the use of aspirin-like agents); and uncommonly, decreased titers of clotting factors, possibly the result of vitamin K malabsorption or deficiency. Compounding the uremic patient's difficulties, administration of heparin to maintain the patency of the dialysis apparatus may enhance the bleeding tendency, leading to subdural hematomas, hemorrhagic pleural effusions, and retroperitoneal bleeding.[100]

Several ways have been suggested to control bleeding to uremic patients, including transfusion of cryoprecipitates,[101] or infusion of DDAVP (Sternate), 0.3 μg/kg body weight, intravenously over a 30-minute span.[102] A more lasting effect may be obtained by oral or intravenous administration of conjugated estrogens, 10 to 50 mg/day for 5 to 10 days[103–105] or by correction of the patients' anemia by transfusion of red blood cells or administration of erythropoietin.[106–108]

BLEEDING ASSOCIATED WITH THROMBOCYTOPENIA

Thrombocytopenia from whatever cause makes a patient susceptible to abnormal bleeding. Cutaneous ecchymoses are usually frightening to the patient but rarely cause major problems. Cutaneous petechiae are ordinarily harmless, but oral petechiae may give the appearance of "blood blisters" when thrombocytopenia is sufficiently severe, and these lesions may bleed. Severe thrombocytopenia may be implicated in intracranial hemorrhage, intraocular bleeding, and bleeding almost anywhere else in the body; in women, menorrhagia is a frequent and distressing symptom.

The treatment of the patient with thrombocytopenia depends in large measure on the pathogenesis of this abnormality (i.e., on whether it is due to decreased production of platelets, to their premature consumption or destruction, or to the dilution of peripheral blood upon infusion of platelet-depleted plasma or other fluids).[109] The differential diagnosis of thrombocytopenia has been dealt with in many current monographs and will not be repeated here except to emphasize the need for a close examination of bone marrow.

Impaired production of platelets is part of the symptom complex of hypoplastic or aplastic anemia. Although the resulting thrombocytopenia may be sufficiently severe that the patient has bleeding problems, this is usually not the

Patients with thrombocytopenia who have platelet counts of 50,000/μl or higher are unlikely to benefit from a platelet transfusion if thrombocytopenia is the sole abnormality.

case. As was concluded at the National Institutes of Health Consensus Conference,[110] it is unlikely that a patient with a platelet count of 50,000/μl or higher will benefit from a platelet transfusion if thrombocytopenia is the sole abnormality. Much more commonly encountered in hematologic practice is the patient in whom platelet production is impaired either as an integral part of neoplastic disease, as in the acute leukemias, or as the result of antineoplastic therapy. In such patients significant spontaneous bleeding is unusual when the platelet count is above 20,000/μl, but other concurrent abnormalities, such as sepsis and DIC, may enhance the risk.[111] Perhaps because of this a wide difference of opinion exists concerning proposed therapeutic regimens for the patient with impaired platelet production. If at all possible, the use of any medication likely to suppress platelet formation should be discontinued. Some authors suggest that prophylactic platelet transfusions are appropriate when the platelet count falls to 5,000 to 10,000/μl, others put the threshold higher (e.g., 20,000/μl), and still others see no need for transfusion in the patient with uncomplicated impaired platelet production. An appropriate starting dosage is 1 unit of platelet concentrate per 10 kg body weight raising the platelet count by 5,000 to 10,000/μl per unit infused as measured 1 hour later[112,113]; other regimens have been proposed. Platelet transfusions are then repeated as needed, perhaps several times a week. If active bleeding is taking place or if surgical procedures are contemplated, more vigorous platelet transfusion therapy may be required. Unfortunately, sooner or later patients receiving platelet transfusions become refractory because of alloimmunization, so that the expected increment does not occur. To minimize these risks, various expedients have been tried, including use of a single, matched donor who is subjected to plateletpheresis, as well as attempts to deplete platelet concentrates of leukocytes.

Thrombocytopenia may also be the result of immune destruction of platelets and their removal from the bloodstream. In such cases examination of the marrow demonstrates the presence of normal or even increased numbers of megakaryocytes, but these cells often appear to be bereft of their normal cytoplasm. A common cause of this syndrome, particularly in adults, is sensitization to one or another medication or chemical (e.g., thiazide diuretics, quinine, or quinidine). Therefore definitive diagnosis cannot be made in an adult until the use of possibly antigenic medications has been discontinued; remission is usual within 1 week. In other patients the disorder appears to have an autoimmune basis, sometimes in association with such other conditions as a variety of neoplasms[92] or systemic lupus erythematosus, in which the thrombocytopenia may run a protracted course, often lasting many years. A similar syndrome has now emerged in patients with AIDS.

A special example of drug-induced thrombocytopenia is that induced by heparin therapy.[114] In some cases the thrombocytopenia is mild, with platelet counts remaining over 100,000/μl; in others, thrombocytopenia can be of great severity and may well be of immunologic origin, although this view is by no means universal.[115–118] Heparin therapy should be discontinued immediately, as severe or fatal thromboembolism may ensue.[119]

Treatment of chronic immune (idiopathic) thrombocytopenic purpura (ITP) in adults is less than ideal. If the platelet count is below about 60,000/μl or there is evidence of a bleeding tendency beyond cutaneous petechiae, oral prednisone, 1 mg/kg/day, will induce a significant rise in platelet count in one-third to one-half of patients.[120] Once remission has occurred, the dosage of prednisone is reduced in weekly steps by 10 mg/day. If thrombocytopenia is frighteningly severe, high-dosage methylprednisolone may be tried,[121] but intravenous γ-globulin, as described below, is probably a wiser choice. A typical regimen is 0.4 to 1.0 g/kg/day of IgG for 2 or more days. Unfortunately, the remissions achieved by glucocorticoids or γ-globulin are usually not sustained, and in many adults splenectomy must be performed. Although the platelet count fails to return to normal in one-third or more of such splenectomized patients, bleeding symptoms may nonetheless be ameliorated; in some patients who do not respond to splenectomy, subsequent treatment with prednisone may be helpful. In other patients with unremitting thrombocytopenia, a variety of approaches have been tried with varying success, including administration of vincristine, danazol, colchicine, or azathioprine.[122]

Snyder and his colleagues[123] have reported the beneficial effect of removing IgG and circulating immune complexes from the plasma of patients with ITP by filtration of plasma, usually separated by an apheresis apparatus, through columns of staphylococcal protein A. Although the response was variable, a significant number of patients achieved remissions of thrombocytopenia that lasted at least 4 weeks. Unfortunately, however, a number of patients had side effects, often suggesting a hypersensitivity-type reaction. This form of therapy is in its infancy and may well find a niche when it becomes clearer in which patients a response can be expected. In contrast to adults, in whom the pathogenesis of thrombocytopenia is usually unclear, the acute ITP of infants and children often seems to be the result of a viral infection, not always more closely defined. Stuart and Kelton[124] summarized some pertinent features of childhood acute ITP. In most children the disorder becomes evident because ecchymoses and petechiae suddenly appear. Other hemorrhagic manifestations may ensue, including nosebleeds and, less often, gingival, oral mucosal, and gastrointestinal bleeding. These authors point out that splenomegaly occurs at about the same rate as in normal children (i.e., in 5 to 10 percent). In their series the platelet count was usually less than 40,000/μl. The prognosis is usually excellent, with complete recovery in 70 to 90 percent of children, most within 1 month of the onset of their illness, and a mortality rate of less than 1 percent.[125] Those who do not respond within 6 months are said to have chronic ITP, but even some of these patients may undergo spontaneous remission. As in adults, intracranial bleeding occurs almost exclusively in patients with a platelet count below 20,000/μl, but this complication is much rarer than is often believed.[124]

Treatment of the child with acute ITP, as in adults, begins with discontinuance of any drug that might be responsible for pathogenesis of the disorder or that might aggravate bleeding (e.g., aspirin). Some pediatric hematologists do not initiate treatment on the basis of the degree of thrombocytopenia alone, relying on the usually benign course of the disorder. If, however, mucosal or other bleeding suggests imminent danger, treatment with glucocorticoids is begun; a typical course is 2 mg/kg/day of prednisone for 2 weeks, with a maximum dose of 80 mg/day, after which the dose is tapered over 1 week; if bleeding is severe, Stuart and Kelton[124] give twice this amount. Alternatively, or if the bleeding is alarming, the patient is additionally given intravenous immunoglobulins, 0.4 to 1 g/kg/day for 2 or more days, as suggested by Imbach et al.[126] and Bussel et al.[127] This procedure may induce a remission lasting as long as 3 months.[128] Among various hypotheses to explain the efficacy of intravenous γ-globulin, one that seems most attractive is that the protein, directly or adsorbed to red blood cells, binds to Fc receptors on monocytes or macrophages so that these cells can no longer remove antibody-coated platelets from the bloodstream.[129] Another mode of therapy, derived from this hypothesis, is to administer anti-D immunoglobulin to those ITP patients who are Rh-positive. The red cells, coated in this way, induce reticuloendothelial cell blockade in a more targeted way than does intravenous γ-globulin.[130]

In patients with immune or autoimmune thrombocytopenic purpura, the transfusion of platelets is usually futile because of their rapid destruction and removal from the circulation. Nonetheless when bleeding seems otherwise uncontrollable, as in the infant who has acute ITP and uncontrollable epistaxis or the adult woman with severe menorrhagia, addition of platelet transfusion to the basic regimen may provide needed if only transient hemostasis.

ACKNOWLEDGMENTS

Otherwise unattributed observations were made with the support of grant HL01661 from the National Heart, Lung and Blood Institute, the National Institutes of Health, U.S. Public Health Service, and by grants from the American Heart Association and its Northeast Ohio affiliate.

References

1. Lane S: Hemorrhagic diathesis. Successful transfusion of blood. Lancet 1:185, 1840
2. Feissly R: Beiträge zur Wesen und zur Therapie der Hämophilie. Jahrb Kinderheilk 110:297, 1925
3. Roberts HR, Penick GD, Brinkhous KM: Intensive plasma therapy in the hemophilias. JAMA 190:546, 1964
4. Patek AJ Jr, Stetson RH: Hemophilia. I. The abnormal coagulation of the blood and its relation to the blood platelets. J Clin Invest 15:531, 1936
5. Patek AJ Jr, Taylor FHL: Hemophilia. II. Some properties of a substance obtained from normal plasma effective in accelerating the clotting of hemophilic blood. J Clin Invest 16:113, 1937
6. Edsall JT, Ferry RM, Armstrong SH Jr: Chemical, clinical and immunologic studies on the products of human plasma fractionation. XV. The proteins concerned in the blood coagulation mechanism. J Clin Invest 23:557, 1944
7. Pool JG, Hershgold EJ, Pappenhagen A: High-potency antihaemophilic factor concentrate prepared from cryoglobulin precipitate. Nature 203:312, 1964
8. Ness PM, Perkins HA: Cryoprecipitate as a reliable source of fibrinogen replacement. JAMA 241:1690, 1979
9. Wagner RH, McLester NG, Smith M et al: Purification of antihemophilic factor (factor VIII) by amino acid precipitation. Thromb Haemost 11:67, 1964
10. Webster WP, Roberts HR, Thelin GM et al: Clinical use of a new glycine-precipitated antihemophilic fraction. Am J Med Sci 250:643, 1965
11. Zimmerman TS: Purification of factor VIII by monoclonal antibody affinity chromatography. Semin Hematol 25:suppl. 1, 25, 1988
12. White GC II, McMillan CW, Kingdon HS, Shoemaker CB: Use of recombinant antihemophilic factor in the treatment of two patients with classic hemophilia. N Engl J Med 320:166, 1989
13. Schwartz RS, Abildgaard CF, Aledort LM et al: Human recombinant DNA-derived antihemophilic factor (factor VIII) in the treatment of hemophilia A. N Engl J Med 323:1800, 1990
14. Mannucci PM, Teconi PM, Castaman G, Rodeghiero F: Comparison of four virus-inactivated plasma concentrates for treatment of von Willebrand's disease: a cross-over randomized trial. Blood 79:3130, 1992
15. Didisheim P, Loeb J, Blatrix C et al: Preparation of a human plasma fraction rich in prothrombin, proconvertin, Stuart factor and PTC and a study of its activity and toxicity in rabbits and man. J Lab Clin Med 53:322, 1959
16. Bidwell E, Booth JM, Dike GWR et al: The preparation for therapeutic use of a concentrate of factor IX containing also factors II, VIII and X. Br J Haematol 13:586, 1967
17. Kelleher JF Jr, Gomperts E, Davis W et al: Selection of replacement therapy for patients with severe factor VII deficiency. Am J Pediatr Hematol Oncol 8:318, 1986.
18. O'Leary DS, Ruymann FB, Conrad ME: Therapeutic approaches to factor X deficiency with emphasis on the use of a new clotting-factor concentrate (Konyne). J Lab Clin Med 77:23, 1971
19. Kasper CK: Postoperative thromboses in hemophilia B, letter. N Engl J Med 289:160, 1973
20. Gruppo R, Bove KE, Donaldson VH: Fatal myocardial necrosis associated with prothrombin-complex-concentrate therapy in hemophilia A, letter. N Engl J Med 309:242, 1983

21. Kim HC, McMillan CW, White GC et al: Clinical experience with a new monoclonal antibody purified factor IX: half-life, recovery, and safety in patients with hemophilia B. Semin Hemat 27:suppl 2, 30, 1990
22. Goldsmith JC, Kasper CK, Blatt PM et al: Coagulation factor IX: successful surgical experience with a purified factor IX concentrate. Am J Hematol 40:210, 1992
23. Hedner U, Kisiel W: Use of human factor VIIa in the treatment of two hemophilia A patients with high-titer inhibitors. J Clin Invest 71:1836, 1983
24. Macik BG, Hohneker J, Roberts HR, Griffin AM: Use of recombinant activated factor VII for treatment of a retropharyngeal hemorrhage in a hemophilic patient with a high titer inhibitor. Am J Hematol 32:232, 1989
25. Mortimer PP, Luban NLC, Kelleher JF, Cohen BJ: Transmission of serum parvovirus-like virus by clotting-factor concentrates. Lancet 2:482, 1983
26. Gordon EM, Ratnoff OD, Saito H et al: Studies on some coagulation factors (Hageman factor, plasma prekallikrein and high molecular weight kininogen) in the normal newborn. Am J Pediatr Hematol Oncol 2:213, 1980
27. Mannucci PM, Ruggeri ZM, Pareti FI, Capitanio A: 1-Deamino-8-arginine vasopressin. A new pharmacologic approach to the management of hemophilia and von Willebrand's disease. Lancet 1:869, 1977
28. Warrier I, Lusher JM: DDAVP: a useful alternative to blood components in moderate hemophilia A and von Willebrand's disease. J Pediatr 102:228, 1983
29. Mannucci PM: Desmopressin (DDAVP) for treatment of disorders of hemostasis. Prog Hemost Thromb 8:19, 1986
30. Mannucci PM: Desmopressin: a nontransfusional form of treatment for congenital and acquired bleeding disorders. Lancet 2:782, 1988
31. Lethagen S, Harris AS, Sjorin E et al: Intranasal and intravenous administration of desmopressin: effect on fVIII/vWf, pharmokinetics and reproducibility. Thromb Haemost 58:1033, 1987
32. De la Fuente B, Kaspar CK, Rickles FR, Hoyer LW: Response of patients with mild and moderate hemophilia A and von Willebrand's disease to treatment with desmopressin. Ann Internal Med 103:6, 1985
33. Rose EH, Aledort LM: Nasal spray desmopressin (DDAVP) for mild hemophilia A and von Willebrand's disease. Ann Intern Med 114:563, 1991
34. Lowe GDO: Vascular disease and vasculitis. p. 532. In Ratnoff OD, Forbes CD (eds): Disorders of Hemostasis, 2nd WB Saunders, Philadelphia, 1991
35. McNicol GP, Fletcher AP, Alkjaersig N, Sherry S: The use of epsilon aminocaproic acid, a potent inhibitor of fibrinolytic activity, in the management of postoperative hematuria. J Urol 86:829, 1961
36. Gardner FH, Helmer RE III: Aminocaproic acid: use in control of hemorrhage in patients with amegakaryocytic thrombocytopenia. JAMA 243:35, 1980
37. Bartholomew JR, Salgia R, Bell WR: Control of bleeding in patients with immune and nonimmune thrombocytopenia with aminocaproic acid. Arch Intern Med 149:1959, 1989
38. Ben-Bassat I, Douer D, Ramot B: Tranexamic acid in acute myeloid leukemia. Possible reduction of platelet transfusions. Eur J Haematol 45:85, 1990
39. Silverstein A: Intracranial bleeding in hemophilia. Arch Neurol 3:141, 1960
40. Forbes CD, Madhok R: Genetic disorders of blood coagulation. p. 141. In Ratnoff OD, Forbes CD (eds): Disorders of Hemostasis. 2nd Ed. WB Saunders, Philadelphia, 1991
41. Gilchrist GS, Piepgras DG, Roskos RR: Neurologic complications in hemophilia. p. 45. Hilgartner M, Pochedly D (eds): In Hemophilia in the Child and Adult. 3rd Ed. Raven Press, New York, 1989
42. Mammen CF: Congenital coagulation disorders. Semin Thromb Hemost 9:1, 1983
43. Andes WA, Wulff K, Smith WB: Head trauma in hemophilia. A prospective study. Arch Intern Med 144:1981, 1984
44. Eyster ME, Gill FM, Blatt PM et al: Central nervous system bleeding in hemophiliacs. Blood 51:1179, 1978
45. Sandler E, Gross S: Prevention of recurrent intracranial hemorrhage in a factor X-deficient infant. Am J Pediatr Hematol Oncol 14:163, 1992
46. Endo Y: Congenital factor X deficiency and incomplete transverse paralysis. JAMA 246:1708, 1981
47. Silverstein A: Neuropathy in hemophilia. JAMA 190:554, 1964
48. Douglas AS, McAlpine SG: Neurologic complications of haemophilia and Christmas disease. Scott Med J 1:270, 1956

49. Gill GC, Thometz J, Scott JP, Montgomery RR: Muskuloskeletal problems in hemophilia. p. 27. In Hilgartner M, Pochedly C (eds): Hemophilia in the Child and Adult. 3rd Ed. Raven Press, New York, 1989
50. Kisker CT, Burke C: Double-blind studies on the use of steroids in the treatment of acute hemarthrosis in patients with hemophilia. N Engl J Med 282:639, 1970
51. Hougie C, Barrow EM, Graham JB: Stuart clotting defect. I. Segregation of an hereditary hemorrhagic state from the heterogeneous group heretofore called "stable factor" (SPCA, proconvertin, factor VII) deficiency. J Clin Invest 36:485, 1957
52. Owen CA Jr, Amundsen MA, Thompson JH Jr et al: Congenital deficiency of factor VII (hypoconvertinemia). Am J Med 37:71, 1964
53. Davidson CS, Epstein RD, Miller GF, Taylor FHL: Hemophilia. A clinical study of 40 patients. Blood 4:97, 1949
54. Prentice CRM, Lindsay RM, Barr RD et al: Renal complications in haemophilia and Christmas disease. Q J Med 40: 47, 1971
55. Greer IA, Lowe GDO, Yogarajah S et al: Haematuria in patients with haemostatic defects. Br Med J 290:1648, 1985
56. Walsh PN, Rizza CR, Matthews JM et al: Epsilon-aminocaproic acid therapy for dental extraction in haemophilia and Christmas disease: a double blind controlled trial. Br J Haematol 20: 463, 1971
57. Carron DB, Boon TH, Walker FC: Peptic ulcer in the haemophiliac and its relation to gastrointestinal bleeding. Lancet 2:1036, 1965
58. Forbes CD, Barr RD, Prentice CRM et al: Gastrointestinal bleeding in haemophilia. Q J Med 42: 503, 1973
59. Dumont M-D, Tapon-Bretaudiere J, Fischer AM et al: Prothrombin Poissy: a new variant of human prothrombin. Br J Haematol 66:239, 1987
60. Margolius A Jr, Jackson DP, Ratnoff OD: Circulating anticoagulants: a study of 40 cases and a review of the literature. Medicine (Baltimore) 40:145, 1961
61. Kasper CK, Aledort LM, Counts RB et al: A more uniform measurement of factor VIII inhibitors letter. Thromb Haemost 34:869–872, 1975
62. Poon M-C, Wine AC, Ratnoff OD, Bernier GM: Heterogeneity of human circulating anticoagulants against antihemophilic factor (factor VIII). Blood 46:409, 1975
63. Verbruggen HW, Novakova IRO, Wessels JMC et al: Frequency of inhibitors in haemophiliacs letter. Lancet 339:1301, 1992
64. Roberts HR, Gross GP, Webster WP et al: Acquired inhibitors of plasma factor IX. A study of their induction, properties and neutralization. Am J Med Sci 251:43, 1966
65. Theodorsson B, Hedner U, Nilsson IM, Kisiel W: A technique for specific removal of factor IX alloantibodies from human plasma: partial characterization of the alloantibodies. Blood 61: 973, 1983
66. Kasper CK: Treatment of factor VIII inhibitors. pp. 58–86. In Coller BS (ed): Progress in Hemostasis and Thrombosis. Vol. 9. WP Saunders, Philadelphia, 1989
67. Bennett B, Ratnoff WD: Immunologic relationships of antihemophilic factor of different species detected by specific human and rabbit antibodies. Proc Soc Exp Biol Med 143:701, 1973
68. Hultin MB, Hennessey J: The use of polyelectrolyte-fractionated porcine factor VIII in the treatment of a spontaneously acquired inhibitor to factor VIII. Thromb Res 44:51, 1989
69. Kernoff PBA, Thomas ND, Lilley PA et al: Clinical experience with polyelectrolyte fractionated porcine factor VIII concentrate in the treatment of hemophiliacs with antibodies to factor VIII. Blood 63:31, 1984
70. Brettler DB, Forsberg AD, Levine PH et al: The use of porcine factor VIII concentrate (Hyate: C) in the treatment of patients with inhibitor antibodies to factor VIII. A multicenter US experience. Arch Intern Med 149:1381, 1989
71. Kurczynski E, Penner JA: Activated prothrombin concentrate for patients with factor VIII inhibitors. N Engl J Med 291:164, 1974
72. Lusher JM: Management of patients with factor VIII inhibitors. Transfusion Med Rev 1:123, 1987
73. Lusher JM: Factor VIII inhibitors. Etiology, characterization, natural history, and management. Ann N Y Acad Sci 509:89, 1987
74. Gringeri A, Santagostino E, Mannucci PM: Failure of recombinant activated factor VII during surgery in a hemophiliac with high-titer factor VIII antibody. Haemostasis 21:1, 1991
75. Stein SF, Duncan A, Cutler D, Glazer S: Disseminated intravascular coagulation (DIC) in a hemophiliac treated with recombinant factor VIIa. Blood 76:438a, 1990

76. Slocombe GW, Newland AC, Colvin MP, Colvin BT: The role of intensive plasma exchange in the prevention and management of hemorrhage in patients with inhibitors to factor VIII. Br J Haematol 47:577, 1981
77. Apter B, McCarthy V, Shapiro SS, Ballas SK: Successful preoperative apheresis of factor VIII antibody using factor VIII concentrate as a replacement fluid. J Clin Apheresis 3:140, 1986
78. Francesconi M, Korninger C, Thaler E et al: Plasmapheresis: its value in the management of patients with antibodies to factor VIII. Haemostasis 11:79, 1982
79. Kasper CK: Complications of hemophilia A treatment: factor VIII inhibitors. Ann N Y Acad Sci 614:97, 1991
80. Gordon EM, Mango R, Goldsmith JC: Lingual hemorrhage in a patient with hemophilia A complicated by a high titer inhibitor: management by continuous infusion of monoclonal antibody-purified factor VIII. Am J Pediatr Hematol Oncol (submitted for publication)
81. Nilsson IM, Jonsson S, Sundqvist S-B et al: A procedure for removing high titer antibodies by extracorporeal protein-A-Sepharose adsorption in hemophilia: substitution therapy and surgery in a patient with hemophilia B and antibodies. Blood 58:38, 1981
82. Négrier C, Dechanvanne M, Alfonsi F, Tremisi PJ: Successful treatment of acquired factor VIII antibody by extracorporeal immunoadsorption. Acta Haematol (Basel) 85:107, 1991
83. Nilsson IM, Freiburghaus C, Sundqvist S-B, Sandberg H: Removal of specific antibodies from whole blood in a continuous extracorporeal system. Plasma Ther Transfusion Technol 5:127, 1984
84. Shapiro SS, Siegel JE: Hemorrhagic disorders associated with circulating inhibitors. p. 245. In Ratnoff OD, Forbes CB (eds): Disorders of hemostasis. 2nd Ed. WB Saunders, Philadelphia, 1991
85. Sultan Y, Kazatchkine MD, Nydegger U et al: Intravenous immunoglobulin in the treatment of spontaneously acquired factor VIII:C inhibitors. Am J Med 91:suppl. 5A, 35S, 1991
86. Todd AAM, Yap PL: Applications of intravenous immunoglobulin in haematology. Blood Rev 6:105, 1992
87. Ratnoff OD: Disseminated intravascular coagulation during pregnancy. p. 117. In Greer IA, Turpie AGG, Forbes CD (eds): Haemostasis and Thrombosis. Chapman & Hall, London, 1992
88. Phillips LL, Sciarra JJ: Hypofibrinogenemia with a dead fetus treated with intravenous heparin. Am J Obstet Gynecol 93:1161, 1965
89. Lerner R, Margolin M, Slate WG et al: Heparin in the treatment of hypofibrinogenemia complicating fetal death in utero. Am J Obstet Gynecol 97:373, 1967
90. Bonnar J: Haemostasis and coagulation disorders in pregnancy. p. 570. In Bloom AL, Thomas DP (eds): Haemostasis and Thrombosis. 2nd Ed. Churchill Livingstone, Edinburgh, 1987
91. Weiner CP: Treatment of coagulation and fibrinolytic disorders. p. 314. In Ketty DC (ed): Hematologic Problems in Pregnancy. Medical Economics Books, Oradell NJ, 1987
92. Ratnoff OD: Hemostatic emergencies in malignancy. Semin Oncol 16:561, 1989
93. Baker WG, Bang NU, Nachman RL et al: Hypofibrinogenemic hemorrhage in acute myelogenous leukemia treated with heparin with autopsy findings of widespread intravascular coagulation. Ann Intern Med 61:116, 1964
94. Gralnick HR, Marchesi S, Givelbar H: Intravascular coagulation in acute leukemia. Clinical and subclinical abnormalities. Blood 40:709, 1972
95. Tallman MS, Kwaan HC: Reassessing the hemostatic disorder associated with promyelocytic leukemia. Blood 79:543, 1992
96. Ratnoff OD: Hemostatic defects in liver and biliary tract disease and disorders of vitamin K metabolism. p. 459. In 2nd Ed. Ratnoff OD, Forbes CB (eds): Disorders of Hemostasis. WB Saunders, Philadelphia, 1991
97. Burns ER: Clinical Management of Bleeding and Thrombosis. Blackwell Scientific, Boston, 1987
98. Shearer MJ: Vitamin K metabolism and nutriture. Blood Rev 6:92, 1992
99. Donaldson VH: Hemorrhagic disorders of neonates. p. 423. In Ratnoff OD, Forbes CD (eds): Disorders of Hemostasis. 2nd Ed. WB Saunders, Philadelphia, 1991
100. Saito H: Hemostatic disorders associated with renal disease. p. 480. In Ratnoff OD, Forbes CB (eds): Disorders of Hemostasis. 2nd Ed. WB Saunders, Philadelphia, 1991
101. Janson PA, Jubelirer SJ, Weinstein MJ et al: Treatment of the bleeding tendency in uremia with cryoprecipitate. N Engl J Med 303:1318, 1980
102. Mannucci PM, Remuzzi G, Pusineri F et al: Deamino-8-D-arginine vasopressin shortens the bleeding time in uremia. N Engl J Med 308:8, 1983

103. Liu YK, Kosfeld RE, Marcum SG: Treatment of uraemic bleeding with conjugated oestrogen. Lancet 2:887, 1984
104. Livio M, Mannucci PM, Vigano G et al: Conjugated estrogens for the management of bleeding associated with renal failure. N Engl J Med 315:731, 1986
105. Bronner MH, Pate MB, Cunningham JT et al: Estrogen-progesterone therapy for bleeding gastrointestinal telangiectasis in chronic renal failure. Ann Intern Med 105:371, 1986
106. Livio M, Gotti E, Marchesi D et al: Uraemic bleeding. Role of anaemia and beneficial effect of red cell transfusions. Lancet 2:1013, 1982
107. Fernandez F, Goudable C, Sie P et al: Low haematocrit and prolonged bleeding time in uraemic patients: effect of red cell transfusions. Br J Haematol 59:139, 1985
108. Moia M, Mannucci PM, Vizzotto L et al: Improvement in the haemostatic defect of uraemia after treatment with recombinant human erythropoietin. Lancet 2:1227, 1987
109. Ratnoff OD: Bleeding Syndromes. Charles C, Springfield IL, 1960
110. Aster RH, Bartolucci AA, Collins JA et al: National Institutes of Health Consensus Conference. Platelet transfusion therapy. JAMA 257:1777, 1987
111. Lee VS, Tarrasenko L, Bellhouse BJ: Platelet transfusion therapy: platelet concentrate preparation and storage. J Lab Clin Med 111:371, 1988
112. Marcus AJ: Platelets and their disorders. p. 75. In Ratnoff OD, Forbes CD (eds): Disorders of Hemostasis. 2nd Ed. WB Saunders, Philadelphia 1991
113. Jackson DP: Management of thrombocytopenia. p. 530. In Colman RW, Hirsh J, Marder VJ, Salzman W (eds): Hemostasis and Thrombosis. 2nd Ed. JB Lippincott, Philadelphia, 1987
114. Bell WR, Tomasulo PA, Alving BM, Duffy TP: Thrombocytopenia occurring during the administration of heparin. A prospective study in 52 patients. Ann Intern Med 85:155, 1976
115. Green D, Harris K, Reynolds N et al: Heparin immune thrombocytopenia: evidence for a heparin-platelet complex as the antigenic determinant. J Lab Clin Med 91:167, 1978
116. Chong BH, Pitney WR, Castaldi PA: Heparin-induced thrombocytopenia: Association of thrombotic complications with heparin-dependent IgG antibody that induces thromboxane synthesis and platelet aggregation. Lancet 2:1246, 1982
117. Sheridan D, Carter C, Kelton JG: A diagnostic test for heparin-induced thrombocytopenia. Blood 67:27, 1986
118. Bell WR: Heparin-associated thrombocytopenia and thrombosis. J Lab Clin Med 111:600, 1988
119. Weismann RE, Tobin RM: Arterial embolism during systemic heparin therapy. Arch Surg 76: 219, 1958
120. McMillan R: Chronic idiopathic thrombocytopenic purpura. N Engl J Med 304:1135, 1981
121. Berchtold P, McMillan R: Therapy of chronic idiopathic thrombocytopenic purpura in adults. Blood 74:2309–2317, 1989
122. Collins PW, Newland AC: Treatment modalities of autoimmune blood disorders. Semin Hematol 29:64, 1992
123. Snyder HW Jr, Cochran SK, Balint JP Jr et al: Experience with protein A-immunoadsorption in treatment-resistant adult immune thrombocytopenic purpura. Blood 79:2237, 1992
124. Stuart MJ, Kelton JG: The platelet: quantitative and qualitative abnormalities. I. Quantitative abnormalities. p. 1343. In Nathan DG, Oski FA (eds): Hematology of Infancy and Childhood 3rd Ed. WB Saunders, Philadelphia, 1987
125. Lilleyman JS: Management of childhood idiopathic thrombocytopenic purpura. Br J Haematol 54:11, 1983
126. Imbach P, Barandun S, d'Apuzzo V et al: High-dose intravenous gammaglobulin for idiopathic thrombocytopenic purpura in childhood. Lancet 1:1228, 1981
127. Bussel JB, Goldman A, Imbach P et al: Treatment of acute ITP of childhood with intravenous infusions of gammaglobulin. J Pediatr 106:886, 1985
128. Firkin BG, Hunt HA, Hane SM: Management of refractory idiopathic thrombocytopenia. Blood Rev 2:149, 1988
129. Bussel JB: Modulation of Fc receptor clearance and antiplatelet antibodies as a consequence of intravenous immune globulin infusion in patients with immune thrombocytopenic purpura. J Allergy Clin Immunol 84:566, 1988
130. Salama A, Kiefel V, Amberg R, Mueller-Eckhardt C: Treatment of autoimmune thrombocytopenic purura with rhesus antibodies (anti-Rh_0(D)). Blut 49:29, 1984

2

ACUTE HEMOLYTIC DISORDERS

KATHLEEN A. LEONARD
HARVEY G. KLEIN

Hemolytic disorders are characterized by shortened survival of circulating red cells, reticulocytosis, and the absence of bleeding. Acute hemolysis may be mild, difficult to diagnose, and short-lived or fulminant, life-threatening, and prolonged over several days or weeks. Both conditions may presage a hematologic emergency for the critical care physician. A wide variety of conditions can be associated with hemolysis. Mechanistically, all are linked by a common premature disruption of the red cell membrane, with intravascular or extravascular release of free hemoglobin. This premature destruction of red cells can occur in the setting of hereditary disease due to intrinsically abnormal red cells or as a result of acquired disease due to deleterious factors affecting red cell membrane integrity.[1] There are several approaches to the diagnosis and classification of hemolytic anemias, including (1) the site of red cell destruction (intravascular or extravascular); (2) the site of the etiologic defect (intracellular (red blood cell) or extracellular/extrinsic factor); and (3) the nature of the defect (hereditary or acquired). Table 2-1 lists hemolytic disorders based on both the site of the defect and its genetic nature.

Although there are major exceptions, in general acute hemolytic disorders are acquired and due to extracellular factors. Hemolysis may be intravascular or extravascular. Intravascular hemolysis, in which red cells are destroyed in the circulation, occurs in the setting of toxins, physical and chemical trauma, immune-mediated processes, and infections that directly affect red cell membrane integrity. The relatively few causes of significant intravascular hemolysis are listed in Table 2-2. Extravascular hemolysis, in which sensitized or less deformable red cells are destroyed by the reticuloendothelial system, is more common.[2]

Acute hemolytic disorders are generally acquired, not hereditary, and are due to extrinsic factors such as antibodies, drugs, mechanical trauma, or infections.

The different diagnosis for a patient presenting with acute hemolysis is extensive; general considerations in-

TABLE 2-1. Classification of Hemolytic Anemias

- Inherited
  - Erythrocyte membrane defects
    - Hereditary spherocytosis
    - Hereditary stomatocytosis
    - Hereditary elliptocytosis
    - Hereditary pyropoikilocytosis
  - Hemoglobin defects
    - Thalassemia
    - Sickle cell anemia
    - Unstable hemoglobins
  - Enzyme deficiencies
    - G-6-PD deficiency
    - Pyruvate kinase deficiency
- Acquired
  - Erythrocyte membrane defects
    - Spur cell anemia
    - Paroxysmal nocturnal hemoglobinuria
  - Extracellular factors
    - Immune hemolysis
      - Alloimmune
        - Hemolytic transfusion reactions
        - Hemolytic disease of the newborn
      - Autoimmune
        - Warm autoimmune hemolytic anemia
        - Cold hemagglutinin disease
        - Paroxysmal cold hemoglobinuria
      - Drug-related
    - Toxins
    - Infection
    - Microangiography
    - Metabolic disorders
    - Physical/chemical agents

Abbreviation: G-6-PD, glucose-6-phosphate dehydrogenase.

TABLE 2-2. Intravascular Hemolysis

Immunologic	Hemolytic transfusion reaction Drug-induced hemolytic anemia, severe Autoimmune hemolytic anemia, severe Paroxysmal cold hemoglobinuria
Infectious	Clostridial sepsis Malarial blackwater fever Babesiosis
Toxins	Brown recluse spider bite Cobra bite
Erythrocyte defects	G-6-PD deficiency Paroxysmal nocturnal hemoglobinuria
Metabolic	Hypophosphatemia
Microangiopathic	All
Physical/chemical agents	All

Abbreviation: G-6-PD, glucose-6-phosphate dehydrogenase.

clude infections, toxins, physical or chemical trauma, microangiopathies, immunologic processes, and metabolic disorders, alone or in combination with intrinsic red cell defects. Acute hemolysis may be suggested by common laboratory screening tests such as hemoglobin and blood smears and a few nonspecific physical findings such as pallor, jaundice, and splenomegaly. Diagnosis is generally made on the basis of meticulous history taking and further laboratory testing. Treatment is usually disease-specific, with transfusion support as needed.

LABORATORY TESTS

Laboratory tests commonly used to evaluate hemolysis include the reticulocyte count, peripheral smear, serum haptoglobin, LDH, bilirubin, plasma hemoglobin, urinalysis, urine hemosiderin, and direct antiglobulin tests.

Abnormalities in common laboratory tests often first suggest the presence of acute hemolysis—progressive anemia with elevated reticulocyte count, bilirubin, and lactate dehydrogenase (LDH). These typical findings, however, will result from widely differing causes of hemolysis. Once the diagnosis has been suggested, the laboratory can be essential in both confirming hemolysis and arriving at a specific diagnosis. Several red cell tests are helpful in establishing the presence of hemolysis by providing evidence of red cell destruction and bone marrow response and by providing information about the underlying cause of hemolysis.

Red Cell Tests

Patients with hemolysis may vary widely in their degree of anemia, depending on the severity of the red cell destruction and the ability of the bone marrow to respond. Red cell production can increase four- to eightfold over baseline levels, and if the erythropoietic response keeps pace with red cell destruction, a compensated hemolysis with stable hemoglobin levels will result. While partially compensated hemolysis is less common in the acute setting, it may mislead the clinician.

The peripheral blood smear may provide further evidence of hemolysis, clues to the cause of the red cell destruction, and occasionally a specific diagnosis. The blood smear may also provide evidence of reticulocytosis before a reticulocyte count is available. On standard Wright-Giemsa stained blood smears, reticulocytes may be detectable by their bluish orange staining and larger size, known as *polychromatophilia*. With more severe hemolysis and anemia, prematurely released *shift reticulocytes* will show basophilic stippling; nucleated red cells may also be seen. Red cell morphology will vary considerably, depending on the cause of hemolysis. For example, agglutinated cells may be seen with autoimmune hemolytic anemia (AIHA) particularly cold agglutinin disease. Spherocytes may be seen with many different hemolytic states, including hemolytic transfusion reactions, infections, burns, and warm AIHA. High percentages of spherocytes suggest hereditary spherocytosis. Erythrophagocytosis may be seen with AIHA and paroxysmal cold hemoglobinuria.[3,4] Schistocytes are seen in microangiopathic processes and in some forms of red cell trauma.[5] Intracellular organisms can be seen and occasionally will result in the difficult and unsuspected diagnosis of malaria, babesiosis, or bartonellosis.

The reticulocyte count is usually elevated, often significantly; in certain situations, such as transfusion-related hemolysis, reticulocytosis may be minimal. The rise in the reticulocyte count may not be immediate and may lead to a misdiagnosis of a hypoproliferative anemia.[6] In acute hemolysis, within 12 to 24 hours iron utilization increases, within 48 hours the bone marrow shows increased erythropoiesis, and within 72 hours the reticulocyte count increases.[7] With massive red cell loss, reticulocytosis may appear earlier.[8] With AIHA, despite a markedly active erythropoietic bone marrow, reticulocytes may be absent, and a rapidly progressive anemia may result.[6,9,10] The mechanism of the reticulocytopenia is unclear, but it has been speculated that in at least some forms of AIHA autoantibody may have a greater affinity for reticulocytes than for red cells.[11] Additionally, in both hereditary spherocytosis and several forms of acquired hemolytic anemia, superimposed parvovirus B19 infections have resulted in aplastic crises with low reticulocyte counts.[12]

Chromium 51 radiolabeling studies provide the most direct measure of red cell survival but are more commonly used in suspected cases of delayed hemolysis. Bone marrow aspirate and biopsy are typically markedly erythroblastic, with normoblastic maturation.[5] Neither test is generally necessary in making a diagnosis of acute hemolysis or helpful in determining the cause.

Serum, Plasma, and Urine Tests

Extravascular hemolysis is more common than intravascular hemolysis but may be more difficult to confirm. Both forms may be present simultaneously.

Several serum, plasma, and urine tests are helpful in confirming the presence of hemolysis by providing evidence of increased hemoglobin catabolism. Laboratory test results will vary, depending on the site of hemolysis, the rate of hemolysis, and the amount of blood destroyed. In certain cases it may not be possible to distinguish intravascular from extravascular hemolysis, and both may occur simultaneously.[5]

With intravascular hemolysis, hemoglobin is released into plasma, causing hemoglobinemia. The free hemoglobin is bound by haptoglobin, an α_2-globulin. The haptoglobin-hemoglobin complex is rapidly cleared by the reticuloendothelial system of the liver. With significant hemolysis, haptoglobin synthesis in the liver will lag behind haptoglobin clearance, and haptoglobin levels will fall and may become undetectable.[7] Intravascular lysis of as little as 20 ml of whole blood or 10 ml of packed red cells may decrease the serum haptoglobin level significantly.[13] Haptoglobin is an acute-phase reactant protein; very high levels seen with stress states may mask increased hemoglobin binding in hemolysis and may not be diagnostically helpful. Conversely, extremely low levels may be present with severe liver disease and also will not be diagnostically helpful.

When haptoglobin levels are depleted, hemoglobin may be visible in the plasma, serum, and urine. Hemoglobinemia may be present only transiently, and urine hemoglobin and urine hemosiderin tests may be diagnostically helpful after an acute episode. At plasma hemoglobin levels of 20 mg/dl, the plasma will be amber, at levels of 50 to 100 mg/dl it will be reddish brown, and at levels above 200 mg/dl it will be cherry red. If hemoglobinemia is present for more than 1 hour, free hemoglobin will be oxidized to methemoglobin, and methemalbumin, which has a characteristic brown color, will appear. Free plasma hemoglobin will be filtered by glomeruli, absorbed by the cells of the renal tubule, and metabolized to hemosiderin. Tubular epithelium is gradually sloughed off, and urine hemosiderin can be detected for up to 5 to 10 days following hemolysis by staining the urinary sediment with Prussian blue and noting intracellular hemosiderin granules. After haptoglobin stores are depleted and the tubular cells have been saturated by hemoglobin, free urinary hemoglobin will be detectable. Hemoglobinuria is generally indicated by dark red or cola-colored urine and can be distinguished from hematuria by the absence of intact red cells on urinalysis.[5,7]

While the features of a fulminant hemolytic transfusion reaction are rarely misdiagnosed, these reactions may present with subtle features, especially in a comatose or anaesthetized patient. Dark urine, fever, or inappropriate increment in hemoglobin posttransfusion should alert the clinician to take appropriate diagnostic steps.

With extravascular hemolysis, confirming hemolysis may be considerably more difficult, as there generally will be no hemoglobinemia, hemoglobinuria, or urine hemosiderinuria. The affected red cells are removed from the circulation by the liver and spleen and destroyed in situ. Although no significant hemoglobin is released directly into the circulation, haptoglobin levels may be reduced, particularly with ongoing hemolysis. With severe extravascular hemolysis, plasma hemoglobin levels may be elevated.[5]

With intravascular and extravascular hemolysis, serum levels of both the released red cell enzymes LDH and serum glutamate oxaloacetate transaminase (SGOT) and unconjugated bilirubin, the metabolic product of released hemoglobin, will often be elevated. However, the degree of elevation is variable, particularly with extravascular hemolysis, and these are nonspecific findings. With both intravascular and extravascular hemolysis in the absence of hepatobiliary disease, serum levels of conjugated or direct bilirubin will be normal. Additionally, because the circulating unconjugated bilirubin is bound to albumin and cannot be filtered through the glomeruli, bilirubin will not be present in the urine even with severe intravascular hemolysis, which is a helpful differential diagnostic finding.[5,14]

The direct antiglobulin test (DAT) or direct Coombs test is essential for evaluating immunologic causes of hemolysis. A positive DAT indicates that there has been an in vivo coating of red cells by the immunoglobulins IgG or IgM and/or complement. Whenever a transfusion reaction or autoimmune hemolysis is suspected, the DAT should be performed. Positive DAT results may be seen with autoimmune disorders, with certain medications, and with several nonhemolytic conditions in the absence of red cell destruction. However, in a clinical setting consistent with hemolysis with supportive laboratory data, a positive DAT strongly suggests an immune hemolysis.

The indirect antiglobulin test (IAT), or indirect Coombs test is helpful in evaluating suspected alloimmune causes of hemolysis. A positive result indicates that the patient has circulating alloantibodies or autoantibodies directed against specific red cell antigens. Alloantibodies are produced in response to foreign red cells introduced by a previous pregnancy or transfusion. Often such antibodies are incidental findings found on transfusion screening and do not cause hemolysis. However, in certain settings such as hemolytic disease of the newborn and hemolytic transfusion reactions, alloantibodies may cause severe hemolysis.

CAUSES OF ACUTE HEMOLYTIC DISORDERS

Acute hemolytic disorders occur in widely diverse settings and do not lend themselves to simple classification. One practical classification system divides the disorders on the basis of cause. Possible causes of acute hemolysis include infections, physical and chemical trauma, toxins, microangiopathies, immune processes, metabolic disorders, and intrinsic red cell defects. Table 2-3 lists the acute hemolytic disorders on the basis of the underlying etiology.

Infectious Agents

A wide variety of infectious agents can cause acute hemolysis. There are several mechanisms of infectious hemolysis, including direct invasion of the erythrocyte by organisms, stimulation of the immune system with production of antibodies directed against red cells, development of a microangiopathy, and elaboration of toxins that disrupt the red

TABLE 2-3. Causes of Acute Hemolysis

Immune Hemolytic Disorders
- Autoimmune hemolysis
  - Warm autoimmune hemolytic anemia
  - Cold hemagglutinin disease
  - Paroxysmal cold hemoglobinuria
- Alloimmune hemolysis
  - Hemolytic disease of the newborn
  - Hemolytic transfusion reactions
- Drug-induced hemolytic anemia
  - Penicillins
  - Cephalosporins
  - α-Methyldopa
  - Hydrochlorothiazide

Infections
- Parasitic
  - Malaria
  - Babesia
- Bacterial
  - Clostridial sepsis
  - Bartonellosis
  - *Mycoplasma pneumoniae*
  - *Escherichia coli*
  - *Yersinia enterocolitica*
  - *Hemophilus influenzae* type b
- Viral
  - Cytomegalovirus
  - Epstein-Barr virus
  - Hepatitis A
  - Hepatitis B
  - Non-A, non-B hepatitis
- Fungal
  - *Aspergillus fumigatus*

Microangiopathic Processes
- Primary
  - Thrombotic thrombocytopenic purpura
  - Hemolytic uremic syndrome
- Secondary
  - Disseminated cancer
  - Chemotherapy induced
  - Pre-eclampsia/HELLP syndrome

Physical/Chemical Agents
- Thermal
  - Microwave
  - Iatrogenic/blood warming
  - Burn injury
  - Inadvertent freezing of blood units
  - Improper thawing of frozen red cells
  - Autologous marrow infusion
- Oncotic
  - Hypotonic saline
  - Dextrose solutions
  - Glycerol infusion
  - Angiographic contrast dye
  - Transurethral prostate resection irrigant
  - Hysteroscopic metroplasty irrigant
  - Drowning
- Physical trauma
  - March hemoglobinuria
  - Prosthetic valve dysfunction
  - Intravascular prosthetic grafts
  - Extracorporeal blood processing instruments
  - Intravenous catheter
  - Single-needle dialysis

Toxic Agents
- Poisons
  - Arsine
  - Copper
  - Chloramine
  - Formaldehyde
  - Sodium chlorate
  - Hydrogen peroxide
  - Lead
  - Gasoline
  - Bromate
- Venoms
  - Wasp
  - Hornet
  - Portugese man-of-war
  - Cobra
  - Brown recluse spider
  - Scorpion
- Drugs
  - Dimethyl sulfoxide
  - Hyperbaric oxygen

Inherited Erythrocyte Disorders
- Enzyme deficiencies: G-6-PD deficiency
- Hemoglobin disorders: Unstable hemoglobins

Metabolic Processes
- Hypophosphatemia
- Wilson's disease

Acquired Membrane Defects
- Paroxysmal nocturnal hemogloginuria
- Spur cell anemia: liver disease

Abbreviations: HELLP, hemolysis, elevated liver enzymes, low platelet count; G-6-PD, glucose-6-phosphate dehydrogenase.

Acute hemolysis may occur with a number of infectious agents but is most severe with malaria, babesiosis, bartonellosis, and clostridial sepsis. Often the diagnosis can be suspected from the history and confirmed on a blood smear.

cell membrane. The classic examples of infectious hemolysis include malaria, babesiosis, bartonellosis, and clostridial sepsis, in which toxins or organisms act directly on the red cells, and hemolysis may be the cardinal manifestation of infection. With other infectious agents, particularly those with an immune basis, hemolysis may be less common and less life-threatening. Although intravascular hemolysis is almost invariably seen with clostridial sepsis, with other forms of infection both intravascular and extravascular red cell destruction may occur, but extravascular hemolysis tends to predominate. Infections that do not affect normal erythrocytes may cause acute hemolysis in patients with inherited red cell defects, such as glucose-6-phosphate dehydrogenase (G-6-PD) deficiency. This association will be discussed separately.

Direct Invasion of Red Cells

Malaria. On a worldwide basis malaria is one of the most important causes of acute hemolysis, although rarely considered in the United States, where, however, between 1975 and 1983 the incidence of imported cases of falciparum malaria, the most severe form of the disease, increased sharply.[15] Transfusion-acquired malaria has also been reported.[16] Clinically, patients present with fever, anemia, and hepatosplenomegaly. The most severe cases are seen in nonimmune individuals, and the disease should therefore always be considered both in nonresident travelers to endemic areas and in young resident children after loss of protective maternal antibodies.[17] The anemia varies considerably in degree and is multifactorial in etiology, occurring primarily as a result of extravascular hemolysis with hypersplenism. There is also a variable component of intravascular hemolysis, which roughly correlates with the degree of parasitemia, and an ill-defined suppression of erythropoiesis.[18–21] Positive DAT results may be seen, with both IgG and complement coating,[22] and immune hemolysis of both parasitized and nonparasitized red cells has been described.[19] With *Plasmodium falciparum* massive intravascular hemolysis may occur, giving rise to "blackwater fever," with prominent hemoglobinuria. The cause is obscure and only in some patients is related to quinine therapy, with a drug-induced hemolysis.[18]

Diagnosis of malaria is made by examination of the peripheral blood smear for both intraerythrocytic and extracellular parasite forms; in cases of minimal parasitemia, a thick smear preparation may be necessary and should be performed when serologic testing is not available. Treatment of an acute attack of malaria usually consists of specific drug therapy and supportive transfusion.[23] Exchange transfusion has also been advocated for severe cases,[24] but its importance remains controversial.[25,26]

Babesiosis. Babesiosis, caused by the protozoon *Babesia microti*, is transmitted by the northern deer tick, *Ixodes dammini*. Most cases have occurred along coastal areas of the northeastern United States, although a case has been reported in Wisconsin.[27] Transfusion-acquired babesiosis has also been reported.[28,29] Clinically, babesiosis varies from asymptomatic to an acute febrile illness with moderate to severe hemolytic anemia with hemoglobinuria. There may be a gradual onset, with a prodrome of malaise and fatigue followed by fevers, rigors, myalgias, and arthralgias.[30,31] The disease appears to be more severe in splenectomized or immunocompromised patients.[31,32] Diagnosis is made by examining the peripheral smear and noting the intraerythrocytic parasites. Treatment consists of combination therapy with quinine preparations and clindamycin. Exchange transfusion has also been reported.[31,32]

Bartonellosis. Human bartonellosis, also known as Oroya fever and Carrion disease, is caused by the small, motile, pleomorphic gram-negative organism *Bartonella bacilliformis*. The disease occurs only in the western Andes of Peru, Ecuador, and Columbia, where it is transmitted by *Phlebotomus* sandflies.[19] Clinically, there are two distinct stages of illness. The acute febrile hemolysis, Oroya fever, is followed in survivors by a chronic cutaneous verrucous process known as *verruca peruana*. Diagnosis is made on the peripheral smear by demonstrating the presence of rod-shaped organisms, singly or in clusters, within or on the surface of red cells and is confirmed by blood culture. Large numbers of red cells (up to 80 to 100 percent) may be affected. Reticulocytosis may be marked, and normoblasts may be present on the peripheral smear.[33,34] Treatment is with penicillin, aminoglycosides, chloramphenicol, or tetracyclines.[19,35]

Toxin Production

Clostridial Sepsis. Clostridia are anaerobic, spore-forming, gram-positive bacilli found in the gastrointestinal and female genital tracts. *Clostridium perfringens* (formerly *welchii*) sepsis may be associated with sudden massive hemolysis.[36] *C. perfringens* produces a number of toxins, the best characterized of which is the α-toxin, a lecithinase. The mechanism of hemolysis is generally thought to involve the effect of the α-toxin on red cell membranes[18]; however, in 1991 a θ-toxin-mediated colloid-osmotic red cell lysis was described.[37] Classically, clostridial infections occurred postpartum or in postabortal infection and wound gas gangrene, but recently hematologic and colonic malignancies have provided a more typical clinical setting, with a gastrointestinal portal of entry.[38] Patients frequently develop massive intravascular hemolysis, often with the hematocrit falling to 5 percent or lower, and with prominent hemoglobinemia and hemoglobinuria. The peripheral smear reveals microspherocytosis, and intact red cells may be difficult to find. Multisystem failure, leukocytosis, and disseminated intravascular coagulation (DIC) are common. Diagnosis is made by noting the characteristic club-shaped organisms on a fluid or tissue smear, by positive blood cultures, or by assaying for the α-toxin of *C. perfringens*. Treatment involves high-dose penicillin, surgical debridement if feasible, and hyperbaric oxygen for gangrene of the extremities.[39]

Escherichia coli *Infection.* *Escherichia coli* urinary tract infection has been reported in association with acute intravascular hemolysis in an immunocompromised individual. The mechanism of the hemolysis is not entirely clear, however. Lupus erythematosus was the underlying disease state, and the direct antiglobulin test was positive, with an IgG autoantibody with anti Rh(e) specificity. The patient's red cells were type A, Rh positive, and Rh(e) positive as well. Although an immunologic basis is possible, the lack of response to steroids was believed to be inconsistent with purely immune destruction. High-titer antibodies directed against the *E. coli* α-hemolysin were demonstrated, and there was complete resolution of hemolysis with appropriate antibiotic therapy, which suggests that hemolysis was due to a direct effect of α-hemolysin on red cells.[40]

Other Infections. Acute hemolysis has been reported with a wide variety of other infections, generally as a relatively uncommon occurrence. Acute hemolysis believed to be related primarily to marked hypersplenism has been reported with miliary tuberculosis, subacute bacterial endocarditis, infectious mononucleosis, infectious hepatitis, and psittacosis.[41] A microangiopathic state, which can occur in DIC seen with any number of bacterial infections or septicemic states, particularly *Neisseria meningitidis* infection,[42] will cause intravascular red cell destruction in fibrin webs in the microvasculature. The degree of hemolysis is generally mild, and coagulopathy is the major manifestation. Acute severe hemolysis with a microangiopathic picture has been reported with *Aspergillus fumigatus* infection.[43] Diagnosis of the microangiopathic state is generally made by noting schistocytes and other red cell fragments on the peripheral smear.

Acute hemolysis with an immune basis has been reported in a number of bacterial and viral processes. Although the exact cause of red cell destruction is not entirely clear, a number of mechanisms have been proposed, including alteration of red cell surface by organisms; immunization by cross-reactive antigens on the infectious agent, with production of red cell autoantibodies; and infection-mediated alterations in B- and T-cell responses, with production of antibodies against red cells.[44,45] With this heterogeneous group of disorders, the infectious manifestations will often predominate over the hemolytic findings, and diagnosis generally rests upon identifying the infectious agent and/or documenting the appropriate serologic response. The DAT will be helpful in detecting warm autoantibodies and cold agglutinins. The peripheral smear may show shift reticulocytosis and spherocytosis, but aside from revealing the presence of red cell agglutination which suggests an immunologic etiology for the hemolysis, it generally will not be diagnostically helpful.

Paroxysmal cold hemoglobinuria (PCH), or Donath-Landsteiner hemolytic anemia, is a classic example of an acute hemolytic process associated with infectious agents; although in years past PCH was associated with syphilis, viral prodromes are now far more common.[46] This is discussed in detail in subsequent sections. Reported associations with acute hemolytic episodes include Epstein-Barr virus with infectious mononucleosis,[47,48] cytomegalovirus,[49] hepatitis A,[50] hepatitis B,[51] non-A, non-B hepatitis,[52] *Mycoplasma pneumoniae*,[53] *Yersinia enterocolitica*,[54] and *Haemophilus influenzae* type b. With *H. influenzae* it has been shown that the capsular polysaccharide is absorbed onto the red cell surface, and an immunologic destruction of sensitized erythrocytes is suggested.[55]

Metabolic Disorders

A number of metabolic disorders have been associated with acute hemolysis as a relatively uncommon manifestation. Acute intravascular hemolysis was noted in a case of acute mountain sickness.[56] Acute, severe hemolysis has been reported in profound hypophosphatemia[57,58]; hemolysis was extravascular and reversible with phosphate supplementation. Laboratory studies demonstrated microspherocytic changes on peripheral smear, markedly reduced red cell adenosine triphosphate (ATP) levels, increased red cell rigidity, and shortened red cell survival.[57]

Acute hemolysis of mild to moderate severity with transient stomatocytosis of 23 to 33 percent has been reported as a complication directly related to acute ethanol intoxication. The destruction was consistent with extravascular hemolysis and resolved with cessation of ethanol intake.[59]

Wilson's disease has been associated with acute hemolysis in periods of copper accumulation, both antedating the diagnosis and occurring with disease exacerbations. Clinically, it manifests as a moderate to severe hemolytic anemia, without hemoglobinemia or hemoglobinuria. The peripheral smear may show polychromatophilia but no change in red cell morphology. Studies have shown increased erythrocyte copper, ceruloplasmin, and hypercupriuria, and other studies have demonstrated that hemolysis occurs as a result of oxidative stress caused by copper accumulation in red cells. Penicillamine is the treatment of choice.[60,61]

Acquired Erythrocyte Membrane Defects

Spur Cell Anemia

Anemia is a common finding in alcoholic liver dysfunction and may be related to several factors, including hypersplenism, nutritional deficiencies, and ethanol-related bone marrow suppression. A chronic mild extravascular hemolysis with target cell formation occurs, with significant cirrhosis and hypersplenism. Spur cell anemia is a more severe hemolytic process, which also occurs in patients with cirrhosis and hypersplenism, especially in association with alcoholic liver disease. Clinically there is moderate to severe red cell destruction, with increasing jaundice and reticulocytosis as prominent signs. The onset may be subacute. The key diagnostic feature is the presence of spiculated "spur" cells on peripheral smear; the spur cells may account for up to 80 to 90 percent of red cells. These spur cells have a markedly increased cholesterol content in the cell membrane, with an abnormal morphology, and undergo extravascular hemolysis by splenic destruction. The development of spur cell anemia is a poor prognostic sign, generally seen in the last few months of life.[62–65]

Paroxysmal Nocturnal Hemoglobinuria

Paroxysmal nocturnal hemoglobinuria (PNH) is an acquired stem cell disorder resulting in varying degrees of episodic hemolysis. In PNH an abnormal clone of stem cells proliferates, producing erythrocytes that are extremely susceptible to complement-mediated membrane damage and lysis, as well as abnormal platelets and granulocytes. Pathophysiologically, the hemolysis appears to be related to erythrocyte membrane deficiencies of a number of regulatory proteins, including at least two complement regulatory proteins that inhibit both classical and alternative complement pathways. Red cell clones lacking these control proteins are abnormally susceptible to hemolysis.[66,67] Clinically, the presentation and symptomatology are variable, and considerable delays in diagnosis are not uncommon. The disease occurs most commonly in adults. Hemolytic anemia, mild thrombocytopenia and granulocytopenia, venous thrombosis, episodic hemoglobinuria, infection, and painful crises are seen. The degree of anemia is extremely variable, and hemoglobinuria may be absent. Episodes of hemolysis may be precipitated by infection or anesthesia. Bone marrow failure may develop, particularly in children and adolescents.[68]

The diagnosis is based on demonstration of increased susceptibility to complement-mediated lysis by the Ham test (acid hemolysis test) or by the sucrose hemolysis test. Supportive laboratory data include reticulocytosis, a low alkaline phosphatase level, and urine hemosiderin. The peripheral smear may show microcytic, hypochromic red cell changes, due to iron loss in the urine, and polychromatophilia; there are no specific morphologic changes. The hemolytic component is treated with prednisone, with iron supplementation as needed. Androgens are used for bone marrow failure. Prophylactic splenectomy and anticoagulation are of little benefit.[68,69] Bone marrow transplantation has been successful[70] and is particularly useful in younger patients with a tendency to bone marrow aplasia.[68] Transfusions, generally necessary to support patients, will on occasion exacerbate hemolysis and may mimic an acute hemolytic transfusion reaction; washed products have been advocated but are probably not absolutely necessary if group-specific (ABO-identical) blood and blood products are used.[71]

Inherited Red Cell Defects

Inherited intrinsic red cell defects include the membrane defects, red cell enzyme deficiency states, and the hemoglobinopathies, as listed in Table 2-1. The clinical features of each of these disorders vary considerably, and the degree of ongoing hemolysis ranges from subclinical or minimal to severe and transfusion-dependent. The family history will often be helpful, and splenomegaly at some point in the disease course is common but not invariable. With all three defect types, regardless of the baseline disease in any given patient, acute hemolytic episodes have been reported, particularly in stress states such as infection with splenomegaly and fever. The etiology of the acute hemolysis may be obscure, particularly in patients with previously subclinical disease. In any case of unexplained acute hemolysis, especially in the setting of drugs, infection, or fever, inherited red cell defects should be suspected.

When acute hemolysis occurs in the setting of infection or medication in the absence of serologic findings, an underlying red cell defect should be suspected.

Hemoglobinopathies

The unstable hemoglobins are a group of rare hemoglobin variants in which altered amino acid sequencing decreases the stability of the hemoglobin molecule, causing a congenital nonspherocytic hemolytic process. The hemoglobin undergoes denaturation and precipitation in the red cell, which may be visible on peripheral smear as Heinz bodies. The red cells are damaged as the Heinz bodies are removed in transit through the spleen.[72] There are more than 100 unstable hemoglobins, and the clinical picture varies from completely asymptomatic to severe hemolytic anemia. Patients with otherwise mild disease may present with acute, primarily intravascular, hemolysis,[73] usually in the setting of infection, particularly viral upper respiratory tract infections, fever, and certain drugs. Redox-active drugs, especially sulfonamides and phenazopyridine (Pyridium), are problematic. The exact mechanism of hemolysis is not understood; in addition to the splenic "pitting" damage with removal of Heinz bodies, a direct oxidant drug effect on the altered hemoglobin may be operative.[72,74] Diagnosis of an unstable hemoglobin is generally made by using either of two screening tests, the isopropranol instability test and the heat precipitation test. These may not be sensitive enough to detect all subclinical, mildly unstable hemoglobins; more elaborate heat precipitation tests may be required. The brillant cresyl blue test will cause Heinz body formation in the presence of unstable hemoglobins.[73] Other laboratory data will be consistent with extravascular hemolysis, and the peripheral smear may show hypochromia, poikilocytosis, and polychromasia; Heinz bodies are present in splenectomized patients. Reticulocytosis may be marked.[74] Treatment is generally supportive, with nutritional supplementation as required.

Membranopathies

There are four types of inherited membrane defects, each with abnormalities of the red cell membrane cytoskeleton and an altered erythrocyte morphology causing congenital hemolytic anemia. The degree of hemolysis is variable, and patients may reach adulthood before experiencing any clinical evidence of hemolysis. Some degree of splenomegaly is usual. Acute hemolytic episodes, with laboratory values indicative of both intravascular and extravascular hemolysis, have been reported with infection in hereditary spherocytosis (HS)[75,76] and with both infection and pregnancy in hereditary elliptocytosis (HE).[77] Diagnosis of the underlying disorder is made by noting both polychromasia and the characteristic red cell morphology on peripheral smear, with numerous microspherocytes or elliptocytes. A negative DAT should be documented, as microspherocytes may be numerous with immune-mediated hemolysis as well. The confirmatory osmotic fragility test is generally positive in HS but may be negative in HE. Splenectomy is the treatment of choice in HS and HE with significant ongoing hemolysis, as this removes the site of red cell destruction.[75,76]

Enzymopathies

A number of red cell enzyme deficiencies have been described, by far the most prevalent of which is G-6-PD deficiency. More than 300 variants of G-6-PD deficiency have been described, not all of which are clinically significant. Individuals with G-6-DP:A, found in 20 percent of black Americans, do not have significantly reduced enzyme levels and are not at risk for hemolysis. G-6-PD:A(−) is the classic mild deficiency state, found in 11 percent of black Americans; affected individuals are at risk for intravascular hemolysis only as neonates and in the settings of infection, exposure to napthalene (mothballs), and certain types of drug therapy.[78,79] Approximately 10 percent of residual G-6-PD activity is retained, mostly in reticulocytes and in young red cells; the result of this heterogeneity is that upon oxidant exposure, acute hemolysis occurs but is self-limited to only the older erythrocytes. G-6-PD-Med is the classic severe deficiency, with barely detectable enzyme levels. Acute hemolytic episodes, induced by infection, napthalene or fava bean exposure, or certain drugs, will be much more severe, as virtually all red cells are G-6-PD-deficient.[78,79] Hypoglycemia-induced hemolysis has also been reported.[80] Drugs implicated in hemolysis with G-6-PD deficiency include sulfamethoxazole, primaquine, phenazopyridine, nitrofurantoin, niridazole, nalidixic acid, methylene blue, doxorubicin, and acetanilide.[79] Acute intravascular hemolysis has also been reported following endoscopic variceal sclerotherapy[81] and anesthesia.[82] Dapsone, which has been used as combination therapy with trimethoprim for *Pneumocystis carinii* pneumonia, has also been noted to induce hemolysis in both G-6-PD-deficient and nondeficient patients.[83] Some degree of caution is warranted when using this drug in ethnic groups at risk for G-6-PD.[84]

According to classic clinical descriptions of G-6-PD oxidant stress, acute intravascular hemolysis and hemoglobinuria generally develop within 48 hours of exposure, with precipitous anemia and with Heinz bodies and blister cells found on peripheral smear. Much less obvious presentations, with mild to moderate anemia and no hemoglobinuria, are common, and recent reports indicate that at least some proportion of G-6-PD-mediated hemolysis is extravascular.[85] Diagnosis of the G-6-PD state is generally made by using the quantitative assay for G-6-PD, a fluorescent assay that measures generation of reduced nicotinamide adenine dinucleotide phosphate (NADPH). A false negative result may be obtained after acute hemolysis in a mildly deficient variant such as G-6-PD:A(−), with all the G-6-PD-deficient older cells having been destroyed. Other available tests include dye-linked reduction of NADP and measures of oxidant-induced Heinz body formation in erythrocytes. Treatment consists of avoiding known oxidant drugs, but in fact most cases are induced by infection. Prophylactic testing for G-6-PD deficiency in certain patient populations has been advocated.[86]

Toxic Agents

Toxins

A wide variety of toxic agents can cause acute hemolysis, including chemical poisons, insect and snake venoms, and medications. The mechanism of red cell injury varies, but many common toxins cause oxidation, leading to membrane damage and intravascular hemolysis. Severe intravascular hemolysis on an immune basis has been reported following ingestion of *Paxillus involutus* mushrooms.[87] Among chemicals causing acute intravascular hemolysis are arsine,[88] copper,[89,90] formaldehyde,[91] chloramines,[92] sodium chlorate,[93] hydrogen peroxide,[94] lead,[95] gasoline,[96] and bromate[97]; several of these agents have been discovered as complications of hemodialysis.[89,91,92,94] Diagnosis is based on clinical or toxicologic identification of the toxic agent, and treatment is substance-specific.

Medications

Medication-related acute nonimmunologic intravascular hemolysis is classically seen with G-6-PD deficiency or related states but can occur in non-G-6-PD deficient patients as well.[98,99] Association of hyperbaric oxygen with acute hemolysis has been reported; this may have been related to a superimposed vitamin E deficiency.[100] Dimethyl sulfoxide (DMSO), used to reduce intracranial pressure, has caused acute intravascular hemolysis.[101] Unconventional intravenous therapy with hydrogen peroxide for esophageal carcinoma[102] and with calcium 2-aminoethanol phosphate for multiple sclerosis[103] resulted in both cases in massive intravascular hemolysis. Calcium 2-aminoethanol phosphate, which is not approved by the Food and Drug Administration (FDA), has been used in Germany for autoimmune disorders and brought into the United States illegally. Treatment involves stopping administration of the offending drug and supportive therapy.

Insect/Snake Venom

Envenomations associated with acute intravascular hemolysis include those caused by the cobra,[104] scorpion,[105] common wasp,[106] hornet,[107] Portugese man-of-war,[108] and brown recluse spider.[109,110] Severe skin lesions at the site of the sting or bite are common. Peripheral smear may show polychromasia and spherocytosis, but there are no specific findings. Treatment is based on the underlying etiology, with supportive therapy and possibly venom antisera.

Physical and Chemical Agents

Thermal

Rarely, acute hemolysis may be seen with the use of frozen, deglycerolized red cell products. Techniques for freezing units of blood require glycerol, a cryoprotective agent, and minimal hemolysis occurs even with long-term storage.[111] When the blood is needed, the units are thawed and washed to remove the glycerol, as liquid glycerol is hyperosmolar and will lyse erythrocytes. Transfusion of thawed but inadequately washed units of frozen red cells[112] or of frozen autologous red cells[113] have resulted in intravascular hemolysis. In this setting the red cell destruction occurs in the blood unit itself, but infusion of the unit causes signs and symptoms of an acute hemolytic transfusion reaction, with intravascular hemolysis and hemoglobinuria. Accidental freezing of liquid whole blood or packed red cells stored in standard preservative media without a cryoprotective agent causes severe red cell destruction. Infusion of an accidentally frozen unit of autologous red blood cells has been reported to result in a clinical picture of intravascular hemolysis with acute renal failure.[114] Autologous bone marrow undergoes a number of processing steps prior to storage, including red cell depletion and stem cell cryopreservation with DMSO. Transient elevations in serum lactate dehydrogenase, and acute hemoglobinemia and hemoglobinuria have been reported with reinfusion of autologous marrow; whether this hemolysis is related to destruction of residual red cells in the marrow upon freezing and thawing or is related to an in vivo toxic effect of DMSO is not clear.[115,116]

Red cells should be transfused as soon as the unit is released from the transfusion service. Storage in inadequately monitored refrigerators and inadvertent freezing or heating may result in transfusion of a hemolyzed unit.

Excess heat will cause acute hemolysis in several situations. Severe third-degree burns over at least 50 percent of the body surface area are associated with acute hemolysis, hemoglobinuria, renal failure, and spherocytes on peripheral smear.[117] Iatrogenic hemolysis following use of warmed units of whole blood or packed red cells has also been reported. Here again, the hemolysis occurs in vitro in the blood unit and upon infusion produces a clinical picture of acute intravascular hemolysis with hemoglobinemia. This has been reported with use of conventional heat transfer blood warmers[118] and waterbaths,[119] as well as with microwave blood warmers.[120,121] It has been shown that with microwave blood warmers, which are no longer marketed in the United States and were designed primarily to warm whole blood units,[122] significant hemolysis is more likely to occur with the smaller volumes and higher hematocrits of packed cells and also in units heated above 46.8°C.[123] Red cell components should be warmed only with systems that have been designed specifically for that purpose and are routinely quality-controlled.

Oncotic

Acute hemolysis with hemoglobinuria and hemoglobinemia can occur with near drowning in fresh water,[124] as well as on exposure to hypertonic and hypotonic solutions. Administration of packed cells with 0.45 percent saline will cause a clinical picture of an acute hemolytic transfusion reaction.[125] Both intravenous 20 percent glycerol solution[126] and angiographic contrast dye[127] have resulted in intravascular hemolysis. Use of hypotonic irrigating solutions in transuretheral resection of the prostate and in hysteroscopic metroplasty has been reported to cause acute intravascular hemolysis in both applications.[128,129]

Mechanical Trauma

Severe mechanical trauma to red cells results in intravascular hemolysis and may occur in the settings of intravenous catheters or extracorporeal blood circuits, excessive running or marching, and cardiac valves or prosthetic grafts. *Macroangiopathic hemolytic anemia* is a term used to describe this condition.

Extracorporeal membrane oxygenation both in neonates and in cardiac surgery patients is known to cause hemolysis, particularly with bubble oxygenators[130]; the incidence and severity of hemolysis may decline as membrane oxygenators become more widely used.[131] It should be noted that some episodes of hemolysis occurring with cardiopulmonary bypass may be related to complement activation and immune destruction rather than to direct red cell trauma.[132] Technical difficulties with an intraoperative autologous transfusion blood processor have caused traumatic intravascular hemolysis with acute renal failure.[133] Single-needle hemodialysis,[134,135] platelet apheresis with partially occluded blood tubing,[136] and exchange transfusion with catheter trauma[137] have all been associated with acute mechanical hemolysis. In these cases intravascular hemolysis develops during or shortly following the procedure, and the peripheral smear shows schistocytes and irregular red cell fragments.

Physical trauma to red cells during running or marching may lead to acute intravascular hemolysis (often called *march hemoglobinuria* or *runner's* or *foot strike hemolysis*). This generally presents as transient hemoglobinuria shortly after exertion, with laboratory values consistent with acute intravascular hemolysis with hemoglobinemia.[138,139] Several authors have noted morphologic changes on peripheral smear, including macrocytosis[139] and echinocytosis of up to 10 percent, possibly related to hemoconcentration.[140] The mechanism may be related to destruction of the oldest subset of red cells in the vasculature of the foot; the amount of hemolysis can be reduced by shortening the distance covered and possibly by increasing protection of the foot.[139] Variants of march hemoglobinuria have been reported, with intravascular hemolysis occurring after karate exercises,[141] conga drum playing,[142] and repetitive head banging.[143]

With the increasing use of extracorporeal treatment and prosthetic devices in the circulation, mechanical hemolysis should be suspected. A blood smear demonstrating schistocytes is a quick screening test.

In traumatic cardiac hemolytic anemia, red cell destruction is due to physical trauma in the arterial circulation, usually related to the presence of a mechanical prosthetic value[144,145] or graft.[146] The damage is thought to occur upon contact with unendothelialized surfaces or to be due to valve malfunction involving either thrombi or small-volume, high-velocity leaks.[144–146] Less commonly, annuloplasty ring,[147] ruptured chordae tendinae repair,[148] porcine valvular dysfunction,[149,150] or vegetative endocarditis[151] is the cause of hemolysis. Severe intravascular hemolysis with hemoglobinuria may appear immediately postoperatively or may be delayed for years.[144] Schistocytes with markedly irregular, triangular red cell fragments are characteristic, and reticulocytosis is generally present. Diagnosis of the exact cardiac pathology may be difficult, and Doppler echo ultrasound is often not able to detect the small-volume leaks. Specialized techniques such as left ventriculography are generally necessary. However, even with cardiac catheterization small leaks may not be detectable, and the diagnosis must be based on the finding of hemolytic anemia with schistocytes in a patient with a prosthetic valve or graft. In cases of severe hemolysis, valve replacement is generally required.[144,152]

Microangiopathic Hemolytic Anemia

In microangiopathic hemolytic anemia (MAHA), red cells are fragmented by fibrin webs, microthrombi, and abnormal endothelium partially occluding arterioles and precapillaries, which gives rise to the characteristic schistocyte and red cell fragments. DIC, in which fibrin thrombi form in the microvasculature, is the mildest form of MAHA; schistocytes are seen in only approximately one-third of cases, and clinically evident hemolysis is unusual.

Primary Thrombotic Microangiopathy

Primary thrombotic microangiopathy includes thrombotic thrombocytopenic purpura (TTP) and hemolytic uremic syndrome (HUS). The cardinal manifestations are MAHA, thrombocytopenia, and thrombotic changes in the microvasculature. Pathologically the findings are identical, with hyaline or fibrin-platelet thrombi in the arteriolar and capillary network. The etiology is unknown; in children there is often a prodromal viral or bacterial illness. The usual age range and pattern of organ involvement are variable, and the distinction between TTP and HUS has been unclear, with some authors considering the two disorders to be the same. Alternative terms such as thrombotic microangiopathy and TTP-HUS emphasize the spectrum of disease.[153,154]

TTP, an uncommon disorder, usually presents in the fourth decade but can be seen at any age. There is a 3:2 female/male predominance. The major presenting manifestations stem from hemolysis, thrombocytopenia, and thrombotic dysfunction of various organ systems, particularly neurologic. Clinically, the classic pentad of thrombocytopenia, MAHA, fluctuating neurologic dysfunction, fever, and renal insufficiency is seen in 40 percent of cases, with the last two findings being inconstant. Laboratory values show thrombocytopenia in the range of 20,000/μl and intravascular hemolysis. LDH, hemoglobin, and reticulocyte counts are used to follow the course of the disease. The peripheral smear characteristically shows schistocytosis and large platelets, with polychromatophilia and other evidence of bone marrow response. In contrast to most acute hemolytic disorders, in which bone marrow biopsy may provide little additional information, in TTP the characteristic microvascular lesion with fibrin-platelet thrombi will be demonstrated in about 35 percent of cases. Laboratory clotting tests, with the exception of platelet counts, will be normal, and renal function studies will vary with the severity of renal involvement. The DAT is negative, which is occasionally important in differentiating these disorders from Evans syndrome, autoimmune hemolytic anemia with thrombocytopenia. The diagnosis is based on the combination of anemia with schistocytosis, thrombocytopenia, and fever in the setting of renal or neurologic dysfunction.[153]

Treatment usually consists of combination therapy with prednisone and plasma exchange,[155] which has been reported to be superior to plasma infusion therapy.[156] Vincristine and intravenous γ-globulin have also been used.[157,158] Platelet transfusions have been associated with increased hemorrhage and renal failure. Splenectomy, antiplatelet agents, maintenance plasma infusion therapy, and maintenance steroid therapy have been found to be ineffective. Relapse is common, occurring in 77 percent of patients, mostly within 2 months of diagnosis. Mortality has been reduced to 9 percent by using plasma exchange and corticosteroids.[155]

HUS is more commonly seen in children and generally presents as a single episode of thrombocytopenia, hemolytic anemia, and renal insufficiency. Atypical HUS, with prominent neurologic involvement, has a poor prognosis. Infections associated with HUS include verotoxin-producing *E. coli*, *Shigella*, and *Streptococcus pneumoniae*.[159–161] Fevers are infrequent and usually transient.[162] Hemolysis is not as prominent as with TTP, possibly because the distribution of the microangiopathic vessels is not as widespread. Spontaneous complete recovery is seen in 64 percent of cases, and in 16 percent there are only mild sequelae; however, 14 percent of patients progress to end-stage renal disease, and 6 percent die acutely. Plasma infusion and exchange are used rarely, generally only in cases of progressive disease with renal and neurologic deterioration.[160] The prognosis is significantly worse in adults than in children, with a mortality rate of 18 to 62 percent. Treatment is with plasma exchange and immunosuppressive agents.[162]

Secondary Thrombotic Microangiopathy

Secondary thrombotic microangiopathy or MAHA encompasses a number of distinctly different disorders that share thrombotic microangiopathy as a rare complication of the primary disease, which may not be active or evident at the time of complication. Secondary thrombotic microangiopathy occurs in a number of settings, including cancer, pregnancy, infection, transplantation, drugs, and immune complex and collagen vascular disorders. Unlike classic TTP-HUS, the severity of secondary thrombotic microangiopathy varies considerably, from mild to fulminant, and the factor responsible for the endothelial damage, such as a specific infection or drug, can usually be identified. Disease progression can be halted or reversed upon removal of the etiologic agent. Platelet transfusion is generally contraindicated, and the usefulness of other therapeutic interventions such as plasma exchange and antiplatelet agents remains unclear. Two of the more common forms of secondary thrombotic microangiopathy, which are associated with pregnancy and carcinoma, are discussed below.[163]

Malignancy-Associated Thrombotic Microangiopathy. Thrombotic microangiopathy associated with malignancy occurs in two forms. The first, carcinoma-associated MAHA, is mostly seen with widely metastatic mucin-producing adenocarcinomas of the stomach, breast, and lung, gastric adenocarcinomas accounting for 52 percent of reported cases. The usual presentation is that of an acute hemolytic anemia, with fatigue and pallor. Neurologic symptoms are frequent, especially headache. Laboratory evaluation reveals a severe hemolytic anemia with characteristic schistocytes and irregular red cell fragments[164] and microspherocytes.[165] Reticulocytosis, thrombocytopenia, and a leukoerythroblastic peripheral smear are common findings. Other laboratory data are consistent with hemolysis. The plasma hemoglobin may be elevated, urine hemoglobin may be detectable,[166] and the DAT is negative. Renal insufficiency is not a prominent finding. Coagulation studies may show evidence of a consumptive coagulopathy, but this aspect of the disorder is less well defined. The prognosis of carcinoma-associated MAHA is dismal, and most patients die within a few weeks of diagnosis. Reducing the tumor burden is the only reliable means of improving the hemolysis. Unlike the situation with other forms of thrombotic microangiopathy, platelet transfusions are not associated with clinical deterioration and should not be withheld.[164]

The second form of thrombotic microangiopathy associated with malignancy is a chemotherapy-related HUS, which usually occurs in patients in remission after treatment with a number of antineoplastic drugs, most notably mitomycin C and bleomycin. The pathogenesis is unclear, but may be related to chemotherapy toxicity combined with circulating immune complexes. The stomach, colon, and breast are the most common primary sites. There is a striking female predominance of almost 2:1. Clinically, patients present with a moderate to severe MAHA, thrombocytopenia, and renal insufficiency 1 to 2 months following completion of chemotherapy. Hypertension and pulmonary edema may develop, but neurologic abnormalities are uncommon. Laboratory findings are typical of MAHA and similar to those seen in carcinoma-associated MAHA, except that coagulation abnormalities and leukoerythroblastic peripheral smears are not seen. Evidence of renal failure is routine, and up to one-third of patients will require dialysis. Chemotherapy-related HUS carries a poor prognosis, with 75 percent of patients dying within 4 months. Steroids and plasma exchange have been tried, but there is no effective treatment. Transfusion should be avoided, as even washed products will exacerbate the syndrome.[164]

Acute hemolysis may occur in pregnancy when eclampsia/pre-eclampsia is complicated by the presence of the HELLP syndrome [characterized by intravascular hemolysis, (H), elevated liver enzymes, (EL) low platelet count (LP)]. The HELLP syndrome occurs in the mid to late third trimester and is associated with significant maternal and fetal mortality. Patients usually present with abdominal pain, nausea, and vomiting and have marked diastolic hypertension.[167–169] Laboratory data reveal evidence of MAHA, thrombocytopenia with platelet counts averaging 50,000, and moderate elevations in transaminase levels. Prothrombin time (PT) and partial thromboplastin time (PTT) are generally normal.[169,170] Haptoglobin and LDH have been used for early detection of the HELLP syndrome in eclamptic patients, with improved outcomes.[171] The only effective treatment is believed to be immediate delivery by cesarean section regardless of the gestational age of the fetus. Plasma exchange has been used postpartum to facilitate recovery.[172]

Immune Hemolysis

Immune hemolysis is characterized by antibody-mediated red cell destruction. According to the type of antibody involved, immune hemolysis can be divided into three main categories—alloimmune, autoimmune, and drug-induced.

Red Cell Antigens

The red cell membrane contains several hundred different red cell antigens, or alloantigens. The presence or absence of these antigens is genetically determined and varies somewhat by ethnic group. Related red cell antigens define a number of blood group systems, the most familiar being the AB and Rh systems. These antigens determine the blood group O, A, B, or AB and the Rh status, positive or negative, respectively. Other examples of blood group antigen systems include those of Kell, Kidd, and Duffy, which are important in alloantibody reactions. A limited number of the 400 red cell antigens are involved in hemolytic reactions.

Red Cell Antibodies

Red cell antibodies may be classified as naturally occurring, alloantibody, or autoantibody. Naturally occurring antibodies, anti-A and anti-B, develop during the first 6 to 12 months of life and are directed against the red cell antigens not present on the red cells. Type AB individuals have no naturally occurring antibodies, and type O individuals have both anti-A and anti-B. Red cell antigens and naturally occurring antibodies provide the basis for blood typing procedures.

Alloantibodies are circulating antibodies in the plasma that are produced in response to foreign red cell alloantigens introduced into the circulation by blood transfusion or pregnancy, as when an Rh(D)-negative mother produces anti-D during pregnancy with an Rh(D)-positive fetus. These antibodies are directed against specific red cell antigens, and the specificity of such antibodies can be determined by serologic testing with commercial panels of red cells of known antigenic type. These are detected by the indirect antiglobulin test and may cause alloimmune hemolysis, including hemolytic disease of the newborn and hemolytic transfusion reactions.

Red cell autoantibodies are produced as a result of disordered immune surveillance and are directed against antigens present on one's own red cells. Autoantibodies are generally present in vivo on the surface of red cells and in plasma as well. Unlike alloantibodies, which react only with red cells of corresponding antigenic type, autoantibodies if present in the plasma may show a nonspecific panagglutination reaction with all red cells, leading to difficulties in cross-matching units of blood for transfusion. Autoantibodies are detected by a positive DAT and may cause autoimmune hemolysis (AIH).

Alloimmune Hemolysis

Most fatal transfusion reactions are caused by clerical errors in which blood is transfused to the wrong patient. Most cases occur in emergencies (in the emergency room, operating room, or intensive care unit) and are related to ABO incompatibility.

In an acute hemolytic transfusion reaction (AHTR), intravascular red cell destruction is mediated by naturally occurring antibodies, anti-A or anti-B, or by alloantibody directed against specific antigens present on the donor red cells. The overall incidence of AHTR is unclear, but one large study at the Mayo Clinic showed one reaction for every 11,167 transfusions given, with a 17 percent fatality rate.[173] The risk of a fatal AHTR appears to be low, with 158 cases reported to the Food and Drug Administration (FDA) in over 100 million transfusions given during a 10-year period, but it is likely that the true number is underreported. Most fatal reactions were seen in emergency settings, such as the emergency room, operating room, and intensive care unit, and were the result of clerical errors in identifying the patient, the cross-match sample, or the unit of blood. Most fatalities involved incompatibility in the ABO system.[174] AHTRs show a marked female preponderance, largely owing to sensitization during pregnancy and the presence of preformed antibodies.[173] The most severe AHTRs are generally seen with ABO incompatibility.[175]

Clinically, the most common manifestations of an AHTR are fever, back pain, and dyspnea, followed by hemoglobinuria, hypotension, and possibly DIC, and renal failure.[174,176] Fatal reactions have been noted to occur after transfusion of as little as 30 ml of blood.[174] In the anesthetized, comatose, or severely ill intubated patient, many of the signs and symptoms may be obscured, and the diagnosis depends on a high index of suspicion following detection of hemoglobinemia and hemoglobinuria. Laboratory findings indicate massive intravascular hemolysis, with hemoglobinemia and hemoglobinuria, and peak total bilirubin and LDH values usually occurring 5 to 8 hours posttransfusion. Peripheral smear may show spherocytosis. Serologic investigation includes a DAT, which is usually positive, as residual surviving red cells are coated by the offending antibody, and a positive IAT, which reveals evidence of the circulating alloantibody.[176] Antibodies capable of fixing complement, especially anti-A and anti-Jka, are more likely to be associated with massive intravascular hemolysis.[173] In certain cases all transfused red cells may be almost immediately destroyed, and the DAT will be negative. Evidence of DIC and thrombocytopenia may be noted as well.

Therapy of massive intravascular hemolysis/acute hemolytic transfusion reaction is supportive and based on demonstrated toxicity. Maintenance of renal blood flow and urine output is critical. Mannitol is no longer recommended for diuresis.

Treatment of an AHTR or of any case of massive intravascular hemolysis is largely supportive and based on demonstrated toxicity. Owing to the rarity of AHTRs, few individuals have extensive experience with management of such patients, and there have been no controlled studies to compare treatment regimens. General measures involve discontinuing the transfusion and replacing the entire tubing set without removing the catheter so that venous access is maintained at all times but no additional blood is infused. Emphasis should be placed on maintaining renal blood flow and urine output by cautious use of low- or renal-dose dopamine and furosemide (Lasix). Heparin has been recommended for post-transfusion DIC, but this remains controversial. Mannitol is no longer recommended for diuresis.[177]

Variations from the usual clinical and serologic picture of AHTR occur for reasons that are not entirely clear. Occasionally an AHTR occurs with minimal symptoms of only fever and chills and failure to increase hemoglobin. Possible explanations are related to the quantity and binding avidity of the antibody present and the amount of red cells given.[173,176] In other rare instances noted in only 13 reports in the literature, massive hemoglobinemia and hemoglobinuria have occurred without other symptoms or sequelae, and extensive serologic workup has failed to reveal any evidence of antibodies. Technetium-99m red cell survival studies have demonstrated rapid hemolysis of red cells with certain antigen compositions, especially in the Rh group.[178]

Acute intravascular hemolysis has also occurred following transfusion with ABO-incompatible platelets, usually owing to the presence of high-titer anti-A present in the plasma. Volume reduction techniques to remove most of the plasma can be used for out-of-group platelet transfusions to minimize the risk of such a reaction.[179–181] Acute hemolysis has also been reported following minor ABO-mismatched liver,[182] kidney,[183,184] and allogeneic bone marrow transplants[185] as a result of the development of an anti-A or anti-B of donor origin. Plasma exchange has been used in such cases to acutely reduce the antibody titer.[185] Acute intravascular hemolysis has also been reported following administration of intravenous γ-globulin[186–188] and antithymocyte globulin,[189,190] owing to the presence of passively acquired alloantibodies anti-A, anti-B, and anti-D.

Polyagglutination is a rare phenomenon in which red cell antigens can be altered by a number of factors, most commonly by the action of microbial enzymes in the setting of severe infection. Usually this gives rise to in vitro laboratory abnormalities but has been reported in association with massive intravascular hemolysis.[191,192]

Autoimmune Hemolysis

AIH occurs in a number of settings, all characterized by red cell destruction and autoantibody formation leading to a positive DAT. AIH can be primary or secondary and associated with drug therapy or systemic illness. The degree of hemolysis depends on several factors, including the type of autoantibody, the presence or absence of complement fixation, and the capacity of the reticuloendothelial system to clear sensitized red cells. The autoantibodies are designated *warm* if they react with red cell antigens at body temperature and *cold* if lower temperatures are required for antibody binding.[3,44,193]

AIH is most commonly seen after age 40 and has a slight female predominance. Warm antibody hemolysis is by far the most common form and usually has a drug or disease association.[3,194] Although acute hemolysis may be seen, chronic hemolytic courses are more common and usually parallel the activity of the underlying disease process. Clinically evident intravascular hemolysis is uncommon, being seen only in severe cases, and is usually associated with cold antibody formation, especially in PCH. Laboratory values are generally consistent with extravascular hemolysis, but as described previously, reticulocytosis may be absent.

AIH can be divided into four main categories: (1) warm AIHA; (2) cold AIHA, or cold agglutinin disease (CAD); (3) PCH; and (4) drug-induced hemolysis. Multiple autoantibodies with both warm and cold characteristics can occur in the same patient, and the term *mixed autoimmune hemolysis* has been used to describe these cases.[194]

Warm Autoimmune Hemolytic Anemia. This form of AIH is mediated by IgG autoantibodies, which show maximal reactivity at 37°C and may or may not fix complement. Approximately 50 percent of warm IgG autoantibodies are directed against Rh antigens. Hemolysis, which may be abrupt in onset, is extravascular, with splenic sequestration of coated red cells.[44] Warm AIHA may be primary but is more typically seen as a manifestation of a number of systemic conditions, including chronic lymphocytic leukemia, lymphoma, and systemic lupus erythematosus.[175] Laboratory values will usually be consistent with extravascular hemolysis, and both spherocytosis and splenomegaly may be prominent. The DAT is reactive with IgG and C3 antiglobulin reagents (67 percent), IgG alone (20 percent), and less commonly, C3 alone (10 percent).[195] Extensive serologic testing may be required to ensure that an underlying alloantibody is not masked. Autoantibodies generally agglutinate not only the red cells of the patient but donor red cells as well. Cross-matching will generally show varying degrees of serologic incompatibility, and units of blood released for transfusion are designated *least incompatible.* It is for this reason that caution must be used in transfusing warm AIHA patients; transfusions should be given when necessary[196] and should never be withheld in the setting of life-threatening anemia.[10] Treatment approaches are aimed at reducing antibody production by using corticosteroids until the DAT becomes negative or by eliminating the site of red cell destruction by splenectomy. If remission is not achieved with splenectomy, immunosuppressive therapy with azathioprine or cyclophosphamide has been recommended.[44,175]

With autoimmune hemolytic anemia, particularly warm AIHA, the crossmatch will generally show some degree of serologic incompatibility. Transfusions should be given cautiously but should not be withheld when anemia is life-threatening.

Cold Hemagglutinin Disease. Cold hemagglutinin disease (CHD) is mediated by IgM autoantibodies, which react best at low temperatures, maximally at 0°C, and which characteristically fix complement. *Thermal amplitude,* which refers to the temperature range at which a particulat autoantibody is active, will vary greatly between patients and is clinically important. A cold agglutinin active up to 34°C, a temperature easily reached in the peripheral circulation of the extremities, will generally cause more severe hemolysis than one active only up to 25°C. The specificity of the autoantibody varies but is commonly anti-I or anti-i.[197] CHD may be primary or secondary and may be associated with lymphoma, or with viral or *M. pneumoniae* infections. Acute hemolysis may occur, especially with infection, but the red cell destruction tends to have an insidious onset and a chronic course. Occasionally patients with cold agglutinins will not show evidence of hemolysis until exposed to cold in a hospital setting; there are case reports of hemolysis occurring when a cooling mattress was used[198] and during cardiac surgery with induced hypothermia and cardioplegia.[199] Intravascular hemolysis is occasionally seen in severe cases. Laboratory studies reveal a DAT reactive with C3 only, as the IgM antibody dissociates after fixing complement. The peripheral smear typically reveals agglutination of red cells in smears dried at room temperature. Splenic destruction is not prominent in CHD, and spherocytosis is not usually seen on peripheral smears.[44,195] Cold agglutinin titers are significantly elevated, and other laboratory data are consistent with hemolysis, usually extravascular. To facilitate cross-matching and other hematologic testing, all specimens should be drawn and maintained at 37°C. Therapy is aimed at avoiding cold and treating the underlying malignancy or infection to eliminate antibody production. Cyclophosphamide is the preferred agent, along with plasmapheresis and steroids. All intravenous fluids and blood products should be warmed. Splenectomy is of no benefit, as with IgM-mediated hemolysis red cells are not preferentially destroyed in the spleen.[44,197]

Paroxysmal Cold Hemoglobinuria. PCH, or Donath-Landsteiner hemolytic anemia, is mediated by a cold-reacting IgG autoantibody known as a *biphasic hemolysin* because it requires a sequence of cold temperature for red cell antibody sensitization followed by warm temperatures for complement-mediated hemolysis.[195] The Donath-Landsteiner autoantibody is almost always directed against the P red cell antigen. PCH occurs in three settings, as (1) chronic syphilitic PCH, occurring in both adults (late-stage syphilis) and children (congenital syphilis); (2) acute postviral PCH, usually seen in children; and (3) chronic idiopathic or autoimmune PCH, usually seen in adults. Although PCH is said to be the least common form of AIH, the acute postviral form may represent between 32 and 40 percent of pediatric AIH cases.[46,200,201]

Clinically, acute postviral PCH presents as an acute-onset hemolytic anemia, with hemoglobinuria and constitutional symptoms that include abdominal, back, and leg pain, chills, and fever. Laboratory data are consistent with intravascular hemolysis. Peripheral smear may show erythrophagocytosis and red cell agglutination and less commonly, spherocytosis. The diagnostic test is the Donath-Landsteiner test, used to distinguish biphasic hemolysis from monophasic hemolysis, which occurs with testing at a single temperature. This test is performed by incubating three sets of complement-enriched patient serum with reagent red cells: one set at 0°C, one set at 37°C, and one set at 0°C followed by 37°C. The test is positive and diagnostic of PCH if hemolysis is seen only when the temperature is raised from 0° to 37°C.[46] The DAT is typically positive for C3 only but may occasionally show both C3 and IgG.[46,200] Acute PCH usually consists of one self-limited episode, and treatment consists of supportive measures such as keeping the patient warm and transfusing all warmed fluids. Red cell units negative for the P antigen are extremely rare, available only from frozen blood stores at large reference centers. As long as warming measures are taken, transfusion of P-negative red cells is not usually necessary. Steroids and splenectomy have been tried. In an uncommon disease that often has a transient course regardless of therapy, it is difficult to assess treatment effect, but the benefit of treatment may be minimal.[46]

Drug-Induced Immune Hemolysis

Drug-induced immune hemolysis (DIH) has been reported with many different drugs, but the vast majority of cases have been due to α-methyldopa and penicillin.[195,202,203] DIH is usually gradual in onset and relatively mild; however, acute, life-threatening hemolysis may occur. Treatment generally consists of withdrawing the drug. There are three mechanisms of DIH; in some cases more than one may be operative.[204,205]

When either chronic or episodic hemolysis is unexplained, a careful history of medication ingested is warranted. Occasionally a change of medication is the only way to confirm the diagnosis of drug-induced hemolysis.

Drug-Induced Warm AIHA. Drug-induced warm AIHA is caused by warm reacting antibodies; α-methyldopa is the prototype but hemolysis with L-dopa, mefenamic acid, and procainamide has been reported as well.[203] This type of autoantibody reacts only with red cells and has no activity against the offending drug. Clinically, the syndrome is identical to warm AIHA, with positive DAT results indicating IgG coating of red cells. The antibody is often directed against antigens of the Rh system. Laboratory data are consistent with extravascular hemolysis. The anemia is usually gradual in onset, but may be severe.[206] Hemolysis resolves upon discontinuation of the drug, but the positive DAT may persist for some time.[203]

Drug Adsorption on Red Cells. Hemolysis involving drug adsorption on red cells is also known as the *hapten mechanism*, in which high-dose intravenous drugs such as penicillins[207] and cephalosporins[208,209] bind directly to red cell membranes. Intravenous amoxicillin[210] and cis-platinum[211] have also been reported to react in this manner. Antibodies with specificity for drug-related antigens, not red cell antigens, are produced. Antibody can be removed from the patient's red cells and shown to react only with penicillin-treated red cells. Anemia develops after 7 to 10 days of therapy and may be severe. The DAT is positive for IgG, and occasionally for complement. Laboratory values are consistent with extravascular hemolysis with spherocytosis. Treatment consists of withdrawing the drug.[203]

Immune Complex Formation. In the type of hemolysis also known as the innocent bystander mechanism, an immune complex is formed between the drug molecule and IgM or IgG plasma protein. Quinidine is the prototype drug. Although the largest number of case reports and a variety of drugs have been associated with this type of hemolysis, it is still the rarest mechanism to occur.[202] Amphotericin B–induced hemolysis[212] has recently been described. In theory, the immune complex binds to the red cell, with complement fixation. The immune complex then dissociates from the cell, and the innocent bystander red cell undergoes either extravascular or intravascular hemolysis. For patients with immune complex-mediated hemolysis, clinical and laboratory findings differ substantially from those of patients with DIH due to the other two mechanisms. The hemolysis may be massive and fulminant,[213] with prominent hemoglobinemia and hemoglobinuria and ensuing renal failure. The DAT is usually positive for complement but not for IgG. Treatment involves discontinuation of the offending drug and supportive therapy.[203]

References

1. Ballas SK: The pathophysiology of hemolytic anemias. Tran Med Rev 4:236, 1990
2. Garraty G: Mechanisms of immune red cell destruction, and red cell compatibility testing. Hum Pathol 14:204, 1983
3. Dacie JV, Worrledge SM: Auto-immune hemolytic anemias. Prog Hematol 66:82, 1969
4. Hernandez JA, Steane SM: Erythrophagocytosis by segmented neutrophils in paroxysmal cold hemoglobinuria. Am J Clin Pathol 81:787, 1984
5. Vilpo JA, Talvensaari KK, Mortensen E: Hemolysis—which laboratory investigations and when. Scand J Clin Lab Invest Suppl 200:10, 1990
6. Leisveld JL, Rowe JM, Lichtman MA: Variability of the erythropoietic response in autoimmune hemolytic anemia. Analysis of 109 cases. Blood 69:820, 1987
7. Jandl JH: Hemolytic anemias. Introduction. p. 179. In Beck WS (ed): Hematology. 4th Ed. MIT Press, Cambridge, MA 1985
8. Miale JB: Laboratory Medicine: Hematology. CV Mosby, St Louis, 1982
9. Conley CL, Lippman SM, Ness P: Autoimmune hemolytic anemia with reticulocytopenia. A medical emergency. JAMA 244:1688, 1980
10. Crosby WH, Rappaport H: Reticulocytopenia in autoimmune hemolytic anemia. Blood 11: 929, 1956
11. Wolach B, Heddle N, Barr RD et al: Transient Donath-Landsteiner haemolytic anaemia. Br J Haematol 48:425, 1981
12. Anderson L: Role of parvovirus B19 in human disease. Pediatr Infect Dis J 6:711, 1987
13. Fink DJ, Petz LD, Black MB: Serum haptoglobin. JAMA 199:109, 1967
14. Berlin NI, Berk PD: Quantitative aspects of bilirubin metabolism for hematologists. Blood 57: 983, 1981
15. Lobel HO, Campbell CC, Schwartz IK et al: Recent trends in the importation of malaria caused by *Plasmodium falciparum* into the United States from Africa. J Infect Dis 152:613, 1985
16. Guerrero EC, Weniger BC, Schultz MG: Transfusion malaria in the United States, 1972–1981. Ann Intern Med 99:221, 1983
17. Kazura JW: Hematologic manifestations of parasitic diseases. p. 1781. In Hoffman R, Benz RJ, Shattil SJ et al (eds): Hematology. Basic Principles and Practice. Churchill Livingstone, New York, 1991
18. Beutler E: Hemolytic anemia due to infections with microorganisms. p. 663. In Williams WJ, Beutler E, Erslev AJ, Lichtman MA (eds): Hematology. 4th Ed. McGraw-Hill, New York, 1990
19. Jandl JH: Blood Pathophysiology. Blackwell Scientific Publishing, Boston, 1991

20. Fleming AF: Haematologic manifestation of malaria and other parasitic diseases. Clin Haematol 10:983, 1981
21. Perrin LH, Mackey LJ, Miescher PA: The hematology of malaria in man. Semin Hematol 19: 70, 1982
22. Abdalla S, Weatherall DJ: The direct antiglobulin test in *P. falciparum* malaria. Br J Haematol 51:415, 1982
23. White NJ: Drug treatment and prevention of malaria. Eur J Clin Pharmacol 34:1, 1988
24. Miller KD, Greenberg AE, Campbell CC: Treatment of severe malaria in the United States with a continuous infusion of quinidine gluconate and exchange transfusion. N Engl J Med 321:65, 1989
25. Exchange transfusion in falciparum malaria, editorial. Lancet 335:324, 1990
26. Saddler M, Barry M: Treatment of severe malaria by exchange transfusion, letter. N Engl J Med 322:58, 1990
27. Steketee RW, Eckman MR, Burgess EC et al: Babesiosis in Wisconsin. A new focus of disease transmission. JAMA 253:2675, 1985
28. Smith RP, Evans AT, Popovsky M et al: Transfusion acquired babesiosis and failure of antibiotic treatment. JAMA 256:2726, 1986
29. Jacoby GA, Hunt JV, Kosinski KS et al: Treatment of transfusion-transmitted babesiosis by exchange transfusion. N Engl J Med 303:1098, 1980
30. Ruebush TK, Cassaday PB, Marsh HJ et al: Human babesiosis on Nantucket Island. Clinical features. Ann Intern Med 86:6, 1977
31. Gombert ME, Goldstein EJ, Benach JL et al: Human babesiosis: clinical and therapeutic considerations. JAMA 248:3005, 1982
32. Rosner F, Zarrabi MH, Benach JL et al: Babesiosis in splenectomized adults. Review of 22 reported cases. Am J Med 76:696, 1984
33. Reynafarje C, Ramos J: The hemolytic anemia of human bartonellosis. Blood 17:562, 1961
34. Ricketts WE: Bartonella bacilliformis anemia (Oroya fever). Blood 3:1025, 1948
35. Gordon-Smith EC, Hows J: Acquired haemolytic anaemias. p. 183. In Hoffbrand AV, Lewis SM, (eds): Postgraduate Haematology. 3rd Ed. Heinemann Professional Publishing, Oxford, 1989
36. Dean HM, Decker CL, Baker LD: Temporary survival in clostridial hemolysis with absence of circulating red cells. N Engl J Med 277:700, 1967
37. Harris RW, Sims PJ, Tweten RK: Evidence that *Clostridium perfringens* theta-toxin induces colloid osmotic lysis of erythrocytes. Infect Immun 59:2499, 1991
38. Tsai IK, Yen MY, Ho IC et al: *Clostridium perfringens* septicemia with massive hemolysis. Scand J Infect Dis 21:467, 1989
39. Clinicopathologic case conference: Abdominal pain, total intravascular lysis and death in a 53 year old woman. Am J Med 88:667, 1990
40. Emody L, Molnar L, Kellermayer M et al: Urinary *Escherichia coli* infection presenting with jaundice. Scand J Infect Dis 21:579, 1989
41. Jandl JH, Jacob HS, Daland GA: Hypersplenism due to infection. A study of five cases manifesting hemolytic anemia. N Engl J Med 264:1063, 1961
42. McGehee WG, Rapaport SI, Hjort PF: Intravascular coagulation in fulminant meningococcemia. Ann Intern Med 67:250, 1967
43. Robboy SJ, Salisbury K, Ragsdale B et al: Mechanism of Aspergillus-induced microangiopathic hemolytic anemia. Arch Intern Med 128:790, 1971
44. Rosse WF: Autoimmune hemolytic anemia. Hosp Prac [Off] 120:105, 1985
45. Bird GWG: Paroxysmal cold hemoglobinuria. Brit J Haematol 37:167, 1977
46. Heddle NM: Acute paroxysmal cold hemoglobinuria. Tran Med Rev 3:219, 1989
47. Thurm RH, Bassen F: Infectious mononucleosis and acute hemolytic anemia; report of two cases and review of the literature. Blood 10:841, 1955
48. Tonkin AM, Mond HG, Alford FP et al: Severe acute haemolytic anaemia complicating infectious mononucleosis. Med J Aust 2:1048, 1973
49. Horwitz CA, Skradski K, Reece E et al: Haemolytic anaemia in previously healthy adult patients with CMV infections. Scand J Haematol 33:35, 1984
50. Lyons DJ, Gilvarry JM, Fielding JF: Severe haemolysis associated with hepatitis A and normal glucose-6-phosphate dehydrogenase status. Gut 31:838, 1990
51. Ceuppens JL, Stevens E, Fevery J et al: Complete recovery from hepatitis B and associated hemolysis in a patient with underlying T-cell deficiency. Gastroenterology 86:937, 1984

52. Zhai Q, Zhou Y, Liu W: Sporadic acute non-A non-B hepatitis complicated by aplastic anemia and haemolysis. Clin Med J [Engl] 103:959, 1990
53. Fiala M, Myhre BA, Chinh LT et al: Pathogenesis of anemia associated with *Mycoplasma pneumoniae*. Acta Haematol (Basel) 51:297, 1974
54. Von Knorring J, Pettersson T: Haemolytic anaemia complicating *Yersinia enterocolitica* infection. Report of a case. Scand J Haematol 9:149, 1972
55. Shurin SB, Anderson P, Zollinger J et al: Pathophysiology of hemolysis in infections with *Haemophilus influenzae* type b. J Clin Invest 77:1340, 1986
56. Lovlin RE, Rowlands S, Kinnear GR et al: Intravascular hemolysis in acute mountain sickness. Aviat Space Environ Med 51:271, 1980
57. Jacob HS, Amsden T: Acute hemolytic anemia with rigid red cells in hypophosphatemia. N Engl J Med 285:1446, 1971
58. Shilo S, Werner D, Hershko C: Acute hemolytic anemia caused by severe hypophosphatemia in diabetic ketoacidosis. Acta Haematol (Basel) 73:55, 1985
59. Douglass CC, Twomey JJ: Transient stomatocytosis with hemolysis: a previously unrecognized complication of alcoholism. Ann Intern Med 72:159, 1970
60. McIntyre N, Clink HM, Levi AJ et al: Hemolytic anemia in Wilson's disease. N Engl J Med 276:439, 1967
61. Deiss A, Lee GR, Cartwright GE: Hemolytic anemia in Wilson's disease. Ann Intern Med 73: 413, 1970
62. Smith JA, Lonergan ET, Sterling K: Spur cell anemia. Hemolytic anemia with red cells resembling acanthocytes in alcoholic cirrhosis. N Engl J Med 271:396, 1964
63. Silber R, Amorosi E, Lhowe J et al: Spur shaped erythrocytes in Laennec's cirrhosis. N Engl J Med 275:639, 1966
64. Grahn EP, Dietz AA, Stefani SS et al: Burr cells, hemolytic anemia and cirrhosis. Am J Med 45:78, 1968
65. Cooper RA: Anemia with spur cells: a red cell defect acquired in the serum and modified in the circulation. J Clin Invest 48:1820, 1969
66. Wilcox LA, Ezzell JL, Bernshaw NJ et al: Molecular basis of the enhanced susceptibility of the erythrocytes of paroxysmal nocturnal hemoglobinuria to hemolysis in acidified serum. Blood 78:820, 1991
67. Rosse WF, Parker CJ: Paroxysmal nocturnal hemoglobinuria. Clin Haematol 14:105, 1985
68. Ware RE, Hall SE, Rosse WF: Paroxysmal nocturnal hemoglobinuria with onset in childhood and adolescence. N Engl J Med 325:991, 1991
69. Rosse WF: Treatment of paroxysmal nocturnal hemoglobinuria. Blood 60:20, 1982
70. Antin JH, Ginsburg D, Smith BR et al: Bone marrow transplantation for paroxysmal nocturnal hemoglobinuria: eradication of the PNH clone and documentation of complete lymphohematopoietic engraftment. Blood 66:1247, 1985
71. Brecher ME, Taswell HF: Paroxysmal nocturnal hemoglobinuria and washed red cells: a myth revisited. Transfusion 29:681, 1989
72. Winterbourne CC: Oxidative denaturation in congenital hemolytic anemia: the unstable hemoglobins. Semin Hematol 27:41, 1990
73. Ohba Y: Unstable hemoglobins. Hemoglobin 14:353, 1990
74. Zinkham WH, Winslow RM: Unstable hemoglobins: influence of environment on phenotypic expression of a genetic disorder. Medicine (Baltimore) 68:309, 1989
75. Becker PS, Lux SE: Hereditary spherocytosis and related disorders. Clin Haematol 14:15, 1985
76. Palek J: Hereditary elliptocytosis and related disorders. Clin Haematol 14:45, 1985
77. Jensson O, Jonasson T, Olaffson O: Hereditary elliptocytosis in Iceland. Br J Haematol 13: 844, 1967
78. Beutler E: Glucose-6-phosphate dehydrogenase: new perspectives. Blood 73:1397, 1989
79. Beutler E: Glucose-6-phosphate dehydrogenase deficiency. N Engl J Med 324:169, 1991
80. Shalev O, Eliakim R, Lugassy GZ et al: Hypoglycemia-induced hemolysis in glucose-6-phosphate dehydrogenase deficiency. Acta Haematol (Basel) 74:227, 1985
81. Bhatia V, Goenka MK, Kochhar R et al: Intravascular hemolysis following endoscopic variceal sclerotherapy, letter. Am J Gastroenterol 85:1435, 1990
82. Sazama K, Klein HG, Davey RJ et al: Intraoperative hemolysis. The initial manifestation of glucose-6-phosphate dehydrogenase deficiency. Arch Intern Med 140:845, 1980
83. Byrd SR, Gelber RH: Effect of dapsone on haemoglobin concentration in patients with leprosy. Lepr Rev 62:171, 1991

84. Cox G, Roberts MS: Glucose-6-phosphate dehydrogenase deficiency (letter). N Engl J Med 324:1742, 1991
85. Arese P, DeFlora A: Pathophysiology of hemolysis in glucose-6-phosphate dehydrogenase deficiency. Semin Hematol 27:1, 1990
86. Valentine WN, Tanaka KR, Paglia DE: Hemolytic anemias and erythrocyte enzymopathies. Ann Intern Med 103:245, 1985
87. Winkelmann M, Stangel W, Schedel I et al: Severe hemolysis caused by antibodies against mushroom *Paxillus involutus* and its therapy by plasma exchange. Klin Wochenschr 64:935, 1986
88. Jenkins GC, Ind JE, Kazantzis G et al: Arsine poisoning: massive haemolysis with minimal impairment of renal function. Br Med J 2:78, 1965
89. Manzler AD, Schreiner AW: Copper induced acute hemolytic anemia. A new complication of hemodialysis. Ann Intern Med 73:409, 1970
90. Holtzman NA, Elliott DA, Heller RH: Copper intoxication. Report of a case with observations on ceruloplasmin. N Engl J Med 275:347, 1966
91. Orringer EP, Mattern WD: Formaldehyde induced hemolysis during chronic hemodialysis. N Engl J Med 294:1416, 1976
92. Eaton JW, Kolpe CF, Swofford HS et al: Chlorinated urban water: a cause of dialysis-induced hemolytic anemia. Science 181:463, 1973
93. Jackson RC, Elder WJ, McDonnell H: Sodium chlorate poisoning complicated by renal failure. Lancet 2:1381, 1961
94. Gordon SM, Bland LA, Alexander SR et al: Hemolysis associated with hydrogen peroxide at a pediatric dialysis center. Am J Nephrol 10:123, 1990
95. Carton A, Maradona JA, Arribas JM: Acute-subacute lead poisoning. Clinical findings and comparative study of diagnostic tests. Arch Intern Med 147:697, 1987
96. Adler R, Robinson RG, Binkin NJ: Intravascular hemolysis: an unusual complication of hydrocarbon ingestion. J Pediatr 89:679, 1976
97. Gradus (Ben-Ezer) D, Rhoads M, Bergstom LB et al: Acute bromate poisoning associated with renal failure and deafness presenting as hemolytic uremic syndrome. Am J Nephrol 4:188, 1984
98. Gordon-Smith EC: Drug induced oxidative hemolysis. Clin Haematol 9:557, 1980
99. Morse EE: Toxic effects of drugs on erythrocytes. Ann Clin Lab Sci 18:13, 1988
100. Mengel CE, Kann HE, Heyman A et al: Effects of in vivo hyperoxia on erythrocytes. II. Hemolysis in a human after exposure to oxygen under high pressure. Blood 25:822, 1965
101. Samozuk M, Reid ME, Toy PT: Intravenous dimethylsulfoxide therapy causes severe hemolysis mimicking a hemolytic transfusion reaction, letter. Transfusion 23:405, 1983
102. Jordan KS, Mackey D, Garvey E: A 39 year old man with acute hemolytic crisis secondary to intravenous injection of hydrogen peroxide. J Emerg Nurs 17:8, 1991
103. Sauter D, Goldfrank L, Charash BD: Cardiopulmonary arrest following infusion of calcium 2-amino ethanol phosphate. J Emerg Med 8:717, 1990
104. Reid HA: Cobra bites. Br Med J 2:540, 1964
105. Chadha JS, Leviav A: Hemolysis, renal failure and local necrosis following scorpion sting. JAMA 241:1038, 1979
106. Monzon C, Miles J: Hemolytic anemia following a wasp sting. J Pediatr 96:1039, 1980
107. Sakhuja V, Bhalla A, Pereira BJG et al: Acute renal failure following multiple hornet stings. Nephron 49:319, 1988
108. Guess HA, Saviteer PL, Morris CR: Hemolysis and acute renal failure following a portugese man-of-war sting. Pediatrics 70:979, 1982
109. Nance WE: Hemolytic anemia of necrotic arachnidism. Am J Med 31:801, 1961
110. Madrigal GC, Ercolani RL, Wenzl JE: Toxicity from a bite of the brown recluse spider (*Loxosceles reclusus*). Clin Pediatr (Phila) 11:641, 1972
111. Valeri CR, Pivacek LE, Gray AD et al: The safety and therapeutic effectiveness of human red cells stored at −80°C for as long as 21 years. Transfusion 29:429, 1989
112. Bechdolt S, Schroeder LK, Samia C et al: In vivo hemolysis of deglycerolized red blood cells. Arch Pathol Lab Med 110:344, 1986
113. Cregan P, Donegan E, Gotelli G: Hemolytic transfusion reaction following transfusion of frozen and washed autologous red cells. Transfusion 31:172, 1991
114. Lanore JJ, Quarre MC, Audibert G et al: Acute renal failure following transfusion of accidentally frozen autologous red blood cells. Vox Sang 56:293, 1989

115. Gomez S, Nagler A, Naparstek E et al: Transient elevation of serum lactic dehydrogenase following autologous bone marrow transplantation. Bone Marrow Transplant 7:487, 1991
116. Burger J, Gilmore MJML, Jackson B et al: Acute haemoglobinuria associated with the reinfusion of bone marrow buffy coat for autologous bone marrow transplantation. Bone Marrow Transplant 7:322, 1991
117. Shen SC, Ham TH, Fleming EM: Studies on the destruction of red blood cells. III. Mechanism and complications of hemoglobinuria in patients with thermal burns: spherocytosis and increased osmotic fragility of red blood cells. N Engl J Med 229:701, 1943
118. Vaughan RL: Morbidity due to exchange transfusion with heat-hemolyzed blood. Am J Dis Child 136:646, 1982
119. Phillips WA, Pottenger LA, DeWald RL: Extracorporeal hemolysis in orthopedic patients. Report of two cases. Clin Orthop 238:241, 1989
120. Staples PJ, Griner PF: Extracorporeal hemolysis of blood in a microwave blood warmer. N Engl J Med 285:317, 1971
121. McCullough J, Polesky HF, Nelson C et al: Iatrogenic hemolysis: a complication of blood warmed by a microwave device. Anesth Analg 51:102, 1972
122. Iserson KV, Huestis DW: Blood warming: current applications and techniques. Transfusion 31:558, 1991
123. Linko K, Hynynen K: Erythrocyte damage caused by the Haemotherm microwave blood warmer. Acta Anaesthesiol Scand 23:320, 1979
124. Rath CE: Drowning hemoglobinuria. Blood 8:1099, 1953
125. Whitelaw JP: Hemolysis caused by half-physiologic strength saline, letter. Transfusion 30:78, 1990
126. Hagnevik K, Gordon E, Lins LE et al: Glycerol-induced haemolysis with haemoglobinuria and acute renal failure. Lancet 1:75, 1974
127. Rao AK, Thompson R, Durlacher L et al: Angiographic contrast agent induced hemolysis in a patient with hemoglobin SC disease. Arch Intern Med 145:759, 1985
128. Landsteiner EK, Finch CA: Hemoglobinemia accompanying transurethral resection of the prostate. N Engl J Med 237:310, 1947
129. D'Agosto J, Ali NMK, Maier D: Absorption of irrigating solution during hysteroscopic metroplasty. Anesthesiology 72:379, 1990
130. Steihorn RH, Isham-Schopf B, Smith C et al: Hemolysis during long term extracorporeal membrane oxygenation. J Pediatr 115:625, 1989
131. Nilsson L, Bagge L, Nystrom SO: Blood cell trauma and postoperative bleeding: comparison of bubble and membrane oxygenators and observations on coronary suction. Scand J Thorac Cardiovasc Surg 24:65, 1990
132. Lamon EW, Bethard A, Powell TJ et al: Hemolysis after cardiopulmonary bypass, letter. J Thorac Cardiovasc Surg 99:751, 1990
133. Hemolysis and renal dysfunction associated with autotransfusion. Health Dev 19:25, 1990
134. Dhaene M, Gulbis B, Lietaer N et al: Red blood cell destruction in single needle dialysis. Clin Nephrol 31:327, 1989
135. Hombrouckx RO, De Vos JY, Larno LA et al: Atypical symptoms during single needle dialysis. ASAIO Trans 36:M335, 1990
136. Howard JE, Perkins HA: Lysis of donor rbc during plateletpheresis with a blood processor. JAMA 236:289, 1976
137. Bowman JM, Pollock JM: Haemolysis of donor red cells at fetal transfusion due to catheter trauma, letter. Lancet 2:1190, 1980
138. Gilligan DR, Blumgart HL: March hemoglobinuria. Studies of the clinical characteristics, blood metabolism and mechanism: with observations of three new cases, and review of the literature. Medicine (Baltimore) 20:341, 1941
139. Eichner ER: Runner's macrocytosis: a clue to footstrike hemolysis. Am J Med 78:321, 1985
140. Selby GB, Frame DC, Eichner LK et al: Athlete's echinocytes: new cause for exertional hemolysis?, abstracted. Blood, suppl. 70:56a, 1987
141. Streeton JA: Traumatic haemoglobinuria caused by karate exercises. Lancet 2:191, 1967
142. Kaden WS: Traumatic haemoglobinuria in conga-drum players. Lancet 1:1341, 1970
143. Blaser S, Macknin ML: Head banging with subsequent hemoglobinuria and acute renal failure. Clev Clin J Med 50:347, 1983
144. Weiss GB, Nienhuis AW, McIntosh CL et al: Traumatic cardiac hemolytic anemia. A late complication of a Starr-Edwards mitral valve prosthesis. Arch Intern Med 139:374, 1979

145. Wong PHC, Nandi PL, Ho FCS et al: Acute intravascular hemolysis indicating thrombosis of Bjork-Shiley aortic prosthesis. Arch Intern Med 143:1471, 1983
146. Sayed HM, Dacie JV, Handley DA et al: Haemolytic anemia of mechanical origin after open heart surgery. Thorax 16:356, 1961
147. Wilson JH, Rath R, Glaser R et al: Severe hemolysis after incomplete mitral valve repair. Ann Thorac Surg 50:136, 1990
148. Gupta SC, Suryaprasad AG: Mechanical hemolytic anemia after repair of ruptured chordae tendinae of mitral valve apparatus. Angiology 30:776, 1979
149. Enzenauer RJ, Berenberg JL, Cassell PF: Microangiopathic hemolytic anemia as the initial manifestation of porcine valve failure. South Med J 83:912, 1989
150. Rajesh PB, Goiti JJ: Acute renal failure due to profound haemolysis—an unusual complication of cusp rupture in cardiac bioprostheses. Eur J Cardiothorac Surg 2:197, 1988
151. Nishiura T, Miyazaki Y, Oritani K et al: Aspergillus vegetative endocarditis complicated with schizocytic hemolytic anemia in a patient with acute lymphocytic leukemia. Acta Haematol (Basel) 76:60, 1986
152. Lilliehei CW: Hemolysis and the St. Jude medical valve. Eur J Cardiothorac Surg 3:90, 1989
153. Kwaan HC: Clinicopathologic features of thrombotic thrombocytopenic purpura. Semin Hematol 24:71, 1987
154. Case records of the Massachusetts General Hospital (Case 30-1991). N Engl J Med 325:265, 1991
155. Bell WR, Braine HG, Ness PM et al: Improved survival in thrombotic thrombocytopenic purpura–hemolytic uremic syndrome. Clinical experience in 108 cases. N Engl J Med 325: 398, 1991
156. Rock GA, Shumak KH, Buskard NA et al: Comparison of plasma exchange with plasma infusion in the treatment of thrombotic thrombocytopenic purpura. N Engl J Med 325:393, 1991
157. Wong P, Itoh K, Yoshida S: Treatment of thrombotic thrombocytopenic purpura with intravenous gamma globulin, letter. N Engl J Med 314:385, 1986
158. Gutterman L: Treatment of thrombotic thrombocytopenic purpura (TTP) with exchange plasmapheresis (EP), vincristine (VCR) and methylprednisolone (MP): a standardized initial treatment in 11 patients, abstracted. Blood 76:suppl. 1, 509a, 1990
159. Ruggenenti P, Remuzzi P: Thrombotic thrombocytopenic purpura and related disorders. Hematol Oncol Clin North Am 4:219, 1990
160. Kaplan BS, Proesmans W: The hemolytic uremic syndrome of childhood and its variants. Semin Hematol 24:148, 1987
161. Martin DL, MacDonald KL, White KE et al: The epidemiology and clinical aspects of the hemolytic uremic syndrome in Minnesota. N Engl J Med 323:1161, 1990
162. Case records of the Massachusetts General Hospital (Case 16-1988). N Engl J Med 318:1047, 1988
163. Kwaan HC: Miscellaneous secondary thrombotic microangiopathy. Semin Hematol 24:141, 1987
164. Murgo AJ: Thrombotic microangiopathy in the cancer patient including those induced by chemotherapeutic agents. Semin Hematol 24:161, 1987
165. Lohrmann HP, Adam W, Heymer B et al: Microangiopathic hemolytic anemia in metastatic carcinoma. Report of eight cases. Ann Intern Med 79:368, 1973
166. Antman KH, Skarin AT, Mayer RJ et al: Microangiopathic hemolytic anemia and cancer: a review. Medicine (Baltimore) 58:377, 1979
167. Pritchard JA, Weisman R, Ratnoff OD et al: Intravascular hemolysis, thrombocytopenia and other hematologic abnormalities associated with severe toxemia of pregnancy. N Engl J Med 250:89, 1954
168. Weinstein L: Syndrome of hemolysis, elevated liver enzymes, and low platelet count: a severe consequence of hypertension in pregnancy. Am J Obstet Gynecol 142:159, 1982
169. Rath W, Loos W, Kuhn W et al: The importance of early laboratory screening for maternal and fetal outcome in cases of HELLP syndrome. Eur J Obstet Gynecol Reprod Biol 36:43, 1990
170. Gilabert J, Estelles A, Ridocci F et al: Clinical and haemostatic parameters in the HELLP syndrome: relevance of plasminogen activator inhibitors. Gynecol Obstet Invest 30:81, 1990
171. Schrocksnadel H: Haptoglobin and free haemoglobin in pregnancy-induced hypertension. Lancet 336:1594, 1990
172. Martin JN, Files JC, Blake PG et al: Plasma exchange for preeclampsia. I: Postpartum use for

persistently severe preeclampsia/eclampsia with HELLP syndrome. Am J Obstet Gynecol 162: 126, 1990
173. Pineda AA, Brizica SM, Taswell HF: Hemolytic transfusion reaction. Recent experience in a large blood bank. Mayo Clin Proc 53:378, 1978
174. Sazama K: Reports of 355 transfusion-associated deaths: 1976 through 1985. Transfusion 30: 583, 1990
175. Patten E: Immunohematologic disease. JAMA 258:2945, 1987
176. Greenwalt TJ: Pathogenesis and management of hemolytic transfusion reactions. Semin Hematol 18:84, 1981
177. Brecher ME, Taswell HF: Hemolytic transfusion reactions. p. 628. In Rossi EC, Simon TL, Moss GS (eds): Principles of Transfusion Medicine. Williams & Wilkins, Baltimore, 1991
178. Harrison CR, Hayes TC, Trow LL et al: Intravascular hemolytic transfusion reaction without detectable antibodies: a case report and review of the literature. Vox Sang 51:96, 1986
179. Conway LT, Scott EP: Acute hemolytic transfusion reaction due to ABO incompatible plasma in a plateletpheresis concentrate. Transfusion 24:413, 1984
180. Murphy MF, Hook S, Waters AH: Acute haemolysis after ABO incompatible platelet transfusions. Lancet 335:974, 1990
181. Reis MD, Coovadia AS: Transfusion of ABO incompatible platelets causing severe haemolytic reaction. Clin Lab Haematol 11:237, 1989
182. Ramsey G, Nusbacher J, Starzl TE: Isohemagglutinins of graft origin after ABO-unmatched liver transplantation. N Engl J Med 311:1167, 1984
183. Orchard J, Young NT, Smith C: Severe intravascular haemolysis in a renal transplant recipient due to anti-B of donor origin. Vox Sang 59:172, 1990
184. Povlsen JV, Rasmussen A, Hansen HE et al: Acquired haemolytic anaemia due to isohaemagglutinins of donor origin following ABO minor incompatible kidney transplantation. Nephrol Dial Transplant 5:148, 1990
185. Hows J, Beddow K, Gordon-Smith E et al: Donor-derived red blood cell antibodies and immune hemolysis after allogeneic bone marrow transplantation. Blood 67:177, 1986
186. Copelan EA, Strohm PL, Kennedy MS et al: Hemolysis following intravenous immune globulin therapy. Transfusion 26:410, 1986
187. Nicholls MD, Cummins JC, Davies VJ et al: Haemolysis induced by intravenously-administered immunoglobulin. Med J Aust 150:404, 1989
188. Kim HC, Park CL, Cowan JH et al: Massive intravascular hemolysis associated with intravenous immunoglobulin in bone marrow transplant recipients. Am J Pediatr Hematol Oncol 10:69, 1988
189. Marmoni AM, Cerri R, Lercari G et al: Positive direct antiglobulin tests and heteroimmune hemolysis in patients with severe aplastic anemia and pure red cell anemia treated with antilymphocytic globulin. Acta Haematol (Basel) 74:14, 1985
190. Prchal JT, Huang ST, Court WS et al: Immune hemolytic anemia following administration of antithymocyte globulin. Am J Hematol 19:95, 1985
191. Levene NA, Levene C, Gekker K et al: Th polyagglutination with fatal outcome in a patient with massive intravascular hemolysis and perforated tumor of colon. Am J Hematol 35:127, 1990
192. Sayas MJ, Pastor E, Casanova C et al: Severe intravascular hemolysis associated with polyagglutinability. Br J Haematol 75:433, 1990
193. Sokol RJ, Hewitt S, Booker DJ et al: Red cell autoantibodies, multiple immunoglobulin classes, and autoimmune hemolysis. Transfusion 30:714, 1990
194. Sokol RJ, Hewitt S, Stamps BK: Autoimmune haemolysis: an 18 year study of 865 cases referred to a regional transfusion centre. Br Med J 282:2023, 1981
195. Petz LD, Garratty G: Acquired Immune Hemolytic Anemias. Churchill Livingstone, New York, 1980
196. Rosenthal RE, Jagathambal: Transfusion therapy for autoimmune hemolytic anemia. Semin Hematol 13:311, 1976
197. Nyedegger UE, Kazatchkine MD, Miescher PA: Immunopathologic and clinical features of hemolytic anemia due to cold agglutinins. Semin Hematol 28:66, 1991
198. Niejadlik DC, Lozner EL: Cooling mattress induced acute hemolytic anemia. Transfusion 14: 145, 1974
199. Wertlake PT, McGinniss MH, Schmidt PJ: Cold antibody and persistent intravascular hemolysis after surgery under hypothermia. Transfusion 9:70, 1969

200. Gottsche B, Salama A, Mueller-Eckhardt C: Donath-Landsteiner hemolytic anemia in children. A study of 22 cases. Vox Sang 58:281, 1990
201. Sokol RJ, Stamps BK, Hitchen PA: Autoimmune haemolysis in childhood and adolescence. Acta Haematol (Basel) 72:245, 1984
202. Garratty G: Immune hemolytic anemia and/or positive direct antiglobulin tests due to drugs. Beitr Infusionther 21:229, 1988
203. Petz LD: Drug-induced immune haemolytic anaemia. Clin Haematol 9:455, 1980
204. Shulman IA, Arndt PA, McGehee W et al: Cefotaxime-induced immune hemolytic anemia due to antibodies reacting in vitro by more than one mechanism. Transfusion 30:263, 1990
205. Salama A, Mueller-Eckhardt C: The role of metabolite-specific antibodies in nomifensine-dependent immune hemolytic anemia. N Engl J Med 313:469, 1985
206. Woolf DCS, Jacobs P: Methyldopa, intravascular hemolysis and renal disease. S Afr Med J 77:213, 1990
207. Swanson MA, Chanmougan D, Schwartz RS: Immunohemolytic anemia due to antipenicillin antibodies. Report of a case. N Engl J Med 274:178, 1966
208. Gralnick HR, McGinniss M, Elton W et al: Hemolytic anemia associated with cephalothin. JAMA 217:1193, 1971
209. Moake JL, Butler CF, Hewell GM et al: Hemolysis induced by cefazolin and cephalothin in a patient with penicillin sensitivity. Transfusion 18:369, 1978
210. Gmur J, Walti M, Neftel KA: Amoxicillin induced immune hemolysis. Acta Haematol (Basel) 74:230, 1985
211. Getaz EP, Beckley S, Fitzpatrick J et al: Cisplatin-induced hemolysis. N Engl J Med 302:334, 1980
212. Salama A, Burger M, Mueller-Eckhardt C: Acute immune hemolysis induced by a degradation product of amphotericin B. Blut 58:59, 1989
213. Garratty G, Houston M, Petz LD et al: Acute immune intravascular hemolysis due to hydrochlorothiazide. Am J Clin Pathol 76:73, 1981

3

CARE OF PATIENTS WITH SICKLE CELL ANEMIA IN THE ADULT EMERGENCY DEPARTMENT

SAMUEL CHARACHE
MABEL KOSHY
PAUL F. MILNER

The cardinal pathophysiologic features of sickle cell disease include chronic hemolytic anemia and vaso-occlusion by rigid sickle cells, resulting in ischemic tissue injury. The hemolytic anemia results in jaundice, formation of gallstones, and hyperactive bone marrow.

The organs most at risk from vaso-occlusion are those with venous sinuses, such as the spleen and bone marrow, and those with limited terminal arterial blood supply, such as the eyes and the head of the femur. Symptoms of hypoxic injury may be acute, as seen in painful episodes, or they may be insidious in onset as in osteonecrosis of the femoral or humeral head or in sickle retinopathy. Accumulated effects of many vaso-occlusions over a patient's lifetime may lead to chronic dysfunction of the lung, kidney, eye, bone, etc.

MAKING A DIAGNOSIS IN THE EMERGENCY DEPARTMENT

If the diagnosis is unclear, reports of hemoglobin electrophoresis (which is the definitive method for diagnosis) are not returned to the emergency department (ED) promptly enough to be of value. A tentative diagnosis can be made nevertheless. Evaluation of the patient includes, in addition to a carefully obtained clinical history and physical examination, a blood count with red cell indices, a screening test for hemoglobin S, and inspection of the blood smear. A positive screening test, a hemoglobin concentration between 6 and 8 g/dl, and a high reticulocyte count with sickled cells on the peripheral smear are common in sickle cell anemia (Hb SS). A positive screening test, an Hb of 9 to 12, and many target cells on smear suggest hemoglobin sickle cell disease (Hb SC). A positive screen, moderate anemia, target cells, and microcytosis are associated with the presence of α- or β-thalassemia (Hb $SS\alpha^{+}$ or Hb $S\beta^{+}$-Thal, respectively), or rarely, iron deficiency. Patients with sickle cell trait (AS) are not anemic and have normal blood smears although the screening test is positive. *Sickle cell disease* is a generic term, which includes Hb SS, Hb SC, and Hb $S\beta^{+}$-Thal but not AS.

THE EMERGENCY DEPARTMENT SCENARIO

To some extent all encounters between physicians and patients involve a "scenario," which sets limits upon or even determines the actions taken by the "players." Those scenarios are played out in all medical encounters, but in the emergency department the tempo is faster and the contrasts between players more sharply drawn than in other doctor-patient contacts. If those problems are to be dealt with effectively, both patients and medical staff must understand how best to cope with each other before the specifics of the visit are handled.

Teaching Patients How to Cope With Emergency Departments

Patients should be told the basic principles that govern their local ED including its location, whether or not it is useful to have a call from the clinic physician precede their arrival, and the general routine they will encounter. Triage must be explained; most patients can understand why the sickest patients come first, even if they do not like to be second. Patients often say they would like an analgesic first and questions later; discussion with them regarding the necessity for accurate diagnosis prior to analgesic administration is essential. Patients should be told whether or not to expect to see their clinic physician while in the ED, to prevent feelings of abandonment. If there is a rule on duration of an ED visit, it may be helpful to explain it to patients before they encounter its application.

Patient education regarding narcotic-induced respiratory depression, urine retention, and ileus is important, so that patients can understand what prevents the physician from giving them as much drug as they might like. They should have been taught these things before their first visit to the

ED, but that often is not the case, and the task may fall on ED staff.

Teaching ED Staff to Cope With Patients With Sickle Cell Anemia

Only a small proportion of patients with Hb SS are repeat visitors to the ED, and ED physicians will find infrequent visitors to be less manipulative and demanding than the subset of patients who make weekly (or more frequent) visits. Patients may have "bad spells" for several months, during which pain grumbles and flares up, only to have a succeeding spell that is virtually pain-free. As in asthma, myocardial infarction, or inflammatory bowel disease, emotional stress can precipitate acute attacks, and ED personnel should not dismiss a patient's complaints as "psychological" without a discussion with the clinic physician.

Explanations regarding the risk of narcotic dependence are usually resented, and confronting the patient only builds up a wall of antagonism. To discuss patient's "problems" in front of them or in front of aides who may later accuse patients of narcotic seeking, is just as bad. Patients should not be given placebos. If they are given a non-narcotic injection [such as a parenteral nonsteroidal anti-inflammatory drug (NSAID)] they should be told what they have received and why, for some patients are aware of the taste and feel of more usual injections.

PAINFUL EPISODES

Painful events are thought to be due to microscopic infarctions of bones and other tissues. Pain may be local or generalized. Possible precipitating causes include dehydration, infection, psychosocial stress, and physical exertion, but painful events may occur spontaneously without any precipitant. The intensity of pain and the reaction to it vary from individual to individual.

The first treatment decision must be whether the event is an uncomplicated sickle crisis. There is no laboratory test and no diagnostic procedure that can prove that complaints are due to a self-limited vaso-occlusive event. We must rule out all other possible etiologies first, and acute infection is almost always first on the list. As with tissue destruction due to any cause, increased leukocytosis (over the patient's usual value) and low-grade fever may be due to infarction as well as to infection. For most patients a white blood cell count above 25,000 suggests infection. After careful questioning and a thorough physical examination, examination of body fluid (urine, sputum, pus) can be helpful. Cultures are important, but a carefully interpreted Gram stain is

There is no laboratory test and no diagnostic procedure that can prove that complaints are due to a self-limited vaso-occlusive event.

what is most important in the ED. A chest x-ray should be obtained for all patients with chest pain unless the site is clearly in a rib, and measurement of arterial oxygen pressure (PaO_2) or saturation should be considered. Once it is decided that pain is due to an uncomplicated vaso-occlusive episode, the patient should be reassured and treated with fluids and appropriate analgesics.

Treatment of Acute Pain

Table 3-1 lists equivalent doses of oral and parenteral narcotics and some of their pharmacologic properties. One can treat acute crises with potent oral narcotics if one uses enough. There is no real difference between drugs in addiction potential; morphine and codeine may be more likely to produce vomiting, and meperidine can cause seizures. Evidence that various tranquilizers can potentiate narcotic effects is very scant; their major effect may be to induce relaxation and sleep.

Oxygen therapy is essential if the patient is hypoxemic ($PaO_2 < 70$ mmHg). Patients with such low values usually should be admitted promptly (unless the hypoxemia is known to be a chronic condition due to long-standing lung disease). If PaO_2 is above 85 mmHg, oxygen administration is little more than a placebo and may depress erythropoiesis.[1] Fluid administration should be viewed similarly: it is necessary only if the patient is dehydrated or likely to become so. Oral fluids are just as good as parenteral ones if the patient will drink them and if there are sufficient nursing personnel to ensure a 3-L intake per 24 hours. Venous access becomes a big problem in older patients, and use of oral fluids may "save that vein" for a later day.

When it comes time for patients to leave the ED, they should not be given "a shot for the road" . . if they walk

TABLE 3-1. Narcotic Analgesic Equivalents

	Equianalgesic Doses[a]	
Drug	IM (mg)	Oral (mg)
Morphine	10	60
Levorphanol	2	4
Hydromorphone	1.5	7.5
Meperidine	75	300
Codeine	130	200
Oxycodone	—	30
Propoxyphene	—	130

[a] Based on acute short-term use. Chronic administration may alter pharmacokinetics and decrease the oral/parenteral ratio. The morphine oral/parenteral ratio decreases to 1.5 to 2.5 on chronic dosing.

into a truck or fall on their heads, the ED personnel are responsible. It is a good idea to give patients a 3- to 7-day supply of oral analgesic to use at home. Many prescription plans supply only generic drugs, and patients should be reminded of that fact.

CHEST SYNDROME

Chest syndrome refers to development of a new lung infiltrate on chest x-ray, which is usually associated with fever and can range in severity from a small patch of atelectasis to bilateral "white-outs" of the lungs. Both pneumonia and infarction are included in the rubric.

An abnormal lung scan finding in a patient with chest syndrome is most significant if a prior normal scan is available for comparison. Sickle cell disease does not protect one from embolism, and if there is a swollen leg or recent surgery, venograms or Doppler studies should be considered, as well as pulmonary arteriograms.

In patients with a lung infiltrate and fever, infectious and vaso-occlusive etiologies usually cannot be separated, and either can cause hypoxemia. Treatment almost always includes antibiotics, but in adults no organisms are usually isolated (perhaps because routine culture methods used do not detect *Mycoplasm* or *Chlamydia* spp.)[2,3] The etiology in adults is probably pulmonary infarction, due to emboli of aggregated sickle cells, or necrotic bone marrow. The latter diagnosis can be established if fat droplets are found in the urine.[4]

Some of the hemoglobin within sickle cells begins to polymerize when oxygen saturation becomes less than 100 percent, and visible sickling begins when PaO_2 falls below 60 to 70 mmHg. If PaO_2 is that low, the stage is set for generalized sickling, which usually causes widespread organ failure, including profound pulmonary failure. Every effort must be made to raise the PaO_2 in such a situation. If PaO_2 does rise to 80 mmHg or more with relatively simply therapy, transfer to an inpatient unit is appropriate, but the patient must continue to be monitored. Ear or fingertip oximetry works well, especially if a reading is first correlated with blood gas measurements.

Some of the hemoglobin within sickle cells begins to polymerize when oxygen saturation falls below 100 percent, and visible sickling begins when the PaO_2 falls below 60 to 70 mmHg. If PaO_2 is that low, the stage is set for generalized sickling, which usually causes widespread organ failure. Every effort must be made to raise the PaO_2 in such a situation.

As patients age, the effect of repeated infarctions becomes manifest as organ failure. Cor pulmonale is a not uncommon consequence of repeated major and minor attacks of chest syndrome.[5] Development of chronically low PaO_2 and right-sided heart failure are ominous signs and may cause patients to be frequent visitors to the ED. Treatment is supportive and often leads to chronic transfusion therapy.

ANEMIA

In hemolytic anemia the reticulocyte count is an important measurement, as it assesses the degree of compensation by the bone marrow for anemia and evaluates the regulation of erythropoiesis. In Hb SS patients the reticulocyte count is usually between 10 and 20 percent, but it may be lower in Hb SC or Hb Sβ-Thal patients.

Causes of Decrease in Usual Hemoglobin Level

During an acute vaso-occlusive event, it is not unusual for the Hb to fall by as much as 2 g/dl from the steady-state value. This is due to a combination of increased sequestration of red cells, hemolysis, and/or depressed erythropoiesis secondary to infection, fever, or oxygen inhalation. If the patient has no cardiorespiratory distress at rest, this is not a cause for alarm. A low reticulocyte count is not necessarily a cause for admission if patients have no symptoms of anemia and their blood count can be rechecked within a few days.

The classic aplastic crisis with a precipitous fall in hemoglobin to levels around 2 to 3 g/dl is due to temporary erythroid aplasia caused by a virus infection, most commonly the human parvovirus.[6] The reticulocyte count will reach a nadir of less than 1 percent early in the crisis and may not begin to recover for 6 to 10 days. Patients should be transfused to an Hb of about 8 g/dl if they show symptoms of insufficient oxygen transport. All patients with aplastic crises should probably be admitted, for the hemoglobin may continue to fall despite transfusion.

Other Causes of Increased Anemia

Folate or vitamin B_{12} deficiency should be considered when red cells are larger than usual and the reticulocyte count is low. Iron deficiency is uncommon but can occur (particularly in patients using aspirin or NSAIDs) and should be confirmed by measurement of transferrin saturation (< 16 percent) or ferritin level (< 25 μg/ml) before iron therapy is started. As in any patient, the cause of iron deficiency, which is almost invariably bleeding, must be determined.

Blood should not be given to treat uncomplicated vaso-occlusive pain crises or simply to raise the hemoglobin level in an anemic but otherwise stable patient with a good reticulocyte response.

Blood Transfusion

Blood should not be given to treat uncomplicated vaso-occlusive pain crises or simply to raise the hemoglobin level in an anemic but otherwise stable patient with a good reticulocyte response.[7] If transfusion is needed, two to three units of red cells is usually enough to raise the hemoglobin concentration to its previous level.

Transfusion Reactions

An acute febrile reaction can usually be avoided by using a filter in the blood line or by using washed red cells. If it does occur, the transfusion should be stopped and Benadryl, 50 mg administered by intramuscular injection. Delayed transfusion reactions[8] are usually seen about the fifth post-transfusion day, when the patient develops increased jaundice and may complain of headache, fever, breathlessness, and pain resembling a crisis. The Hb will be lower than it was, as all the transfused red cells may have been destroyed, and occasionally the patient's own cells are also destroyed by an autoantibody. If the patient had undergone an exchange transfusion, the resulting fall in hemoglobin concentration may be disastrous. It is important to realize that chronically anemic patients can survive with a very low Hb (<3.0 g) if supported by intensive care.

RIGHT UPPER QUADRANT ABDOMINAL PAIN

Gallstones are very common in adults and children with sickle cell anemia but may remain asymptomatic for many years after they are diagnosed. In the ED the preferred initial examination for acute cholecystitis is abdominal ultrasonography. A technetium-labelled HIDA or diisofenex scan is useful to demonstrate cystic duct obstruction. Both medical and surgical consultation should be obtained, especially when gallstones are discovered during routine assessment (e.g., on a chest x-ray).

Symptoms due to gallstones have to be distinguished from acute hepatitis with a tender swollen liver and hepatic sequestration of sickle cells. A syndrome of hyperbilirubinemia with absent or minimal abdominal symptoms has been described. Total bilirubin may reach 100 mg/dl, most of which is unconjugated (indirect reacting bilirubin). Hyperbilirubinemia usually subsides in a few days. Diagnosis is by exclusion of other causes such as acute viral hepatitis.

Peptic ulceration is quite common in sickle cell anemia. A careful history may distinguish it from cholelithiasis, but the two conditions may coexist.

SURGERY AND ANESTHESIA

Although surgery and anesthesia are not part of ED practice, discussions and decisions regarding them usually take

Hematologic consultation should be sought as soon as possible if surgery is likely, for partial exchange transfusions take some time to organize and complete.

place in the ED. Contrary to popular belief, patients with sickle cell disease tolerate general anesthesia well,[9] and no particular method or agent is contraindicated. The incidence of complications in the postoperative period is increased in sickle cell disease but can be reduced by careful preoperative precautions and careful postoperative nursing care. Patients should be hydrated intravenously for 24 hours prior to surgery, smoking should be curtailed, and instructions should be given in the use of an incentive spirometer. Routine blood tests should always include measurement of PaO_2, since hypoxemia may be an important risk factor for postoperative complications. Hematologic consultation should be sought as soon as possible if surgery is likely because partial exchange transfusions take some time to organize and complete.

NEUROLOGIC COMPLICATIONS

Acute neurologic complications are reported in 6 to 20 percent of children and in approximately 10 to 15 percent of adults. Convulsions, stupor, transient ischemic attacks, and clearly defined strokes can occur in any age group. Since convulsions can occur in neurologically intact persons who do not excrete the meperidine metabolite normeperidine, observation of seizures in a patient being treated with that drug does not necessarily indicate occurrence of a stroke. Diagnosis of a neurologic event may require the use of lumbar puncture, computed tomography (CT), and magnetic resonance imaging (MRI). Arteriography must be considered if other studies suggest a surgically correctable lesion.[10]

THE EYE

Trauma to the eye may produce hyphema, or blood in the anterior chamber. In the aqueous humor sickling not only of red cells from patients with sickle cell disease but also from those with sickle cell trait, is greatly facilitated. If the canal of Schlemm is obstructed by rigid sickled cells, the result is not infarction but increased intraocular pressure (glaucoma) and, not infrequently, secondary occlusion of the central retinal artery. In patients whose red cells can sickle, hyphema should prompt ophthalmologic consultation to evaluate the need for washout or decompression of the anterior chamber. It is not clear whether all patients with hyphema should have emergent testing for the presence of Hb S; prudence may suggest a positive response, but there are no prospectively collected data to substantiate such a practice.

There probably is an increased incidence of occlusion of the central retinal artery or its branches in patients with sickle cell disease. Established treatment does not differ from that of other patients, and spontaneous recovery without recurrence may follow the event.

Vitreous hemorrhage and retinal detachment are serious problems in patients with sickle cell disease. Bleeding comes from fragile neovascularizations, and much as in diabetic retinopathy, photocoagulation may slow or stop progression of the lesions. Emergent ophthalmologic consultation while the patient is in the ED is needed for both diagnosis and management. Vitreous hemorrhage may be one of the very few manifestations of sickle cell disease that can be prevented. If a patient has had a vitreous hemorrhage, regular visits to an ophthalmologist with an interest in retinal vascular disease are a very good idea.

JOINT PAIN

"Arthritis" may be the presenting complaint in patients with Hb SC or Hb $S\beta^+$-Thal. Warm, swollen joints are not uncommon. The most likely cause is an infarct in underlying bone, but synovial infarction has been described in some cases. Often, treatment with indomethacin for 4 to 5 days produces relief.

The problem comes from nonsickling causes of acute arthritis, especially infectious agents. Monarticular arthritis should raise the question of infection by direct extension of osteomyelitis or by hematogenous seeding (gonorrheal arthritis). Mono- or polyarticular lesions also suggest secondary gout, which is seen in only a fraction of patients with high serum urate levels. Joint aspiration is usually indicated, with cell count, Gram stain, examination under polarized light, differential white blood cell count, and description of viscosity. Acute gouty arthritis can be treated with indomethacin, but chronic colchicine therapy may prevent some attacks. The risk/benefit ratio of allopurinol therapy is unclear in sickle cell disease, for not all patients with high serum urate levels develop gout.

Persistent Hip or Shoulder Pain

Patients with sickle cell disease may come to the ED because of *persistent* arthritic pain in the hip or shoulder. The pain is different in quality and duration from that of vaso-occlusive crises and may indicate the onset of osteonecrosis within the femoral or humeral heads. The most sensitive technique to detect the problem at an early stage is MRI. Bed rest and NSAIDs often provide relief.

A patient who returns to the ED because of persistent hip pain in the presence of evidence of early aseptic necrosis should be referred for an orthopedist's opinion. The procedure known as *core decompression* may be indicated, but hip replacement should not be seriously considered until function is severely limited (because the long-term results of hip replacement in Hb SS patients are not entirely encouraging.)[11,12] Shoulder pain may be intolerable, and although anti-inflammatory drugs may provide help, shoulder arthroplasty may be the only way to provide permanent pain relief.

ANKLE ULCERS

Patients my come to the ED because of pain associated with chronic ankle ulcers and occasionally because of spreading cellulitis that originated in an ulcer. There is no specific treatment method for healing sickle cell-related leg ulcers.[13] All healing methods, including transfusion and skin grafts, are associated with similar recurrence rates. Once the patient develops ankle ulcers, aggressive care should include daily cleansing, and application of wet to dry saline or Burow's solution dressings. If cellulitis is not acute, occlusive dressings or Unna boots can be used, but careful follow-up is needed. Topical antibiotics are rarely beneficial. If there is evidence of spreading cellulitis or systemic spread of infection, hospitalization is usually required for intravenous antibiotic therapy, since the usual infecting organisms (*Staphylococcus aureus* and *Pseudomonas aeruginosa*) are usually resistant to orally administered agents).

PREGNANCY

Pregnant patients require meticulous prenatal care, and if a diagnosis of pregnancy is established in the ED, the patient should be referred to a high-risk obstetric clinic with experience in treating women with sickle cell disease.

Patients with sickle cell disease are at increased risk from a variety of complications of pregnancy. Spontaneous abortion, intrauterine growth retardation, and prematurity are known risks to the fetus. Patients require meticulous prenatal care, and if a diagnosis of pregnancy is established in the ED, the patient should be referred to a high-risk obstetric clinic with experience in treating women with sickle cell disease.

Should delivery seem imminent in the ED, labor should be managed with caution as the underlying hemodynamics of anemia with a high cardiac output are accentuated during this period of intrauterine contraction and pain. If cesarean section will be necessary, rapid exchange transfusion can be of benefit; as with any type of major surgery, hematologic consultation should be sought promptly.

PRIAPISM

A painful, persistent penile erection occurs at some time in about 40 percent of men with sickle cell disease. It usually occurs during sleep and wakes the patient because of pain.

In the adult it tends to be of two kinds—an intermittent repetitive event lasting about 30 minutes to 6 hours but resolving with physical exercise or an acute persistent erection continuing for more than 24 hours or several days.

In children the acute form has a good prognosis and is best treated conservatively. In the adult the longer the erection continues, the worse the prognosis for future sexual function. Acute persistent priapism (duration over 24 hours) is best treated by a corpus cavernosum–corpus spongiosum shunt procedure performed through the glans penis,[14] which can be done in an ambulatory care setting without general anesthesia. Patients should always be admitted for observation following the procedure. There is no evidence that blood transfusion or any of a number of nonoperative procedures can reduce the duration of priapism in the adult patient. Given that, it probably is better to proceed early on to a shunt procedure to decongest the organ.

THE FREQUENT VISITOR

If some patients seem to be spending an extraordinary amount of their lives in the emergency room, it may be time to discuss their long-term management with their clinic physician or family practitioner. There are no proven chronic treatments for prevention of sickle cell crises, and of those approaches that have some cachet, placebo effects have not been excluded as explanations for beneficial effects. These measures range from moving to a warmer or less stressful environment to chronic transfusion therapy to administration of a drug such as hydroxyurea. Each of them has drawbacks or toxicities as well as uncertain benefits, and should not be entered upon without discussion, reflection, and the advice of a hematologist with experience in their use.

There are no proven chronic treatments for prevention of sickle cell crises, and of those approaches that have some cachet, placebo effects have not been excluded as explanations for beneficial effects.

References

1. Embury SH, Garcia JF, Mohandas N et al: Effects of oxygen inhalation on endogenous erythropoietin kinetics, erythropoiesis, and properties of blood cells in sickle cell anemia. N Engl J Med 311:291, 1984
2. Shulman ST, Bartlett J, Clyde WA Jr, Ayoub EM: The unusual severity of mycoplasmal pneumonia in children with sickle-cell disease. N Engl J Med 287:164, 1972
3. Miller ST, Hammerschlag MR, Chirgwn K et al: Role of Chlamydia pneumoniae in acute chest syndrome of sickle cell disease. J Pediatr 118:30, 1991
4. Hutchinson RM, Merrick MV, White JM: Fat embolism in sickle cell disease. J Clin Pathol 26: 620, 1973
5. Powars D, Weidman JA, Odom-Maryon T et al: Sickle cell chronic lung disease: prior morbidity and the risk of pulmonary failure. Medicine (Baltimore) 67:66, 1988

6. Kelleher JF, Luben LC, Cohen BJ, Mortimer PP: Human serum parvovirus as the cause of aplastic crisis in sickle cell disease. Am J Dis Child 138:401, 1984
7. Milner PF, Squires JE, Larison PJ et al: Posttransfusion crisis in sickle cell anemia. South Med J 78:1462, 1985
8. Cox JV, Steane E, Cunningham G, Frenkel EP: Risk of alloimmunization and delayed hemolytic transfusion reactions in patients with sickle cell disease. Arch Intern Med 148:2485, 1988
9. Homi J, Reynolds J, Skinner A et al: General anaesthesia in sickle-cell disease. Br Med J 1:1599, 1979
10. Anson JA, Koshy M, Ferguson L, Crowell RM: Subarachnoid hemorrhage in sickle-cell disease. J Neurosurg 75:552, 1991
11. Clarke HJ, Jinnah RH, Brooker AF, Michaelson JD: Total replacement of the hip for avascular necrosis in sickle cell disease. J Bone Joint Surg [B] 71:465, 1989
12. Milner PF: Osteonecrosis of the femoral head in sickle cell disease. N Engl J Med 325:1476, 1991
13. Koshy M, Entsuah R, Koranda A et al: Leg ulcers in patients with sickle cell disease. Blood 74: 1403, 1989
14. Hamre MR, Harmon EP, Kirkpatrick DV et al: Priapism as a complication of sickle-cell disease. J Urol 145:1, 1991

4

IMMUNE THROMBO-CYTOPENIC PURPURA

DIANE J. NUGENT

Platelets play a critical role in the maintenance of normal hemostasis and vascular integrity. Patients with platelet counts of less than 20,000/mm^3 or with dysfunctional platelets develop increased bruising, petechiae, and mucous membrane bleeding. In its most extreme form thrombocytopenia may result in life-threatening intracranial or gastrointestinal bleeding. In the intensive care setting every effort is made to re-establish normal hemostasis and cell counts in thrombocytopenic patients by infusing random donor platelets. In the case of bone marrow failure (i.e., aplastic anemia or postchemotherapy), transfusion alone is usually adequate to restore a normal platelet count. However, thrombocytopenia due to immune destruction is a much more challenging problem for the intensivist because transfused platelets are also rapidly destroyed, often without making any measurable impact on the platelet count.

Petechiae, bruising, and mucous membrane bleeding are hallmarks of thrombocytopenia.

THROMBOCYTOPENIA DUE TO ANTIPLATELET AUTOANTIBODIES

Immune thrombocytopenic purpura (ITP) is one of the most common forms of autoimmune disease affecting both adults and children. Patients with ITP develop autoantibodies, which bind to platelet membrane antigens, mediating the rapid destruction of antibody-coated cells in the reticuloendothelial system, principally the spleen and liver. Clinically, a previously well child is suddenly noted to have an increase in bleeding manifestations. Parents may note a "rash," actually petechiae, on the face following a crying or breath-holding episode. Petechiae may also appear in association with minor trauma or in dependent areas of the limbs (i.e., the lower arms and legs). Almost all thrombocytopenic patients have petechiae and increased frequency and size of bruises—whence the term *purpura* in this syndrome. Many patients also experience nose and oral mucosal bleeding. Approximately 10 to 20 percent patients experience menorrhagia, hematuria, or hematochezia. Fortunately, the incidence of life-threatening bleeding into a major organ such as the brain or gastrointestinal tract is actually rare, occurring in 1 percent of cases or less. However, the devastating nature of these bleeds calls for immediate and aggressive therapy to control the hemorrhage and minimize permanent damage.

The spleen should not be enlarged in ITP.

Apart from the bleeding manifestations described above, the remainder of the examination should be normal. Patients with ITP should *not* have hepatosplenomegaly, diffuse adenopathy, leg or joint pain or swelling, weight loss, or fevers. These findings are more likely to be associated with acute viral infections (Epstein-Barr virus [EBV] or cytomegalovirus [CMV]), malignancy (leukemia or lymphoma), collagen vascular disease (rheumatoid arthritis, systemic lupus erythematosus [SLE], or immune complex disease), or the acquired immunodeficiency syndrome (AIDS). Thrombocytopenia may be a presenting feature in any of these syndromes, but further laboratory examination should clarify the underlying disease process.

The presentation and prognosis of ITP may vary according to age, sex, and familial predisposition to autoimmune disease. Even in uncomplicated ITP there is considerable variation in presentation and prognosis (Table 4-1). Based on the duration of thrombocytopenia, a distinction is made between acute and chronic ITP. Thrombocytopenia lasting less than 6 months is termed acute, and that lasting longer than 6 months is termed chronic. Children are more likely to have the acute form of ITP, in which the thrombocytopenia resolves within 2 to 4 months of diagnosis in 60 to 75 percent of patients regardless of therapy.[1,2] Childhood ITP occurs with equal frequency in boys and girls, is seasonal in nature, and may follow a recent infectious exposure or

TABLE 4-1. Comparison of Childhood and Adult Forms of ITP

Childhood Form
- Onset is acute
- Thrombocytopenia < 6 months
- Male/female ratio 1:1
- Incidence is seasonal: winter > fall > spring > summer
- Peak age 2–5 years

Adult Form
- Onset usually chronic
- Thrombocytopenia > 6 months
- Male/female ratio 3:1
- Incidence is the same year-round
- Positive family history of other autoimmune diseases

immunization, which suggests a role for viral or bacterial antigens in triggering antiplatelet autoantibodies.[3] There is no familial predisposition in the acute form of childhood ITP. The peak age for acute ITP is 2 to 5 years, coinciding with the time during which children experience the greatest frequency of viral infections.

Chronic ITP is the more common course in the adult (75 to 85 percent of adult cases) and like other autoimmune diseases, occurs more frequently in women (3:1 female/male ratio). Chronic ITP is *not* seasonal in nature and may be associated with autoantibodies to nonplatelet antigens (e.g., antinuclear antigen [ANA] or anti-ds DNA). Furthermore, chronic ITP is more likely to occur in families in which there is an increased incidence of other autoimmune diseases.[4,5] The latter pattern suggests an underlying, perhaps inherited, immune dysregulation. Unlike SLE or diabetes mellitus, however, the genetic predisposition for ITP has not been linked to histocompatibility antigens such as HLA class I or HLA class II DR, DP, or DQ antigens.[6–8] Like other syndromes, ITP may occur as an isolated phenomenon or in association with other conditions such as SLE, pregnancy, or EBV and similar infections.

Laboratory Evaluation

Over the years ITP has been defined by the triad of thrombocytopenia, decreased platelet survival, and increased platelet production based on increased bone marrow megakaryocytes. An initial laboratory evaluation should include a complete blood count, reticulocyte count, chemistry panel with liver enzymes, erythrocyte sedimentation rate, and bone marrow aspiration to evaluate megakaryocyte number and rule out occult malignancy, dysmyelopoiesis, or early marrow failure. Some centers include viral serology to rule out human immunodeficiency virus (HIV), EBV, and CMV as well. Laboratory findings should include:

- Platelet count below 100,000
- Normal white cell count and differential
- Normal hemoglobin
- Smear possibly showing slight increase in platelet size
- No red cell fragments seen
- Chemistry panel normal
- Bone marrow showing increased number of megakaryocytes

The complete blood count should be normal apart from the decreased platelet count. If the hemoglobin or white blood count is decreased, this may be due to an underlying bone marrow failure as seen with aplastic anemia, or it may be an early sign of a malignancy involving the bone marrow, such as leukemia or lymphoma. The chemistry panel might also provide clues to the underlying diagnosis if the liver enzymes are elevated, as is seen with hepatitis alone, with hepatitis triggering aplastic anemia, or with an elevated uric acid or lactate dehydrogenase (LDH) level as in malignancy. The sedimentation rate may suggest underlying collagen vascular disease or occult malignancy. In the case of an adult or adolescent patient presenting with acute-onset thrombocytopenia, many centers send off studies including anti-DNA binding, ANA, and total complement to rule out collagen vascular disease, which in the early phase may present with isolated thrombocytopenia. Patients with ITP may have occult hematuria due to a low platelet count, but they should *not* have proteinuria, casts in the urine, hypertension, or elevated creatinine or blood urea nitrogen, as is seen in SLE-associated nephritis.

ITP patients with decreased hemoglobin and increased reticulocyte count may have autoimmune hemolytic anemia as well, and a Coombs test should be performed.

The hematocrit may be decreased in ITP patients with significant hemorrhage due to thrombocytopenia. In the acute setting the reticulocyte count may not yet be elevated, and it is necessary to perform a bone marrow aspiration to rule out marrow failure or leukemia. A small number of ITP patients may also have antierythrocyte autoantibodies (Evans syndrome), resulting in hemolytic anemia and an increased reticulocyte count. The Coombs test, both direct and indirect, is positive in this case. Patients with mononucleosis (EBV infection) may also have both antiplatelet and anti-red cell antibodies, but the reticulocyte count may not be so strikingly elevated because the antierythrocyte antibody is directed against i-antigen, which is predominantly expressed on reticulocytes. These cells are then selectively removed, leaving the patient anemic with a "normal" or relatively decreased reticulocyte count.

Because of rapid turnover, ITP platelets are young and "sticky," so the bleeding time is not as long as would be anticipated for the degree of thrombocytopenia.

Histopathologic examination of the bone marrow has been described in both acute and chronic ITP. In the early stages of ITP the bone marrow may appear normal without the expected expansion of platelet precursors. As the bone marrow responds to persistent thrombocytopenia, the megakaryocytes begin to increase in number, particularly the early, less mature cells (ploidy $\leq$ 4N) and the very large megakaryocytes (ploidy $\geq$ 16N). This pattern is more likely to be seen after 4 weeks of thrombocytopenia and may be seen with immune or nonimmune platelet destruction syndromes. The myeloid and erythroid precursors should be *normal* in both number and appearance in ITP. Children with the acute form of ITP who are younger than 4 years of age may have an increased number of small lymphocytes in their bone marrow. Notably, these may account for 20 to 30 percent of nucleated cells in the bone marrow and are often positive for early B-cell markers such as CD10 (CALLA) and CD19 (early B-cell antigen).[9] Eosinophilia may also be associated with childhood ITP but has no prognostic value in predicting the severity or chronicity of the disease.[10,11]

Etiology

In the early 1950s Harrington and co-workers observed that pregnant women with thrombocytopenia often gave birth to infants with profound but transient thrombocytopenia.[12,13] This observation suggested to them that a plasma factor causing maternal thrombocytopenia could cross the placenta and mediate thrombocytopenia in the fetus and newborn. To prove that this factor was indeed present in the plasma of thrombocytopenic patients with increased platelet turnover, Harrington infused himself with plasma from a patient with ITP.[14] He became acutely thrombocytopenic, with bleeding and a brief seizure, necessitating his own admission to the hematology ward for several days until his platelet count recovered. Subsequent studies demonstrated that the antiplatelet activity was found in the γ fraction of ITP plasma,[12] and Harrington isolated the factor in the immunoglobulin fraction of plasma protein. Clinical investigation undertaken in other medical centers confirmed that immunoglobulin G antiplatelet antibodies were responsible for the rapid destruction of circulating platelets in ITP.[15]

There are at least three ways that platelets accumulate immunoglobulin on the surface, thus triggering their removal in the reticuloendothelial system. Most often, autoantibodies bind directly to membrane structures on the platelet surface, which results in rapid destruction of the thrombocyte. A second mechanism of immune clearance involves binding of non-platelet-specific antibodies to a target antigen (such as viral proteins or an ingested drug), which have adhered nonspecifically to the platelet membrane. In the latter circumstance, the antiviral or antidrug antibody mediates clearance of circulating platelets as "innocent bystanders." In addition, immune complexes composed of antigen and immunoglobulin in the circulation may bind via Fc receptors normally expressed on the platelet surface. Again, the platelet is removed in the reticuloendothelial system, which only detects the immunoglobulin- and sometimes complement-coated thrombocyte. Drug-induced antibodies causing thrombocytopenia are represented in all three of these categories—that is, they can induce platelet-specific autoantibodies, bind to drug adherent to the platelet, or bind to drug that is bound specifically to a platelet glycoprotein. A good history of current or past medications is essential to properly manage ITP patients.

The bone marrow responds to a decrease in circulating platelets by increasing megakaryocyte number, size, and ploidy. This in turn results in platelets that are slightly larger than normal and represent a younger than normal population, owing to the rapid turnover of thrombocytes. Thus, the bleeding time in patients with ITP is shortened relative to the absolute number of platelets, and these patients rarely have major bleeding even though the platelet count may fall below 20,000/mm^3.[16] A notable exception to this generalization occurs in the case of autoantibodies that bind to structures on the platelet surface that are critical to normal platelet aggregation or adhesion. In this setting patients present with prolonged bleeding times and hemorrhagic symptoms even though their platelet count is above 50,000/mm^3.

Since Harrington established the immune nature of ITP, originally called *idiopathic* thrombocytopenic purpura, many authors have replaced the term *idiopathic,* with *immune* or *immune-mediated* in discussing the disease. Physicians began to rely on the demonstration of increased platelet-associated immunoglobulin or the presence of circulating antiplatelet antibodies in patient plasma to confirm the diagnosis. Initially, assays focused on quantifying increased levels of platelet-bound IgG, IgM, and complement. The sensitivity of these assays was significantly limited by the fact that platelets, the target tissue, were markedly decreased in number. Moreover, platelets carry an internal pool of serum-derived IgG in their α-granules as the result of uptake by the megakaryocyte and packaging during platelet production.[17,18] The purpose of this α-granule-associated IgG in normal individuals is unknown. However, it complicates the interpretation of test results that show an increase in platelet-associated IgG because with *nonimmune* platelet destruction syndromes, platelet activation may occur and trigger the release of α granules, thus nonspecifically increasing the amount of surface-associated IgG. Therefore increase in platelet-associated IgG alone may support the diagnosis of ITP but does not rule out the possibility of low-grade activation and consumption of platelets due to other etiologies such as hemolytic uremic syndrome, vascular abnormalities (arteriovenous shunts or cavernous hemangiomas), or massive tissue damage such as that seen with burns or head trauma. For these reasons hematologists now rely on the demonstration of free antiplatelet antibody in the serum to clarify the underlying etiology of increased platelet destruction.

Work in the 1960s and 1970s focused on the development of sensitive assays to detect free antiplatelet antibodies in serum, even though autoantibodies are often of low titer and affinity. These new techniques increased the efficiency of antibody screening so that all patients might be evaluated by using indirect binding assays to detect and quantitate the amounts of antibody bound to the platelet and free in the plasma.[19,20] Antiplatelet antibodies of the IgM class can also mediate platelet destruction, particularly when they fix complement.[21–23] Increased platelet-associated complement (C3) levels are found in roughly 30 to 40 percent of chronic ITP patients.[24,25] In children about one-third of the patients have only IgM platelet-reactive antibodies and another 20 to 30 percent have both IgG and IgM. In adults the reported frequency of IgM antiplatelet antibodies is 10 percent or less, which may reflect the relative dominance of chronic ITP in adults.

Treatment

Although the management of the severe, hemorrhagic ITP patient will be discussed throughout this chapter, it should be emphasized that the majority of patients with acute ITP require only minimal intervention. In the absence of an antiplatelet autoantibody, or exposure to aspirin-containing compounds that induce platelet dysfunction, patients may not demonstrate any bleeding manifestation until the count drops below 20,000 to 30,000/mm^3. When aspirin was more widely used, patients presented with bleeding at platelet counts of 30,000/mm^3 or higher. Indeed, many cases of mild to moderate ITP may go undiagnosed these days in the absence of aspirin, because these patients may never develop petechiae or bruising suggestive of thrombocytopenia unless the count falls below 20,000/mm^3. In a safe home environment acute ITP patients can be observed without any treatment until the count recovers. When the platelet count is less than 20,000 to 30,000/mm^3, therapy is initiated in order to minimize the risk of serious hemorrhage from protracted thrombocytopenia.

In ITP the main goal of therapy is to slow down the clearance of antibody-coated platelets by the reticuloendothelial system and block the production of autoantibody by B lymphocytes. In the absence of severe hemorrhage, therapeutic modalities used in acute ITP include corticosteroids and intravenous immunoglobulin. Patients with chronic ITP may also be treated with anti-Rh immunoglobulin, splenectomy, danazol, or immunosuppression with chemotherapeutic drugs such as vincristine or cyclophosphamide. In the severe, hemorrhagic ITP patient, all these modalities may be used in the first few days to weeks of therapy, along with plasmapheresis just to control massive blood loss.

In general, prophylactic platelet transfusions are contraindicated in patients who are not actively bleeding, because the infused platelets are rapidly destroyed and thus a "safe" platelet count can not be maintained. For this reason, physicians should withhold platelet transfusions except when there is evidence of hemorrhage, regardless of the platelet count, or in preparation for and during surgical procedures.

Central nervous system (CNS) and gastrointestinal bleeding may be the presenting features of autoantibody-mediated thrombocytopenia, and patients are often given transfusions in an effort to minimize blood loss and CNS damage. Even though the autoantibody mediates the rapid clearance of the infused platelets, some of the platelets will provide hemostatic effect at the site of hemorrhage, and active bleeding may stop or decrease significantly. Platelet transfusions should be used judiciously along with therapy aimed at reducing autoantibody production and blocking reticuloendothelial cell clearance of antibody-coated cells.

Corticosteroids

For many years, oral corticosteroids were the mainstay of therapy in patients with ITP even though there has been considerable controversy over their efficacy in acute ITP.[1,26] Retrospective studies of clinical trials from 1975 through 1984 suggests that treatment with prednisone (2 mg/kg/day) will shorten the time needed to achieve a "safe" platelet count (usually 40,000 to 50,000/mm^3) as compared with placebo or with no therapy.[1,2,26–33] In addition, some clinical trials also measured bleeding time or induction time of petechiae following application of a tourniquet in order to evaluate improved platelet-vascular wall interaction with prednisone versus placebo.[32,33] Both studies suggest that steroid therapy decreases the skin manifestations of bleeding seen with thrombocytopenia even though the platelet count itself has not changed significantly.

Because prednisone may mask leukemia, bone marrow aspiration must be performed prior to treatment.

All adults and children who are treated with corticosteroids must undergo bone marrow aspiration before beginning therapy. Prednisone is an active agent in lysing malignant cells and may mask the diagnosis of leukemia or lymphoma. In addition, steroids given to patients with untreated leukemia or lymphoma usually trigger a tumor lysis syndrome with hyperkalemia, hypocalcemia, and hyperuricemia, which can cause cardiac arrhythmias, change in mental status, and renal failure if not properly managed with fluids, alkalization, and electrolyte support. If a pediatric patient is diagnosed with ITP in an area where bone marrow aspiration is not available and therapy is indicated, it is preferable to treat with intravenous immunoglobulin (described below), which does not require examination of a bone marrow aspirate if the physical examination and laboratory work data are otherwise normal. Evaluation of an adult patient should always include a bone marrow aspirate because dysmyelopoeisis or preleukemia is much more common in adults.

Mechanism of Action. Corticosteroids have been demonstrated to have multiple sites of action.[34–42] They decrease autoantibody production and may interfere with autoantibody binding to target antigens.[35,36] They also decrease the effective clearance of antibody-coated platelets by the reticuloendothelial system, resulting in increased platelet survival.[34] There is some evidence to suggest that steroids improve endothelial cell function and capillary integrity, thereby decreasing the vascular "leak" and oozing associated with thrombocytopenia when the platelet-vascular interaction is compromised.[37–43] Approximately one-third of the total platelet mass is stored in the spleen even in normal individuals. Corticosteroids mobilize these platelet stores in the spleen, resulting in an increase in circulating platelets. This effect may not be very notable in the early course of the disease, but it does cause anxiety in physicians and parents as the patient is weaned from steroids because the circulating platelet count will drop proportionately as platelets return to the splenic pool.[44] Therefore, a decrease in platelet count should be anticipated during this phase, but the count should not fall to the extremely low levels seen before treatment. When such a drop occurs during steroid withdrawal, the steroids are increased to a level at which the platelet count was stable, and a slower weaning process is reinstituted. If the patient becomes thrombocytopenic again with weaning, the patient has a steroid-dependent form of ITP and may require additional therapy in order to be weaned off corticosteroids entirely. Finally, a patient who does not respond to corticosteroids within 7 to 10 days is categorized as steroid-resistant, and alternate therapy should be instituted.

The usual dose of steroids in a patient without active bleeding is 2 mg/kg/day of prednisone given in two or three divided doses over a 24-hour period. With bleeding or severe thrombocytopenia, some physicians give 4 mg/kg/day for 3 to 4 days and then lower the dose to 2 mg/kg/day. After 2 weeks the patient is slowly weaned from the corticosteroids. Even if there is an immediate response to prednisone, it is generally recommended to continue at the 2 mg/kg/day dose rate for at least 1 week prior to decreasing the dose. Prednisone, 2 mg/kg/day for 2 weeks is the most commonly recommended regimen, but steroids are used extensively for many diseases by pediatric hematology-oncology specialists, so it is not surprising that a number of regimens have been instituted to treat ITP. High-dose steroid therapy has been shown to be effective in patients with acute ITP and in patients who were thought to be steroid-resistant. In this regimen 15 mg/kg/day of methylprednisolone is given intravenously for three consecutive days; this has increased platelet count within 2 to 3 days in 75 percent of the patients. Hypertension and flushing may be serious side effects of this approach, so it has not been widely used, although the original papers describing this protocol reported no "severe" side effects.[45,46] Low-dose steroids have also been used in both adult (n = 223) and pediatric (n = 160) patients with acute, nonhemorrhagic ITP in a prospective randomized trial.[47] Patients were randomly assigned to receive prednisone in either conventional (1 mg/kg/day) or low (0.25 mg/kg/day) dosage. Among children, 60 percent had a platelet count above 30,000/mm^3 after 7 days of treatment with no significant difference between conventional and low-dose steroids. Adult patients, however, did show a significant difference at day 14 of treatment, almost twice as many patients receiving conventional doses having a platelet count greater than 50,000/mm^3 as did those treated with low-dose prednisone. For adults it would appear that higher doses are required for a rapid response.

ITP patients treated with steroids must be closely monitored for hypertension.

Side Effects. Corticosteroids do have side effects, which must be considered in deciding whether or not to treat. Short-term use of steroids will result in weight gain, early signs of cushingoid facies, and behavior changes, particularly in young children. Some patients may develop hypertension, a particularly *dangerous* complication in the setting of thrombocytopenia, which places those patients at increased risk of intracranial hemorrhage (ICH). All thrombocytopenic patients should be monitored very closely for hypertension while receiving steroids. Long-term use of prednisone will result in growth delay, skin and hair thinning, pancreatitis, cataracts, and hyperglycemia.

Intravenous Immunoglobulin

The first therapeutic trial with intravenous immunoglobulin (IVIG) for a disease other than primary immunodeficiency or AIDS was described in 1981 by Imbach et al.[48] in children with ITP. This study was based on the observation by Imbach and others that patients with primary immunodeficiency or agammaglobulinemia and antiplatelet antibodies had a marked reduction in their thrombocytopenia following routine immunoglobulin infusions.[49,50] Imbach et al.'s landbmark paper[48] suggested that IVIG might alter the process of autoantibody-mediated destruction of tissue, in this case circulating platelets. In the ensuing years IVIG has been used successfully in an ever increasing number of autoimmune diseases.[51–57]

The rapid recovery in platelet count observed following infusion of IVIG in ITP patients is thought to be secondary to an immediate effect on the reticuloendothelial system. Clearance of antibody-coated red blood cells is strikingly decreased following an infusion of IVIG, and this effect may last for 4 to 6 weeks.[57] Since the level of circulating autoantibody is not affected immediately following IVIG administration, the early response to therapy must be due to reticuloendothelial blockade.[58,59] One hypothesis rests on the observation that infused IgG can bind to free Fc receptors, thus blocking sites that could be used to remove antibody-coated cells or particles. Fc blockade might also result from the increased number of antibody-coated red cells in individuals with blood types A or B because anti-A and anti-B are present in the pooled immunoglobulin preparations. This contribution must not be a major factor because there is no difference in response to IVIG between type O and type A or B ITP patients.[60] The concentrations of antibodies to minor red cell antigens or major blood groups is not significant enough to result in a positive Coombs test, and thus the hemolysis must be minor component of the Fc blockade. To test this hypothesis, several groups selected ITP patients who were Rh-positive and intentionally administered anti-D (Rhogam, intravenous preparation).[61,62] Although the hemolysis was limited, there was a rise in the platelet count starting 2 to 4 days after administration. The response time was slightly delayed as compared with the response to IVIG, but the effect persisted, lasting 2 to 6 weeks longer than that of immunoglobulin infusions.

Intravenous infusion of anti-D can also be used to treat refractory ITP in Rh-positive patients.

There is general agreement regarding the induction of reticuloendothelial system dysfunction following IVIG, but certain inconsistencies prevent researchers from agreeing that total occupancy of the receptors or even of a subset of receptors is the sole mechanism.[56–59,63] In the case of anti-D administration, the dose of IVIG was 40,000 times as great as the dose of intravenous anti-D IgG, and yet small amount of intravenous Rhogam was as effective as IVIG. The antibody-coated red cells could be detected in the circulation for weeks following Rhogam administration, so it is difficult to imagine that all the Fc receptors were blocked in those patients receiving Rhogam.[64]

Given the large pool of donors that make up each batch of immunoglobulin, some researchers have proposed that anti-idiotypic antibodies block autoantibody binding to circulating blood cells.[65,66] Indeed, the anti-idiotypic antibodies have been demonstrated to block autoantibody binding in vitro.[65] These anti-idiotypic reagents may also have a direct effect on idiotype-bearing regulatory T cells or B cells.[66] Natural killer cell function is also decreased following infusion of immunoglobulin.[67] In future large-scale studies to evaluate the number and function of these immunoregulatory cells following IVIG administration should help to clarify the relative importance of the current in vitro studies. Finally, immunoglobulin infusions may also play a role in the elimination of chronic viral infections that compromise bone marrow production, especially in HIV-positive patients with ITP. Platelet counts will rise significantly with the elimination of CMV, EBV, and Parvovirus infections in the bone marrow.

In the initial work by Imbach et al., 2 g/kg of immunoglobulin was administered intravenously to ITP patients over 5 days.[48] To minimize the cost of hospitalization, physicians began to give larger doses of IVIG over a shorter period of time.[52] IVIG was given 0.800 to 1.0 g/kg/day until the platelet count reached 40,000/mm^3, a level at which there would be minimal risk of ICH. On the average, both previously untreated patients and patients with recurrent thrombocytopenia required only 1.8 g/kg of IVIG per course. Generally, acute ITP patients are now given 0.500 to 1.0 g/kg/day for 2 days, and the platelet count usually continues to rise well above 40,000/mm^3 over the following week. The dosage may vary with chronic ITP patients, who often require 1.0 to 3.0 g/kg of immunoglobulin per course or who may be given additional drugs such as corticosteroids or vincristine in conjunction with IVIG. Following splenectomy, patients who were previously refractory to therapy may respond to immunoglobulin infusions.

Side Effects. The majority of adults and children experience headache and flushing with IVIG. Recently, a new preparation of immunoglobulin has been made available, which can be administered to the patient as a 12.5 percent rather than a 4 percent solution. This decreases the infusion time and total volume of the immunoglobulin preparation, thereby decreasing the incidence of headaches and hypertension in many patients. Owing to sensitization to immunoglobulin allotypes, patients are at risk of allergic reactions or even anaphylaxis in the rare IgA-deficient individual. For this reason baseline immunoglobulin levels of all patients are documented prior to IVIG, and vital signs are closely monitored throughout the infusion. IVIG must be given very slowly (or not at all) to those patients in whom a large protein load with increase in intravascular volume might result in cardiac failure or critical hypertension. As in the case of corticosteroids, the combination of thrombocytopenia and hypertension may predispose to ICH.

As compared with IVIG, prednisone is much more cost-effective (in the average patient the cost is less than $100 for steroids, compared with more than $2,000 for IVIG). The advantage of IVIG for the general practitioner is that it does not require a bone marrow aspirate in the small child. In addition, it appears that patients, especially children, achieve platelet counts of 30,000/mm^3 or higher in a shorter time following IVIG than following conventional doses of corticosteroid, which shortens their hospital stay.[68]

Danazol

Danazol is an attenuated androgen, which has been used alone or in combination with prednisone to maintain a safe platelet count.[69] Its mechanism of action may be similar to that of the corticosteroids in that the number of Fc receptors on monocytes is decreased in patients receiving danazol. This drug is often used with prednisone in the steroid-dependent patient to facilitate the weaning process and minimize prednisone side effects in chronic cases.

Immunosuppressive Agents

Immunosuppressive agents are reserved for adult patients in whom conventional therapy with IVIG, corticosteroids, and splenectomy has failed.[70] In children vincristine may be used in order to avoid splenectomy, particularly in those less than 5 years of age, who are at increased risk of sepsis from encapsulated bacteria following splenectomy. One should be confident that HIV is not the underlying cause of the thrombocytopenia prior to using these agents, as both pediatric and adult patients have immune systems that are already severely compromised in this setting.

Vincristine is one chemotherapeutic agent used in ITP that will not suppress bone marrow production of platelets.

Vincristine is one of the most commonly used immunosuppressive agents in ITP, because it does not decrease bone marrow production of red blood cells. Its toxicity is primarily neurologic, but it may be given two to three times at weekly intervals with very few side effects (e.g., constipation, loss of deep tendon reflexes). Infusions of vincristine over 4 hours may also be given, but one may see more signs of weakness with this regimen, particularly in the older patient. Vinblastine infusions are also used, but myelosuppression is associated with this agent.

Alkylating agents, particularly cyclophosphamide, and the thiopurines have also been shown to be useful. However, bone marrow suppression and increased risk of malignancy with these drugs make them less attractive for prolonged therapy in either children or adults. While the patient is receiving these drugs, the dosage is adjusted to maintain a leukocyte count above 2,000/mm^3, an absolute neutrophil count above 1,000/mm^3, and a platelet count above 50,000/mm^3. A summary of the agents used in refractory ITP and their side effects in adults can be found in a recent review by Berchtold and McMillan.[70]

Splenectomy

Platelets should be given after the clamping of the splenic pedicle if they must be used during splenectomy.

When medical management fails, splenectomy may be required to decreased platelet destruction and autoantibody production. IVIG prior to surgery may obviate the need for platelet transfusion, but in patients who are profoundly thrombocytopenic, platelets may be given to decrease the risk of major bleeding. If possible, platelets should be given after the clamping of the splenic pedicle, as the survival of the transfused platelets will be markedly improved once the splenic circulation is blocked.

Many chronic ITP patients undergo splenectomy, and normalization of platelet count is achieved in approximately 70 to 80 percent of cases. The spleen plays a major role in the removal of antibody-coated cells and is more efficient than the liver in immune destruction of cells because of the relatively slower rate of splenic blood flow. This difference is accentuated by changes in the splenic microcirculatory pathway associated with lymphoid hyperplasia, a common finding in spleens of patients with chronic ITP.[71] These changes result in longer transit time of antibody-coated platelets in areas rich in macrophages.

Besides eliminating the major site of platelet destruction, splenectomy also removes a significant number of antibody-secreting B lymphocytes normally resident in the spleen. Approximately 40 percent of the nucleated cells in the spleen are B cells, the remainder being composed of T lymphocytes, monocytes, and macrophages. Over a period of 4 to 12 weeks the serum antiplatelet autoantibody decreases markedly, and eventually platelet-associated immunoglobin (PAIG) also decreases to normal or near normal levels. It is unclear how splenectomy results in the resolution of ITP. Clearly, B cells prolifrate and respond appropriately to antigenic challenge in sites other than the spleen, because postsplenectomy patients continue to produce adequate amounts of immunoglobulins of all subclasses. Some patients also continue to produce low levels of autoantibody, but in the absence of splenic destruction the bone marrow is able to compensate for the low-grade consumption that remains in the reticuloendothelial system. In patients in whom splenectomy is successful, removal of the spleen may have eliminated the autoantibody-secreting B cells or more importantly, may have disrupted the T- and B-cell dysregulation responsible for the autoimmune reactivity. In the 15 to 20 percent of cases in which immune thrombocytopenia is not resolved by splenectomy, antibody-coated platelets are removed by the liver or may even be destroyed by macrophages in the bone marrow itself.[72]

Emergency Management of the Hemorrhaging Patient

Extraordinary effort is required to control bleeding in the patient with profound thrombocytopenia and bleeding into the CNS (i.e., intracranial, fundal or spinal hemorrhage). In addition, massive blood loss into the abdomen, gastrointestinal tract, or spleen in the thrombocytopenic patient may result in cardiovascular failure or shock and represents a true hematologic emergency. This is one of the rare situations in which platelet transfusions are given to the patient with antiplatelet autoantibody.

Platelet transfusion is most effective if "megapacks," consisting of 10 to 20 random donor units (4 or 5 single donor units) that have pooled and concentrated, can be given as quickly as possible in the hope that some of the platelets will reach sites of bleeding before they are removed by the spleen. High-dose steroids such as methylprednisolone are given intravenously as soon as the diagnosis has been established on the basis of baseline blood and bone marrow aspirate studies. This is followed by lower, more conventional, doses of predisone until the ITP resolves. In addition, IVIG should also be given as soon as possible, with close monitoring of the blood pressure to prevent fluid overload and hypertension, which should be avoided at all costs in the setting of intracranial hemorrhage. If the patient is big enough for central line placement, plasmapheresis may also be used to decrease the amount of circulating autoantibody, even though the effect may be transient unless immunosuppressive agents are used in conjunction with this procedure. The half-life of IgG autoantibody is approximately 4 to 6 weeks, so one may not see the effect of chemotherapy on decreased antibody production for several weeks. Plasmapheresis may only remove a relatively small amount of the IgG autoantibody because most of it is either attached to the platelets or in the extravascular space. Even so, it may be useful as an emergency procedure in controlling hemorrhage. If both plasmapheresis and IVIG are to be used, it should be remembered to apply plasmapheresis *first*; otherwise the infused IgG will be removed along with the offending autoantibody.[73]

Protein A immunoadsorption columns have been used with pheresis to selectively remove autoantibody and Ig-containing immune complexes.

Emergency surgical procedures (splenectomy or craniotomy) may be necessary in the early hours or days of therapy if bleeding cannot be stopped. In this setting platelet megapacks are given prior to and during the procedure to minimize blood loss. As mentioned above in connection with splenectomy, platelets given after the splenic vessels have been clamped will have a longer survival time in the circulation and be more effective in controlling blood loss. Although CNS bleeding is rare in ITP, the long-term neurologic sequelae and risk of death associated with this event warrant these heroic efforts.

THROMBOCYTOPENIA FROM ALLOANTIBODIES

Immunization against platelet alloantigens may occur during pregnancy or following exposure to blood products. Not all patients produce alloantibodies during pregnancy or following a single exposure to blood, but in those who do, these antibodies can cause significant thrombocytopenia and life-threatening bleeding in the clinical syndromes of neonatal alloimmune thrombocytopenic purpura (NATP) and post-transfusion purpura (PTP).

Even during the first pregnancy, maternal antiplatelet alloantibodies can cross the placenta and cause profound thrombocytopenia in the fetus and newborn. The presentation of thrombocytopenia in a *healthy* infant whose mother has a normal platelet count is most often due to maternal alloantibodies. The diagnosis is confirmed with the demonstration of antiplatelet antibody in maternal plasma, which reacts with paternal platelets in the absence of maternal autoantibody. Over 50 percent of the platelet-specific alloantibodies in NATP are reactive with the PlA1 epitope on glycoprotein IIIa.[74] Given that PlA1 alloantibodies predominate in reported cases of NATP, it would appear to be more immunogenic than other alloantigens. This alloantigen is absent in 2 percent of the population (Table 4-2). On the basis of the high probability that these PlA1-negative women would marry PlA1 positive men, it is surprising that the actual incidence of NATP is so low—1 to 4 per 10,000 live births.[75,76] Perhaps mild cases of NATP are missed because these infants usually do not bleed or develop petechiae until the platelet count drops below 20,000/mm^3.

Prenatal Treatment of NATP

The diagnosis of NATP is usually made following the birth of the first thrombocytopenic infant. Women who are then identified as alloimmunized to platelet-specific antigens should be monitored very closely throughout subsequent pregnancies. Intermittent screening of maternal serum should be performed to detect platelet-specific alloantibodies, which is similar to prenatal Coombs testing in women who are Rh-negative. All women in the mother's family should also be evaluated prior to or during pregnancy to

TABLE 4-2. Alloantigen Phenotype and Frequency in Various Populations

Antigen System	Allele	Glycoprotein Association	Phenotype Percentage		
			N. America	Spain	Japan
P1A (Zw)	1 (a)	IIIa	98.0	97.5	100
	2 (b)		28.0	14.0	0.0
Pen (Yuk)	a (b)	IIIa	99.0	99.9	99.9
	b (a)		1.7	0.0	1.7
Ko (sib)	a		—	20.0	27.1
	b		—	96.6	98.0
Bak (Lek)	a	IIb	91.0	93.6	78.9
	b		n.d.	n.d.	n.d.
Br (Zav, Hc)	a	Ia–IIa	21.0	40.0	99.9
	b		—	90.0	5.8
P1E	1	Ib	>99.0	n.d.	n.d.
	2		4.0	n.d.	n.d.
P1T	?	V	>98.0	n.d.	n.d.

Abbreviations: n.d., no data.

determine whether they might also be at risk of alloimmunization. For PlA1-negative women who are also DR3 (DRw52)-positive, prenatal fetal blood sampling is strongly recommended, as these women are at increased risk of alloimmunization, and maternal screening may not be sensitive enough to detect the alloantibody early in pregnancy.[77–79]

Prenatal ICH may result in significant neurologic damage or in intrauterine demise and miscarriage, particularly in women with anti-PlA1 alloantibody, in whom the incidence of prenatal ICH is 10 to 16 percent.[74] Prenatal ultrasonography can be very useful in detection of fetal ICH in women who are known to be sensitized but have not yet borne a child with prenatal ICH. When ultrasound reveals fetal ICH, administration of IVIG and dexamethasone to the mother should be instituted immediately.[80] In those families in which a previous infant has had intrauterine ICH, more aggressive monitoring of fetal platelet count is recommended.[80,81] To treat fetal thrombocytopenia, mothers are given IVIG (1 g/kg/week) with or without dexamethasone. This regimen has been successful in elevating the fetal platelet count in the majority of cases.

Neonatal Treatment of NATP

Because of the high frequency of these alloantigens, random donor platelets are usually ineffective in treating thrombocytopenia in the neonate. When platelets are given, it is best to use washed maternal apheresis platelets, as they lack the alloantigen. *Washing is required* to remove

Maternal platelets must be washed prior to infusion in an infant with NATP.

maternal plasma containing the offending alloantibody. Often maternal platelets may be harvested prior to elective delivery and made available for transfusion shortly after birth. IVIG has also been used successfully in the neonate and is particularly helpful in areas where plateletpheresis and washing is unavailable.[82,83]

Post-Transfusion Purpura

PTP occurs 7 to 10 days following blood produce infusion in a patient who has previously received a transfusion or been pregnant.[76,84] An alloantibody is produced, which destroys not only any transfused platelets but also the patient's platelets, even though they do not express this phenotype. Although extremely rare, PTP occurs most commonly in the fewer than 2 percent of the population who are PlA1-negative.[74] The post-transfusion plasma usually has high-titer anti-PlA1 activity, but the mechanism of autologous platelet destruction is unclear. Hypotheses suggesting a cross-reactive alloantibody that recognizes autoepitopes in close proximity to the PlA1 site have yet to be proven. Reported cases include one with PTP secondary to alloantibody to Bak a, Pen a and two with anti-PlA2 antibodies.[85–87] Among the approximately 100 cases reported since its description in 1959, only four have described men as having PTP.[74] When a series of PTP patients with anti-PlA1 alloantibodies were HLA-typed, over 90 percent were DR3-positive, with the supertype DRw52 predominating in these individuals.[77,78] Patients are usually in their late forties or older, but PTP has been reported in a 16-year-old girl not previously pregnant.[87]

Transfusions should be avoided in PTP; if red cells or platelets are necessary, leukocyte-depleted blood product will minimize chills and febrile reactions.

Platelet transfusions are contraindicated in PTP patients, in whom the treatment of choice is IVIG or plasmapheresis.[84] The frequency of transfusion reaction in these patients is quite high, with 46 percent experiencing chills and fever during blood product infusion. Therefore, red cells should be washed and filtered whenever possible. If platelets must be given for life-threatening hemorrhage, they should be PlA1-negative, washed, and filtered as well. The therapy and possible mechanisms of autologous platelet destruction in PTP have been more thoroughly addressed in a 1989 review of this disorder.[74]

References

1. Lusher JM, Enami A, Ravindranath Y, Warrier AI: Idiopathic thrombocytopenic purpura in children. Am J Pediatr Hematol Oncol 6:149, 1984
2. Walker RW, Walker W: Idiopathic thrombocytopenic purpura, initial illness and long-term follow-up. Arch Dis Child 59:316, 1984

3. Lusher JM, Iyer R: Idiopathic thrombocytopenic purpura in children. Semin Thromb Hemost 3:175, 1977
4. Lippman SM, Arnett FC, Conley CL: Genetic factors predisposing to autoimmune diseases. Am J Med 73:827, 1982
5. Panzer S, Penner E, Graninger W et al: Antinuclear antibodies in patients with chronic idiopathic autoimmune thrombocytopenia followed 2–30 years. Am J Hematol 32:100, 1990
6. Gratama JW, D'Amaro J, deKoning J: The HLA system in immune thrombocytopenic purpura: its relation to the outcome of therapy. Br J Haematol 56:287, 1984
7. Mueller-Eckhardt G, Pawelec G, Haas R: HLA-DP antigens in patients with chronic autoimmune thrombocytopenia (AITP). Tissue Antigens 34:121, 1989
8. Mayr WR, Mueller-Eckhardt G, Krüger M: HLA-DR in chronic ITP. Tissue Antigens 18:56, 1981
9. Cornelius AS, Campbell D, Schwartz E: Elevated common acute lymphoblastic leukemia antigen expression in pediatric immune thrombocytopenic purpura. Am J Pediatr Hematol Oncol 13:57, 1991
10. McClure PD: Idiopathic thrombocytopenic purpura in children: diagnosis and management. Pediatrics 55:68, 1975
11. Lusher JM, Khalifa AS et al: Idiopathic thrombocytopenic purpura in children. Semin Thromb Hemost 3:175, 1977
12. Harrington WJ, Minnich V, Hollingsworth JW et al: Demonstration of a circulating factor in the blood of patients with thrombocytopenic purpura. J Lab Clin Med 38:1, 1951
13. Harrington WJ, Sprague CC, Minnich V et al: Immunologic mechanisms in neonatal and thrombocytopenic purpura. Ann Intern Med 38:433, 1953
14. Altman L: Who Goes First? The Story of Self-Experimentation in Medicine. Random House, New York, 1987
15. Shulman NR, Marder VJK, Weinrach RS: Similarities between known antiplatelet antibodies and the factor responsible for thrombocytopenia in idiopathic purpura. Ann N Y Acad Sci 124: 499, 1965
16. Slicter S: Controversies in platelet-transfusion. Annu Rev Med 31:509, 1980
17. George JN, Saucerman S, Handagama PJ: Immunoglobulin is a platelet alpha granule-secreted protein. J Clin Invest 76:2020, 1985
18. Handagama PJ, George JN, Saucerman S: Incorporation of a circulating protein into megakaryocyte and platelet granules. Proc Natl Acad Sci USA 84:861, 1987
19. McMillan R, Aaui P, Millard F et al: Platelet-associated and plasma antiglycoprotein autoantibodies in chronic ITP. Blood 70:1040, 1987
20. Kiefel V, Santoso S, Weisheit M et al: Monoclonal antibody-specific immobilization of platelet antigens. Blood 70:1722, 1987
21. Kayser W, Mueller-Eckhardt C, Mueller-Eckhardt, G: Complement-fixing platelet autoantibodies in autoimmune thrombocytopenia. Am J Hematol 11:213, 1981
22. Pawha J, Giuliani D, Pocceco M: Platelet-associated IgM levels in thrombocytopenia. Vox Sang 45:97, 1983
23. Cines DB, Wilson SB, Schreiber AD: Platelet antibodies of the IgM class in immune thrombocytopenic purpura. J Clin Invest 75:1183, 1985
24. Hauch TW, Rosse WF: Platelet-bound complement (C3) in immune thrombocytopenia. Blood 50:1129, 1977
25. Cines DB, Schreiber AD, Wilson SB: Immune thrombocytopenia: use of a Coombs' antiglobulin test to detect IgG and C3 on platelets. N Engl J Med 300:106, 1979
26. Dunn NL, Maurer HM: Prednisone treatment of acute ITP of childhood. Am J Pediatr Hematol Oncol 6:159, 1984
27. Lusher JM, Zuelzer WW: Idiopathic thrombocytopenic purpura in childhood. J Pediatr 68:971, 1966
28. Lammi AT, Lovric VA: Idiopathic thrombocytopenic purpura: an epidemiologic study. J Pediatr 83:31, 1973
29. Simons SM, Main CA, Yaish HM et al: Idiopathic thrombocytopenic purpura in children. J Pediatr 87:16, 1975
30. McWilliams NB, Maurer HM: Acute idiopathic thrombocytopenic purpura in children. Am J Hematol 7:87, 1979
31. Benham ES, Taft LI: Idiopathic thrombocytopenic purpura in children: results of steroid therapy and splenectomy. Aust Pediatr J 8:311, 1972
32. Sartorius JA: Steroid treatment of idiopathic thrombocytopenic purpura in children. Preliminary results of a randomized cooperative study. Am J Pediatr Hematol Oncol 6:165, 1984

33. Buchanan GR, Holtkamp CA: Prednisone therapy for children with newly diagnosed idiopathic thrombocytopenic purpura. A randomized clinical trail. Am J Pediatr Hematol Oncol 6: 355, 1984
34. McMillan R, Longmire RL, Yelenosky R et al: In vitro platelet phagocytosis by splenic leukocytes in idiopathic thrombocytopenic purpura. N Engl J Med 290:249, 1974
35. Dixon R, Rosse W: Platelet antibody in autoimmune thrombocytopenia. Br J Haematol 31:129, 1975
36. McMillan R, Longmire RL et al: The effect of corticosteroids on human IgG synthesis. J Immunol 116:1592, 1976
37. Robson HN, Duthie JJR: Capillary resistance and adrenocortical activity. Br Med J 2:971, 1950
38. Labran C: Etude de l'action vaso-constrictrice de la prednisone. Rev Fr Etudes Clin Biol 8:765, 1963
39. Hutter JJ, Hathaway WE: Prednisone-induced hemostasis in a platelet function abnormality. Am J Dis Child 129:641, 1975
40. Alexander M, van den Bogart N, Fondu P: Le pronostic et le traitement du purpura thrombopénique idiopathique de l'enfant. Arch Fr Pediatr 33:329, 1976
41. Johnson SA: Endothelial supporting function of platelets. p. 283. In Johnson SA (ed): The Circulating Platelet. Academic Press, Orlando, FL, 1971
42. Kitchens CS, Weiss L: Ultrastructural changes of endothelium associated with thrombocytopenia. Blood 46:567, 1975
43. Kitchens CS, Weiss L: Amelioration of endothelial abnormalities by prednisone in experimental thrombocytopenia in the rabbit. J Clin Invest 60:1129, 1977
44. Hill-Zobel RL, McCandless B, Kang SA et al: Organ distribution and fate of human platelets: studies of asplenic and splenomegalic patients. Am J Hematol 23:231, 1986
45. Von dem Borne AE, Vos JJ, Pegels JG et al: High dose intravenous methylprednisolone or high dose intravenous gammaglobulin for autoimmune thrombocytopenia. Br Med J 296:249, 1988
46. Del Principe D, Menichelli A, Mori PG et al: Phase II trial of methylprednisolone pulse therapy in childhood chronic thrombocytopenia. Acta Haematol (Basel) 77:226, 1987
47. Bellucci S, Charpak Y, Chastang C et al: Low doses vs conventional doses of corticoids in immune thrombocytopenic purpura (ITP): results of a randomized clinical trial in 160 children, 223 adults. Blood 71:1165, 1988
48. Imbach P, Barandun S, d'Apuzzo V: High dose intravenous gammaglobulin for idiopathic thrombocytopenic purpura in childhood. Lancet 1:1228, 1981
49. Bondolfi R, Hirt A, Barandum S: Autoimmunhaemolytische Anaemie bei congenitaler Agammaglobulinaemie. Behandlungserfolg durch Immunoglobulin-Substitution. Schweiz Med Wochenschr 110:1950, 1980
50. Barandun S, Imbach P, Morell A, Wagner HP: Clinical indications for immunoglobulins. p. 275. In Nydegger UR (ed): Immunotherapy. A guide to Immunoglobulin Prophylaxis and Therapy. Academic Press, Orlando, FL, 1981
51. Arsura E, Bick A, Brunner NG et al: Effects of repeated doses of intravenous immunoglobulin in myasthenis gravis. Am J Med Sci 295:438, 1988
52. Ballow M, Parke A: The uses of intravenous immune globulin in collagen vascular disorders. J Allergy Clin Immunol 84:608, 1989
53. Gelfand EW: The uses of intravenous immune globulin in collagen vascular disorders. J Allergy Clin Immunol 84:613, 1989
54. Rowley AH, Shulman ST: What is the status of intravenous gamma globulin for Kawasaki syndrome? Pediatr Infect Dis J 7:463, 1988
55. Pocecco M, DeCampo C, Cantoni L et al: Effect of high dose intravenous IgG in newly diagnosed diabetic children. Helv Paediatr Acta 42:289, 1987
56. Bussel JB, Goldman A, Imbach P: Treatment of acute idiopathic thrombocytopenia of childhood with intravenous infusions of gammaglobulin. J Pediatr 106:886, 1985
57. Bussel JB: Intravenous immunoglobulin therapy for the treatment of idiopathic thrombocytopenic purpura. Prog Hemost Thromb 8:103, 1986
58. Fehr J, Hofmann V, Kappeler U: Transient reversal of thrombocytopenia in idiopathic thrombocytopenic purpura by high-dose intravenous gammaglobulin. N Engl J Med 306:1254, 1982
59. Barbano G, Saleh MN, Mori PG et al: Effect of intravenous gammaglobulin on circulating and platelet-bound antibody in immune thrombocytopenia. Blood 73:662, 1989
60. Mueller-Eckhardt C, Salama A, Kiefel V: A new concept for the effector mechanism of intravenous immunoglobulin in hemocytopenias. Blut 48:353, 1984

61. Salama A, Kiefel V, Amberg R: Treatment of autoimmune thrombocytopenic purpura with rhesus antibodies (anti-Rho (D)). Blut 49:29, 1984
62. Boughton BJ, Chakraverty T, Baglin TP et al: The treatment of chronic idiopathic thrombocytopenia with anti-D (Rho) immunoglobulin: its effectiveness, safety and mechanism of action. Clin Lab Haematol 10:275, 1988
63. Segal DM, Dower SK, Titus JA: The role of non-immune IgG in controlling IgG-mediated effector function. Mol Immunol 20:1177, 1983
64. Salama A, Mueller-Eckhardt C: Use of Rh antibodies in the treatment of autoimmune thrombocytopenia. Transfus Med Rev 6:17, 1992
65. Berchtold P, Dale GL, Tani P et al: Inhibition of autoantibody binding to platelet glycoprotein gammaglobulin. Blood 74:2414, 1989
66. Newland AC, Macey MG, Veys PA: Cellular changes during the infusion of high dose intravenous immunoglobulin. Blut 59:82, 1989
67. Engelhard D, Waner JL, Kapoor N et al: Effect of intravenous immune globulin on natural killer cell activity: possible association with autoimmune neutropenia and idiopathic thrombocytopenia. J Pediatr 108:77, 1986
68. Imbach P, Wagner HP, Berchtold P: IVIG versus oral corticosteroids in acute immune thrombocytopenic purpura in childhood. Lancet 2:464, 1985
69. Ahn YS, Harrington WJ, Mylvagvnam R et al: Danazol for the treatment of idiopathic thrombocytopenic purpura. N Eng J Med 309:1396, 1983
70. Berchtold P, McMillan R: Therapy of chronic idiopathic thrombocytopenic purpura in adults. Blood 74:2309, 1989
71. Schmidt EE, MacDonald IC, Groom AC: Changes in splenic microcirculatory pathways in chronic idiopathic thrombocytopenic purpura. Blood 78:1485, 1991
72. Ballem PJ, Segal GM, Stratton JR et al: Mechanisms of thrombocytopenia in chronic autoimmune thrombocytopenic purpura. J Clin Invest 80:33, 1987
73. Snyder HW, Cochran SK, Balint JP et al: Experience with protein A-immunoadsorption and treatment-resistance adult immune thrombocytopenic. Blood 79:2237, 1992
74. Kunicki TJ, Beardsley DS: The alloimmune thrombocytopenias: neonatal alloimmune thrombocytopenic purpura and post-transfusion purpura. Prog Hemost Thromb 9:203,1989
75. Blanchette VS, Peters MA, Pegg-Feige K: Alloimmune thrombocytopenia. Review from a neonatal intensive care unit. Curr Stud Hematol Blood Transfus 52:87, 1986
76. Shulman NR, Marder V, Hiller M et al: Platelet and leukocyte isoantigens and their antibodies: serologic, physiologic and clinical. Prog Hematol 4:222, 1964
77. Mueller-Eckhardt C, Mueller-Eckhardt G, Willen-Ohff H et al: Immunogenicity of and immune response to the human platelet antigen Zwa is strongly associated with HLA-B8 and DR3. Tissue Antigens 26:71, 1985
78. DeWall LP, van Dalen CM, Engelfriet CP et al: Alloimmunization against the platelet-specific Zwa antigen, resulting in neonatal alloimmune thrombocytopenia or post-transfusion purpura, is associated with the supertypic DRw52 antigen including DR3. Hum Immunol 17:45, 1986
79. Daffos F, Forestier F, Kaplan C et al: Prenatal diagnosis and management of bleeding disorders with fetal blood sampling. Am J Obstet Gynecol 158:939, 1988
80. Bussel JB, Berkowitz T, McFarland JG et al: Antenatal treatment of neonatal alloimmune thrombocytopenia. N Eng J Med 319:1374, 1988
81. Kaplan C, Daffos F, Forestier F et al: Management of alloimmune thrombocytopenia: antenatal diagnosis and in utero transfusion of maternal platelets. Blood 72:340, 1988
82. Massey GV, McWilliams NB, Mueller DG et al: Intravenous immunoglobulin in treatment of neonatal isoimmune thrombocytopenia. J Pediatr 111:133, 1987
83. Bizzaro N, Dianses G: Neonatal alloimmune amegakaryocytosis. Case report. Vox Sang 54: 112, 1988
84. Mueller-Eckhardt C: Post-transfusion purpura. Br J Haematol 64:419, 1986
85. Taaning E, Morling N, Ovesen H et al: Posttransfusion purpura and anti-Zwb. Tissue Antigens 26:143, 1985
86. Furihata K, Nugent DJ, Aster RH, Kunicki TJ: On the association of the platelet-specific alloantigen, Pen, with glycoprotein IIIa. Evidence for heterogeneity of glycoprotein IIIa. J Clin I 80: 1624, 1987
87. Chapman JF, Murphy MF, Berney SI et al: Post-transfusion purpura associated with anti-Bak a and anti-P1A2 platelet antibodies and delayed haemolytic transfusion reaction. Vox Sang 52:313, 1987

5

DISSEMINATED INTRAVASCULAR COAGULATION

MICHAEL W. LANKIEWICZ
WILLIAM R. BELL

Disseminated intravascular coagulation (DIC) is a clinical and pathologic entity resulting in simultaneous unregulated activation of the coagulation and fibrinolytic pathways. It is a syndrome with serious clinical consequences, which is encountered in all areas of medicine but particularly in the critical care setting.

DIC is the subject of an extensive literature and ongoing investigations. Although the pathophysiology has been understood in general terms for some time, new details have recently been recognized. Despite current understanding, treatment of this process remains difficult and controversial. Historically, the diagnosis and treatment of DIC have been topical for several decades; however, experimental models have existed for perhaps several hundred years. In the experimental laboratory over 150 years ago, intravenous injection of brain tissue was shown to induce lethal diffuse intravascular clotting[1] and over a century ago it was discovered that controlling the rate of such an infusion could prevent thrombus formation and in fact cause the blood to be incoagulable, with subsequent widespread bleeding.[2] Today excellent experimental models such as the generalized Schwartzman reaction and other models facilitate the study of this process.[3–8]

DIC is not a primary disease entity but rather a pathologic process secondary to an underlying illness.

DIC is not a primary disease entity; it is secondary to an underlying, usually severe, and most often systemic illness. DIC is a progressive pathologic process, resulting in diffuse thrombus formation and excessive activity of the fibrinolytic system, and its most prominent clinical feature frequently is bleeding or a bleeding tendency. The process involves many biologic substances, coagulation glycoproteins, mediators/regulators of coagulation and fibrinolysis, and physiologic responses, which activate coagulation, platelet aggregation, and thrombus formation, with subsequent activation of the fibrinolytic system.

PATHOGENESIS

Past and ongoing investigations into the pathogenesis of DIC have resulted in an increased understanding of the complex mechanisms resulting in the clinical and laboratory features of DIC. The hemostatic system is a multifaceted meshwork of biochemical pathways, precisely balanced and regulated by endogenous activators and inhibitors of coagulation, coagulation factor production, clearance of activated factors, and the fibrinolytic pathway. In DIC this balance is severely disrupted; this can occur in a number of ways. A procoagulant substance such as tissue factor may enter the circulation from injured, damaged, or abnormal tissue.[9,10] Tissue factor is a plasma membrane glycoprotein, which functions as a cofactor for factor VII or VIIa, with subsequent activation of the extrinsic pathway of coagulation. Exposure of subendothelial tissues may stimulate platelet aggregation as well as activate the intrinsic pathway of coagulation. Plasmin generation is stimulated via factor XII and the intrinsic pathway, as well as by increased release of endogenous activating substances. Malignant cells of various types may release proteases that act directly on coagulation factors and plasminogen, further activating these systems.

Most features of DIC are attributable to the generation of thrombin or a thromboplastic substance and plasmin from a variety of inciting events.

Although the underlying inciting events vary in different clinical settings, the common result is generation of thrombin and plasmin in an unregulated or abnormally regulated fashion. Most of the clinical features of DIC are attributable to the actions of thrombin or plasmin.

Action of Thrombin

Thrombin's primary function in normal hemostasis is cleavage of fibrinogen to form fibrin,[11] the molecules of which may complex with fibrinogen or polymerize to form fibrin thrombi. Other actions of thrombin include activation of factor XIII, resulting in cross-linking of fibrin polymers; activation of factors VIII and V, resulting in positive feedback for thrombin generation; and activation of platelets, resulting in aggregation, shape changes, and loss of normal function.[12,13] In addition, thrombin participates in activation of protein C, which is often present in decreased amounts in DIC and has direct effects on endothelial cells, inducing production of a variety of mediators such as platelet-activating factor (PAF), prostacyclin, and von Willebrand factor.[14–16] Thrombin may also influence the fibrinolytic pathway by inducing release of both tissue plasminogen activator and plasminogen activator inhibitor from endothelial cells.[17,18] Thus, the actions of thrombin can result in decreased levels of fibrinogen, factors II, V, VIII, and XIII, and protein C, as well as in thrombocytopenia and/or platelet dysfunction.

Action of Plasmin

Plasmin is a nonspecific proteolytic enzyme capable of digesting fibrin and fibrinogen as well as other coagulation proteins. The relative activities of thrombin and plasmin account for the spectrum of presentations in DIC, ranging from thrombus formation without bleeding to excessive fibrinolysis and hemorrhage. Plasmin is formed from plasminogen, its zymogen by the action of endogenous activators such as tissue plasminogen activator, which are released from damaged endothelial cells, or by factor XII and the intrinsic pathway. Neutrophil proteases may also be important in plasminogen activation in some cases.[19,20] When plasmin is generated in adequate amounts, degradative fragments of fibrinogen and fibrin (FDP-fdp) are detectable in the plasma. These fragments have physiologic significance as well as constituting the best laboratory marker for DIC. These degradation products are nonclottable by thrombin and inhibit fibrin formation, fibrin polymerization, and platelet activation, further contributing to the process of DIC. Thus features of DIC attributable to plasmin formation include excess fibrinolysis and hemorrhage; production of degradation products; decreased levels of fibrinogen and factors V, VIII, and IX; and platelet dysfunction.

The spectrum of presentations of DIC is in part related to the relative amounts of thrombin-like substances and plasmin that are generated.

Role of Coagulation Inhibitors

Recently considerable interest has been focused on the role of coagulation inhibitors in the process of DIC. Anti-thrombin III complexes with thrombin, resulting in its neutralization. The activity of antithrombin III is enhanced by the presence of heparin, which accounts for heparin's therapeutic usefulness. Protein C is activated by thrombin and facilitates inactivation of factors Va and VIIIa, resulting in negative feedback on thrombin generation. The levels of these inhibitors are frequently reported as low in the setting of DIC.[21,22] Preparations of both protein C and antithrombin III have been demonstrated to be protective against DIC induced by *Escherichia coli* in animal models.[23,24] These observations have raised questions about the importance of these inhibitors in the pathogenesis of DIC and the possible therapeutic applications of purified preparations.

The levels of protein C and antithrombin III are frequently low in DIC. The significance of these levels in the pathogenesis of DIC is unclear.

Tissue factor pathway inhibitor (TFPI), previously known as extrinsic pathway inhibitor or lipoprotein-associated coagulation inhibitor, inhibits tissue factor/factor VIIa complexes and the extrinsic pathway of coagulation.[25] Immunodepletion of TFPI results in increased sensitivity to

DIC induced by tissue factor in animal models.[26] TFPI probably protects against DIC in the setting of minor illnesses and injuries; however, normal levels have been observed in the setting of DIC, which suggests that depletion or deficiency of TFPI is not important in the pathogenesis of DIC.

Mechanism of Plasmin and Thrombin Generation

Leukocyte proteases are the primary cause of DIC in the setting of promyelocytic leukemia; however, other mechanisms may also be operational.

Generation of plasmin and thrombin is caused by a variety of inciting events, depending on the underlying illness. The direct activity of proteases released from leukemic cells is thought to be the primary mechanism of coagulation activation in DIC associated with acute promyelocytic leukemia (APL).[19,20] However, a 1988 report by Cozzolino et al. suggests that the mechanism may be more complex.[27] They determined that APL cells that were associated with a coagulopathy elaborated interleukin 1, while those not associated with a coagulopathy did not. Furthermore, increased endothelial cell production of tissue factor and decreased expression of thrombomodulin were induced by interleukin 1. These changes were blocked by the addition of anti-interleukin 1 antibodies. Since tissue factor complexes with factor VII to initiate the extrinsic pathway of coagulation and thrombomodulin is an important cofactor in the activation of the coagulation inhibitor protein C, these changes were believed to alter the endothelial properties in favor of thrombosis and contribute to DIC.

Role of Bacterial Endotoxin

In the setting of gram-negative sepsis, endotoxin has long been implicated in the activation of coagulation. Recent studies by Warr and associates suggest that tissue factor may be the primary mediator of DIC in this setting.[28] In a rabbit model of DIC induced by endotoxin, these investigators were able to block or attenuate DIC by administering anti-tissue factor antibodies. Interestingly, endotoxin-induced shock was not affected, which suggests that tissue factor is not important in other aspects of sepsis. Gram-positive organisms cause DIC, albeit less frequently than gram-negative bacteria. Kessler et al. demonstrated that *Staphyloccus aureus* can induce platelet aggregation in vitro, and the degree and rapidity of this response correlated with the severity of DIC in the patients from whom the strains were isolated.[29] Subsequently this group examined the role of various cell wall components in this phenomenon. Peptidoglycan from isolates associated with DIC aggregated platelets more potently than did peptidoglycan from isolated not associated with DIC.[30] A second component of the bacterial cell wall, teichoic acid, blunted this effect and may be a modulator of the ability of peptidoglycan to incite DIC. Peptidoglycan is known to produce localized Schwartzman reactions in rabbits and activate complement in vitro.[31,32] This group postulated that the relative amounts of these components present in the bacterial cell wall may be an important factor in determining the ability of some strains of organisms to produce DIC.

Additional Effects

One study suggests a possible role for PAF in DIC.[33] A specific PAF antagonist attenuated DIC-like changes induced both by endotoxin and by infusion of PAF in a rat model. The relative clinical importance of these mechanisms remains unclear.

Whatever the inciting event, these processes result in severe disruption of the balance and regulation of coagulation and fibrinolysis and consequent reduction in the levels of many coagulation factors. The decreased levels are predominantly due to premature destruction of coagulation proteins by plasmin, the action of which is not specific for fibrin. Consumption of coagulation proteins also plays a minimal role. Since this process is often present in very ill patients with multisystem dysfunction, the process may be further exacerbated by impaired reticuloendothelial function, hepatic function, and renal failure.

CAUSES

DIC is not a disease but rather a pathologic process seen in the setting of one or more primary disease entities. There are many known causes of DIC, and it may be safe to say that any illness could cause this process. Disorders commonly associated with DIC are sepsis, malignancy, obstetric complications, liver disease, and trauma. DIC may be seen in any condition associated with serious metabolic disturbances, acidosis, hypotension, shock, or hypoxemia. These illness and conditions could each potentially promote entrance of a procoagulant substance or a mediator of coagulation into the circulation and subsequent activation of the coagulation and fibrinolytic systems.

DIC is most commonly seen in the setting of sepsis, malignancy, obstetric complications, liver disease, and trauma.

Sepsis

Sepsis is perhaps the most widely recognized cause of DIC. DIC is observed most frequently in the setting of gram-negative sepsis, but it has been described in association with infections of all types, including those due to viruses, fungi, rickettsia, and protozoa. Although initiation of DIC in infection probably has multiple mechanisms, endotoxin is a primary mediator in gram-negative sepsis. As noted earlier, there is evidence that tissue factor is involved and may be the final messenger in this activation process.[28] Bacterial cell wall components are being examined as possible inciting agents in gram-positive infections.[29,30] Factors that may be important regardless of the nature of the infecting organism include initiation or at least modulation of DIC by substances released in the inflammatory reaction, such as proteases from white blood cells, as well as by endogenous mediators of coagulation inappropriately released by damaged endothelial cells and tissue factor from injured tissue.

Malignancy

DIC is often seen in the setting of malignancy. Tumor cells may produce and release tissue factor or other procoagulant substances. In addition, proteolytic enzymes may be produced that act directly on coagulation proteins or plasminogen, resulting in zymogen activation. The classic example of this mechanism is promyelocytic leukemia, which is often associated with DIC. The initiation of DIC has been attributed to release of proteases from the large granules of the leukemic cells. There is some evidence that other mediators such as interleukin 1 may be involved. DIC may appear only after treatment with chemotherapeutic agents; this involves release of procoagulants from damaged tumor (and other) cells, as well as endothelium damage. Attribution of DIC to malignancy requires caution. Such patients are frequently compromised by their disease and/or chemotherapy, and fulminant or occult infection may be present, accounting for the DIC. Any malignancy can cause DIC, but it is seen most frequently with carcinomas of the lung, pancreas, stomach, and prostate.

Attribution of DIC to malignancy requires caution, and concomitant infection should also be considered.

Trousseau Syndrome

Of particular note is the DIC associated with Trousseau syndrome. This subset of DIC is characterized by recurrent venous or arterial thrombosis in the setting of underlying malignancy. When Trousseau syndrome is present, thrombosis is often the presenting problem, with concomitant or subsequent hemorrhage alerting the physician to the occult malignancy.

Trousseau syndrome is characterized by migratory recurrent venous or arterial thrombosis in the setting of malignancy.

Obstetric Complications

DIC has long been known to be associated with obstetric complications including retained placenta, placenta previa, abruptio placentae, dead fetus syndrome, amniotic fluid embolism, and septic and induced abortions. The common thread in this list of obstetric causes of DIC is once again entrance of procoagulant substances into the maternal circulation, usually from the uterus. In the setting of preeclampsia, eclampsia, or so-called HELLP syndrome (hemolysis, elevated liver enzymes, low platelet count), coagulopathy is often present.[34,35] DIC may underlie the coagulation problems, but hepatic synthetic failure must also be considered. One must be cautious not to miss the diagnosis of thrombotic thrombocytopenic purpura-hemolytic uremic syndrome (TTP-HUS), which is also a complication of pregnancy and the postpartum state and shares some features with DIC. Recently a case of DIC has been reported as a complication of hysteroscopy.[36]

When evaluating obstetric patients for DIC, the diagnosis of TTP-HUS should also be considered.

Liver Disease

The presence of liver disease further complicates evaluation of patients for the presence of DIC.

The diagnosis of DIC in the setting of liver disease presents special problems. Since the liver is the site of synthesis of most of the known coagulation factors and many mediators and inhibitors of coagulation, as well as the route of clearance of activated coagulation factors and fibrinolytic degradation products, severe liver dysfunction can significantly alter the normal balance of the coagulation system, even in the absence of true DIC. This difficulty was highlighted by VanDeWater et al., who studied patients with liver disease and elevated FDP-fdp levels by routine assays.[37] Their technique used more specific antibody assays and attempted to identify patients whose elevated FDP-fdp levels were in fact due to the activity of plasmin on fibrin or fibrinogen. A small fraction of these patients were found to have plasmin degradation fragments, and in each of these cases another illness was present that could account for the presence of DIC. This suggests that routine studies for FDP-fdp levels may not be useful in the setting of liver disease. It may also be true that FDP levels are further elevated because of impaired clearance by the liver. Other laboratory features of DIC are affected by the presence of liver dysfunction. Thrombocytopenia, considered a cardinal feature of DIC, may be present in patients with liver disease as a consequence of alcoholism or hypersplenism due to congestive splenomegaly. Hypofibrinogenemia, as well as decreased levels of other coagulation factors, may be present because of synthetic impairment.

Vitamin K deficiency can also cloud the diagnosis of DIC in liver disease. These patients are frequently debilitated, may suffer from nutritional deficiencies, and are often treated with broad-spectrum antibiotics. Antibiotic therapy can affect coagulation by eliminating intestinal flora as a source of vitamin K. Several antibiotics in the cephalosporin family are also significant antagonists of the vitamin K-dependent γ-carboxylation process and can contribute to coagulopathy in compromised patients. In the setting of liver disease routine studies suggestive of DIC may improve with vitamin K administration.[38]

More specific assays for DIC in the setting of liver disease are clearly needed. Decreased levels of TFPI have been suggested by some authors to be a marker for DIC in patients with liver disease, but recent data have not borne this out.[39] To date we are left with routinely available laboratory studies, which must be interpreted with a thorough understanding of the nature of DIC and the pitfalls of these tests. In addition, it is extremely likely that liver disease lowers the threshold for inciting DIC from other causes for all the reasons outlined above.

Trauma

DIC has been recognized as a consequence of trauma. The likely mechanism is entrance of tissue factor and other thromboplastic materials into the circulation from damaged tissues. This process may be further fueled by associated hypoxia and metabolic disturbances. Multitrauma patients may also be susceptible to infection, which adds another means of developing DIC.

Peritoneovenous Shunts

Peritoneovenous shunts of various types are often associated with DIC. In this setting DIC may be initiated by the presence of the foreign body to some extent, but the likely primary mechanism is entrance of collagen and other procoagulants into the circulation from the peritoneal fluid via the shunt. Edney et al. suggest that the absence or disappearance of DIC in patients with peritoneovenous shunts is a marker for shunt failure.[40] This is one situation in which DIC may be chronic and require no intervention.

DIC is frequently identified in the setting of hemangiomas; this association is termed the *Kasabach-Merritt syndrome*. The mechanism of initiation of DIC in this setting is not well understood, but it is thought to be related to damaged or abnormal endothelial cells within the tumor. When the lesion is removed, either by spontaneous involution or by medical or surgical intervention, the DIC resolves.

Additional Causes

A complete list of causes of DIC is not possible; however other less common causes of DIC include heat stroke, ulcerative colitis, collagen vascular diseases, pancreatitis, aortic aneurysms, envenomation by snake or other animal bites, and TTP. DIC has been reported to be caused by administration of therapeutic agents such as hetastarch and quinine[41,42] and has also been reported as a complication of blood product transfusion reactions and administration of activated prothrombin complex preparations.[43] Reports intermittently appear implicating pulmonary embolus as a cause of DIC; however in a large series of patients with angiogram-proven pulmonary emboli, DIC was extremely rare.[44] A thorough search for other causes of DIC is indicated when DIC is detected in the setting of pulmonary embolus.

CLINICAL FEATURES

In general terms the diagnosis of DIC should be entertained in the appropriate clinical setting when there is unexplained bleeding or a tendency to bleed. Since DIC is a systemic process, the bleeding is usually widespread and typically involves multiple organ systems and anatomic sites, including the gastrointestinal, respiratory, and urinary tracts, the skin, the mucous membranes, and often the central nervous system. The extent of bleeding does not necessarily correlate with the level of DIC activity, and thus fulminant DIC may present only as an increased bleeding tendency with minor trauma, venipuncture, or attempted invasive procedures. Additional findings seen with DIC as a result of microthrombosis and end-organ damage are oliguria, renal failure, and hypoxemia. Neurologic manifestations of DIC may be global or focal and can be related to large vessel thrombosis, subarachnoid hemorrhage, or intracerebral hemorrhage, as well as microvasular thrombosis.[45] Several clinical subsets of DIC should be noted.

In DIC with hemorrhage, bleeding is typically from multiple sites, reflecting the systemic nature of the process.

Trousseau Syndrome

Trousseau syndrome, as noted earlier, is a syndrome of clinically apparent arterial or venous recurrent thrombosis, seen in the setting of underlying malignancy.[56] The malignant process is often occult at the time of presentation, and one's suspicion should be raised by thrombosis that is unexplained, located in unusual anatomic sites, or recurrent. The diagnosis should be entertained when patients with thrombosis respond adequately to heparin anticoagulation but relapse or deteriorate in the face of "therapeutic" warfarin anticoagulation when the heparin is discontinued. Intense investigations often fail to identify the underlying process, and in these cases patients must be treated continuously with heparin and periodically reevaluated. It is noteworthy that a significant number of Trousseau patients fail to demonstrate typical laboratory evidence of DIC, and the diagnosis is made on clinical grounds.

Purpura Fulminans

In purpura fulminans the skin lesions appear hemorrhagic; however, microthrombosis is the underlying histologic finding.

Purpura fulminans is a cutaneous manifestation of DIC seen primarily but not exclusively in children in the setting of infection. This syndrome is classically associated with meningococcemia but can be seen with other bacterial or viral infections. The skin lesions initially appear hemorrhagic, as ecchymotic areas, and then progress to demarcated black and/or purple lesions and eventually to dermal necrosis. Histologic examination reveals microvascular thrombosis as the primary pathologic process.[47] Early recognition of this syndrome may have important therapeutic implications.

Hemangiomas

In the Kasabach-Merritt syndrome DIC may mandate intervention not otherwise indicated.

As mentioned above, hemangiomas are sometimes associated with clinical or laboratory evidence of DIC (Kasabach-Merritt syndrome). Since congenital lesions of this nature often involute with time, the presence of DIC may have important therapeutic implications, mandating therapy not otherwise necessary. Absent or mild DIC may allow for an expectant approach, while severe coagulopathy with hemorrhage may mandate supportive measures directed toward correcting the coagulopathy, as well as surgical or medical treatment of the lesion by resection, radiation therapy, or embolization.

Characterization

Some authors find it useful to characterize DIC as acute or chronic. DIC is chronic in approximately 10 percent of described cases; examples of chronic DIC include Trousseau syndrome and Kassabach-Merritt syndrome, as well as DIC in the setting of malignancy, aortic aneurysms, peritoneovenous shunts, and some obstetric complications.

DIAGNOSIS

Diagnosis of DIC can be difficult and requires a firm grasp of the pathophysiology, thorough clinical assessment, and an understanding of the strengths and limitations of routinely available laboratory tools (Table 5-1). Despite ongoing efforts to improve laboratory techniques, no single test that is diagnostic for DIC is readily available.

TABLE 5-1. Diagnostic Studies in DIC

Test	Finding/Comment
Prothrombin time, activated partial thromboplastin	Usually prolonged, may be normal
Specific factor assays	Reduced levels present
Fibrinogen	Usually low, may be normal; decline in level is significant
Fibrinogen/fibrin degradation products	Elevated
D-dimer	Elevated, more specific than FDP-fdp but less sensitive
Platelet count	Low
Blood smear	Thrombocytopenia, red cell fragmentation
Whole blood clotting time	Delayed clotting, rapid lysis
Protein C, antithrombin III, α_2-antiplasmin levels	May be low, not routinely available

Coagulation Studies

The prothrombin and activated partial thromboplastin times may be normal in the setting of DIC.

Although prolongation of the prothrombin time (PT) or activated partial thromboplastin time (aPTT) is often noted as early evidence of DIC in some patients, these tests are frequently not helpful and can be normal in the presence of DIC. Consumption as well as activity of the fibrinolytic system may result in reduced levels of factors II, VII, VIII, IX, X, XI, and XII. Factor assays are not routinely available, which makes them impractical from a diagnostic standpoint. Fibrinogen levels, however, are routinely determined when DIC is suspected. Hypofibrinogenemia is supportive of the diagnosis of DIC in the appropriate setting, but normal fibrinogen levels do not exclude DIC. Fibrinogen is an acute-phase reactant and may be elevated in malignancy, infection, or other inflammatory condition, thereby masking the DIC process. If serial measurements are made, a decline in fibrinogen level at the suspected time of onset of DIC supports the diagnosis.

Demonstration of increased quantities of FDP-fdp remains the most useful method of detecting DIC.

Demonstration of increased quantities of the degradation products of fibrinogen and fibrin, reflecting activity of the plasmin/plasminogen fibrinolytic system, remains the most useful method of detecting DIC. This system is the only endogenous pathway that digests fibrinogen and fibrin; thus, detection of abnormal quantities of FDP-fdp is a direct measure of the activity of this system. Routine assays for FDP-fdp do not discriminate between fragments of fibrinogen and of fibrin. Recent efforts have been directed toward a more specific assay for fragments specific to cross-linked fibrin. The presence of such a fragment is thought to reflect both thrombin production (and its action on fibrinogen) and activity of the fibrinolytic system. Detection of these fragments would constitute a more sensitive assay for DIC. Assays for D-dimer, thought to be a degradation product of cross-linked fibrin only, are now commercially available and are finding widespread use. Comparisons of D-dimer and FDP-fdp suggest that D-dimer may in fact be more specific for DIC, while FDP-fdp appears to be more sensitive.[48] Investigators have suggested that a combination of these assays might be optimal. However, D-dimer has been shown to be elevated in other pathologic states, such as liver disease, malignancy, deep venous thrombosis, myocardial infarction, and complicated pregnancy; therefore it should not be viewed a definitive test for the presence of DIC.[49,50]

Comparisons of D-dimer and FDP-fdp suggest that D-dimer may be more specific for DIC, while FDP-fdp appears to be more sensitive.

An additional consideration when interpreting FDP-fdp results, particularly in the critical care setting, is the presence of heparin, either from line flushes or from parenteral administration. When a routine latex agglutination test is used to detect FDP-fdp, heparin may cause false positive results.[51] Heparin-contaminated samples may be evaluated for the presence of FDP-fdp, but special processing of the specimen is necessary.

Monoclonal antibodies to a variety of fibrin fragments have been produced in the research laboratory. Antibodies to X-oligomer have been proposed as a useful tool to measure true fibrinolysis, since they are unaffected by fragments of fibrinogen or non-cross-linked fibrin.[52] These are the earliest soluble fragments released from cross-linked fibrin by the action of plasmin. The clinical utility of this technique is not yet certain.

Measurements of thrombin and plasmin generation have been proposed as useful in the diagnosis of DIC. Takahashi et al. measured thrombin–antithrombin III complexes and plasmin–α_2-antiplasmin complexes in patients with DIC as a means of quantifying the activity of the respective pathways.[53,54] Both complexes were found to be elevated in DIC. Decreased levels of α_2-antiplasmin have been suggested as markers for excess fibrinolysis in the setting of DIC.[55] At this time such assays are not routinely available.

Platelet Count/Peripheral Blood Smear

DIC is nearly always accompanied by thrombocytopenia, which is at times the presenting feature of the process. Any time that thrombocytopenia is detected, but particularly when DIC is suspected, a peripheral blood smear should be prepared. In addition to confirmation of thrombocytopenia, the blood smear should be evaluated for the presence of red blood cell fragmentation. Microangiopathic hemolytic changes of this nature are seen in 50 to 60 percent of DIC cases and support the diagnosis. When extensive fragmentation is present, one must be cautious to exclude the diagnosis of TTP-HUS.

When extensive red blood cell fragmentation is seen on the peripheral blood smear, TTP-HUS should also be considered.

Additional Studies

A simple bedside test that may be useful is the single-tube clotting time. It can be performed by placing 1 ml of whole blood in a plain glass tube and tilting the tube every 30 seconds. Normally in 4 to 10 minutes a clot should form, which can subsequently be observed for clot retraction, a measure of platelet function, and clot lysis, a reflection of activity of the fibrinolytic system. This simple test can provide crude information about coagulation, fibrinolysis, and platelet number and function.

A single-tube clotting time is a useful bedside test, which can yield information about both the coagulation and fibrinolytic systems.

The eugloblin lysis time is an inexact measure of fibrinolytic activity. It is not believed to be sensitive or reliable for the evaluation of suspected DIC.

TREATMENT

Since DIC is not a primary disease entity, treatment should be directed toward the underlying process causing the disruption (Table 5-2). The key to effective therapy is management of DIC, thus minimizing end-organ damage and hemorrhagic consequences while the underlying illness is identified and treated if possible. If the underlying process cannot be addressed, attempts at such management and avoidance of the consequences of DIC are usually futile. Vital to management of DIC is aggressive medical management of other secondary problems, such as tissue ischemia, hypovolemia, hypotension, hypoxemia, and electrolyte and acid-base disorders. Although these processes may not be primary triggers for DIC, their presence impairs management and may exacerbate the process.

Replacement Therapy

In the setting of DIC with hemorrhage, the initial management step recommended is a trial of factor replacement in the form of fresh-frozen plasma (FFP). This is the logical choice, since multiple factor deficiencies are generally present and FFP contains all plasma proteins. Replacement therapy has historically been used with some hesitancy and has been thought to "fuel the fire" of DIC by providing substrate for generation of additional FDPs, thereby lead-

Blood product replacement in the form of FFP, cryoprecipitate, and platelets is the first line of therapy for DIC.

TABLE 5-2. Treatment of DIC

Treatment Modality	Indication	Comment
Fresh frozen plasma	Factor deficiencies with hemorrhage	Believed by some authors to exacerbate process if not given with heparin
Cryoprecipitate	Hypofibrinogenemia	Not indicated for multiple factor deficiencies
Platelet transfusions	Thrombocytopenia	Continue only if clinical improvement or documented increments in platelet count
Heparin	Prevention of microthrombosis and organ damage	Clearly indicated in some settings, controversial in most (see text)
Antifibrinolytic agents	Hemorrhage despite above measures	Used primarily with heparin; thrombotic complications when used alone (see text)
Antithrombin III concentrates	Low levels of antithrombin III	Experience with and availability limited
Protein C concentrates	Low levels of protein C	Experience with and availability limited

ing to exacerbation of the bleeding tendency. Despite this concern, achievement of hemostasis in the face of severe coagulation protein deficiencies is unlikely, and a trial of replacement therapy is generally accepted as reasonable first-line treatment. When severe hypofibrinogenemia is present, cryoprecipitate is an excellent source of fibrinogen and may be helpful. One should be aware that this product should not be used exclusively to address multiple factor deficiencies. Transfused platelet are rapidly consumed in DIC; however in the face of bleeding and thrombocytopenia, a trial of platelet transfusions may be reasonable. If such a trial is made, platelet counts should be obtained 1 hour after transfusion; if no increase is observed, further platelet transfusions are not indicated.

In the setting of liver disease, where the diagnosis of DIC is particularly difficult, vitamin-K deficiency may masquerade as or exacerbate DIC.[38] In this setting or whenever DIC is suspected, administration of vitamin K should not be considered a trivial intervention.

Heparin

The use of heparin in the treatment of DIC remains controversial in most settings.

The use of heparin in DIC remains controversial but in general has fallen from favor. In fact, little documented clinical evidence remains in support of the efficacy of heparin in DIC. The reluctance to use heparin is further supported by the increased recognition of heparin-induced thrombocytopenia and rarely, thrombosis. Despite the lack of supporting data, many experienced clinicians use heparin in patients with DIC. Its use holds considerable appeal on a biochemical basis, and a cautious trial may be undertaken when deterioration is seen in the face of adequate supportive measures and blood component replacement. Recommendations range from intermittent subcutaneous administration of low doses of heparin to constant intravenous infusion. Decreased levels of antithrombin III are frequently seen in patients with DIC, which may limit the efficacy of heparin therapy.

Some clinicians favor the use of ϵ-aminocaproic acid (EACA) with heparin. This compound is a serine protease inhibitor, which impairs conversion of plasminogen to plasmin, thereby inhibiting the fibrinolytic system. Concurrent therapy with heparin and EACA, aimed at inhibiting both coagulation and fibrinolysis, has considerable appeal; however, clinical experience remains limited. EACA alone is not usually recommended and may result in widespread thrombus formation due to decreased fibrinolytic activity with unchecked coagulation. Recently the use of EACA alone has been advocated by some authors when marked activation of the fibrinolytic system that is out of proportion to coagulation activation is detected.[55]

EACA alone can cause thrombotic events in patients with DIC, and in general should only be used with heparin.

EACA may also be employed in the Kasabach-Merritt syndrome, in which therapy with inhibitors of the fibrinolytic system has been reported to be helpful.[56–60] Addition of cryoprecipitate in the treatment of patients with hypofibrinogenemia has been reported to result in substantial improvement in the coagulopathy and shrinkage of the tumor, presumably owing to intralesional thrombosis. These measures may be considered when expectant therapy is not possible.

EACA may be useful in the management of the Kasabach-Merritt syndrome.

Several exceptions exist in which the indications for heparin is more clear-cut. When Trousseau syndrome is present, heparin is indicated and essential. Prompt response to heparin followed by relapse or deterioration is often the initial evidence of Trousseau syndrome. In patients with purpura fulminans, early intervention with heparin may minimize the extent of dermal necrosis. In patients with dead fetus syndrome or amniotic fluid embolus, heparin therapy may also be on firmer ground.

Use of heparin is more clearly indicated in Trousseau syndrome, purpura fulminans, and certain obstetric complications.

DIC associated with acute promyelocytic leukemia (APL) has been an accepted indication for heparin for some time, and improvement in laboratory measurements of DIC is routinely seen with its use. Goldberg et al., in a recent review of their patients with APL from 1974 to 1985, have questioned the wisdom of this practice.[61] They obtained excellent outcomes in managing patients with FFP and

Although it is widely employed, debate over the benefits of heparin in patients with promyelocytic leukemia is ongoing.

platelet transfusions and cited the risk of historic controls in ascribing improved outcomes to the use of heparin, particularly in light of other improvements in medical management and chemotherapy. Similarly, Rodeghiero et al. retrospectively examined outcomes in 268 consecutive APL patients treated with either heparin, antifibrinolytic agents, or supportive measures alone and found no significant difference in hemorrhagic deaths between groups.[62] Other authors continue to urge use of heparin in this setting.[63,64] APL patients may constitute one subset of DIC in which a prospective trial is feasible to resolve the question of the usefulness of heparin in treatment of DIC.

Other Therapeutic Agents

DIC therapy with preparations of endogenous inhibitors of coagulation such as *antithrombin III* and *protein C* has recently been a growing area of interest. Levels of both protein C and antithrombin III are frequently decreased in the setting of DIC.[21,22] Replacement of physiologic levels of natural inhibitors of coagulation has some appeal. In animal models prophylaxis with antithrombin III prior to administration of endotoxin attenuated DIC and decreased organ damage.[24] Administration of antithrombin III to the animals 1 hour after endotoxin had a similar but less marked effect. In humans some studies show benefit but lack adequate controls.[65] Several patients with purpura fulminans were treated with antithrombin III, and investigators were impressed by the rapid resolution of DIC-associated findings.[66] Similarly, infusion of activated protein C has been shown to be protective against DIC induced by *E. coli* in a baboon model.[23] Therapy of DIC with protein C has been attempted in humans; improvement has been reported in two of three patients given protein C after each had failed heparin therapy.[67] Again, no controls could be cited.

Gabexate is a serine protease inhibitor that exerts anticoagulant effects by several mechanisms and has been used by Umeki et al. to treat DIC.[68] The rationale offered is that unlike heparin, gabexate is not dependent on AT III. Their small study concluded this agent may be as effective as heparin in the therapy of DIC. Recombinant hirudin, a thrombin-specific inhibitor of coagulation, has demonstrated the ability to block or attenuate endotoxin-induced DIC in an animal model.[69]

DIC is frequently seen in association with peritoneovenous shunts. In this setting if the patient is asymptomatic and DIC is mild, usually no intervention is indicated. In an animal model *antiplatelet agents* were shown by Salem et al. to prevent induction of DIC by injection of ascitic fluid.

The same authors treated a small number of patients with antiplatelet agents prior to and after shunt placement and demonstrated some usefulness of this modality, although no controls were cited.[70]

Litt et al. have cited effective therapy with *ketoconazole* of DIC associated with prostatic carcinoma.[71] The result may have been due to suppression of the tumor by decreased testosterone and adrenal steroid production or perhaps to a direct effect of ketoconazole on activators of coagulation or fibrinolysis.

Assessment of Treatment Modalities

The clinical utility of any treatment modality is inherently difficult to assess. The process of DIC is almost always in a state of flux, and hopefully, interventions are made concurrently with aggressive measures addressing the underlying illness. The clinical spectrum of DIC is also very broad. These and other considerations make evaluation of therapy problematic at best.

Some authors cite laboratory measurements as useful tools to quantify relative activation of the fibrinolytic and coagulation pathways and to guide therapeutic interventions. Williams determined levels of α_2-antiplasmin in patients with DIC (and other bleeding diatheses) and concluded that decreased levels indicated excessive fibrinolysis and were correlated with severe bleeding.[55] EACA was used in this setting and observed to improve hemostasis, although no controls were cited or improvement in mortality discussed. Andoh et al. have described an assay for tissue factor activity of leukemia cells and suggested a formula to predict the heparin dose required to control DIC.[72] Takahashi et al. have assessed thrombin and plasmin generation by measuring plasma levels of thrombin–antithrombin III complexes (TAT) and plasmin–α_2-antiplasmin complexes (PAP), respectively.[53,54] Both complexes were markedly elevated in patients with DIC, and the TAT/PAP ratio correlated with different disease categories. Most strikingly, patients with APL had the highest PAP levels and the lowest TAT/PAP ratio. It was suggested that these markers may be helpful in directing or monitoring therapy.

In summary, the cornerstone of therapy for DIC remains aggressive treatment of the underlying disease and associated medical problems. When there is hemorrhage in the setting of DIC, a trial of replacement therapy is usually warranted. With noted exceptions, further intervention must be considered on a patient-by-patient basis, depending on the clinical and laboratory manifestations of DIC. Other agents in the armamentarium include heparin, antifibrinolytic agents, antithrombin III, and protein C. Eventually more refined measures of coagulation activation and fibrinolysis may be available to guide therapeutic interventions.

References

1. De Blainville HMD: Injection de matière cérèbrale dans les veins. Gaz Med Paris p. 524, 1834
2. Wooldrich LC: Über intravasculare Gerinnungen. Arch Anat Physiol p. 397, 1886
3. Levin J, Beck E: A re-appraisal of the role of blood coagulation and platelets in the generalized Schwartzman phenomenon. Thromb Haemost 15:519, 1966
4. Lerner RG, Rappaport SI: Disappearance of fibrinogen-^{131}I after endotoxin: effects of a first and second injection. Am J Physiol 214:532, 1968
5. Forman EN: Generalized Schwartzman reaction: role of the granulocyte in intravascular coagulation and renal cortical necrosis. Br J Haematol 16:507, 1969
6. Corrigan JJ: Effect of anticoagulating and non-anticoagulating concentrations of heparin on the generalized Schwartzman reaction. Thromb Haemost 24:136, 1970
7. Latour J, Prejeau JB, Margaretten W: Corticosteroids and the generalized Schwartzman reaction. Am J Pathol 65:189, 1971
8. Muller-Berghaus B, Obst R: Induction of the generalized Schwartzman reaction in pregnant and non-pregnant rats by colchicine. Am J Pathol 69:131, 1972
9. Rivers RPA, Hathaway WE, Weston WL: The endotoxin induced coagulant activity of human monocytes. Br J Haematol 30:311, 1975
10. Colucci M, Balconi R, Lorenzet A et al: Cultured human endothelial cells generate tissue factor in response to endotoxin. J Clin Invest 71:1893, 1983
11. Baily K, Bettleheim FR, Lorand L, Riddlebrook WR: Action of thrombin in the clotting of fibrinogen. Nature 167:233, 1951
12. Pareti FI, Capitanio A, Mannucci PM: Acquired storage pool disease in platelets during disseminated intravascular coagulation. Blood 48:511, 1976
13. Yamazaki H, Motomiya T, Watanabe C et al: Consumption of larger platelets with decrease in adenine nucleotide content in thrombosis, disseminated intravascular coagulation and postoperative states. Thromb Res 18:77, 1980
14. Weksler BB, Ley CW, Jaffe EA: Stimulation of endothelial cell prostacyclin production by thrombin, trypsin, and the ionophore A23187. J Clin Invest 62:293, 1978
15. Prescott SM, Zimmerman GA, McIntyre TM: Human endothelial cells in culture produce platelet activating factor (1-alkyl-2-acetyl-sn-glycero-3-phosphocoline) when stimulated by thrombin. Proc Natl Acad Sci U S A 81:3534, 1986
16. Levine JD, Harlan JM, Harker LA et al: Thrombin-mediated release of factor VIII antigen from human umbilical vein endothelial cells in culture. Blood 60:531, 1986
17. Gelehrter TD, Sznycer-Laszuk R: Thrombin induction of plasminogen activator inhibitor in cultured human endothelial cells. J Clin Invest 77:165, 1986
18. Dichk D, Quertermous T: Thrombin regulation of mRNA levels of tissue plasminogen activator and plasminogen activator inhibitor-1 in cultured human umbilical vein endothelial cells. Blood 74:222, 1989
19. Egbring R, Schmidt W, Fuchs G, Havemann K: Demonstration of granulocytic proteases in plasma of patients with acute leukemia and septicemia with coagulation defects. Blood 49:219, 1977
20. Gouault-Heilmann M, Chardin E, Sultan C, Josso F: The procoagulant factor of leukemic promyelocytes: demonstration of immunologic cross-reactivity with human brain tissue factors. Br J Haematol 30:151, 1975
21. Marlar RA, Endres-Brooks J, Miller C: Serial studies of protein C and its inhibitor in patients with disseminated intravascular coagulation. Blood 66:59, 1985
22. Lammle B, Tran TH, Ritz R, Duckert F: Plasma prekallikrein, factor XIII, antithrombin-III, C1-inhibitor and alpha 2-macroglobulin in critically ill patients with suspected disseminated intravascular coagulation. Am J Clin Pathol 82:396, 1984

23. Taylor FB, Chang A, Esmon CT et al: Protein C prevents the coagulopathic and lethal effects of *Escherichia coli* infusion in the baboon. J Clin Invest 79:918, 1987
24. Emerson TE, Fournel MA, Redens TB et al: Efficacy of antithrombin III supplementation in animal models of fulminant *Escherichia coli* endotoxemia or bacteremia. Am J Med 87:27S, 1989
25. Rao LVM, Rappaport SI: Studies of a mechanism inhibiting the initiation of the extrinsic pathway of coagulation. Blood 69:645, 1987
26. Sandset PM, Warn-Cramer BJ, Maki SL, Rappaport SI: Immunodepletion of extrinsic pathway inhibitor sensitizes rabbits to endotoxin induced intravascular coagulation and the generalized Schwartzman reaction. Blood 78:1496, 1991
27. Cozzolino F, Torcia M, Miliani A et al: Potential role of interleukin-1 as the trigger for diffuse intravascular coagulation in acute nonlymphoblastic leukemia. Am J Med 84:240, 1988
28. Warr TA, Rao VM, Rapaport SI: Disseminated intravascular coagulation in rabbits induced by administration of endotoxin or tissue factor: effect of anti-tissue factor antibodies and measurement of plasma extrinsic pathway inhibitor activity. Blood 75:1481, 1990
29. Kessler CM, Nussbaum ES, Tuazon CU: In vitro correlation of platelet aggregation with occurrence of disseminated intravascular coagulation and subacute bacterial endocarditis. J Lab Clin Med 109:647, 1987
30. Kessler CM, Nussbaum ES, Tuazon CU: Disseminated intravascular coagulation associated with *Staphyloccus aureus* septicemia is mediated by peptidoglycan-induced platelet aggregation. J Infect Dis 164:101, 1991
31. Rotta J: Endotoxin-like properties of peptidoglycan. Immunobiology 149:230, 1975
32. Verbrugh HA, vanDijk WC, Peters R et al: The role of *Staphylococcus aureus* cell wall peptidoglycan, teichoic acid, and protein A in the process of complement activation and opsonization. Immunology 37:615, 1979
33. Inura Y, Terashita Z, Nishikawa K: Possible role of platelet activating factor in disseminated intravascular coagulation, evidenced by use of a PAF antagonist CV-3988. Life Sci 39:111, 1986
34. Van Dam PA, Renier M, Baekekandt M et al: Disseminated intravascular coagulation and the syndrome of hemolysis, elevated liver enzymes and low platelets in severe preeclampsia. Obstet Gynecol 73:97, 1989
35. Sibai BM: The HELLP syndrome: much ado about nothing? Am J Obstet Gynecol 162:311, 1990
36. Jedeikin R, Olsfanger MB, Kessler I: Disseminated intravascular coagulopathy and adult respiratory distress syndrome: life-threatening complications of hysteroscopy. Am J Obstet Gynecol 162:44, 1990
37. VanDeWater L, Carr JM, Aronson D, McDonagh J: Analysis of elevated fibrin(ogen) degradation product levels in patients with liver disease. Blood 67:1468, 1986
38. Mant MJ, Hirsh J, Pineo GF, Luke KH: Prolonged prothrombin time and partial thromboplastin time in disseminated intravascular coagulation not due to deficiency of factors V and VIII. Br J Haematol 24:725, 1973
39. Warr TA, Rao VM, Rapaport SI: Human plasma extrinsic pathway inhibitor activity. II. Plasma levels in disseminated intravascular coagulation and hepatocellular disease. Blood 74:994, 1989
40. Edney JA, Hill A, Armstrong D: Peritoneovenous shunts palliate malignant ascites. Am J Surg 158:598, 1989
41. Spearing RL, Hickton CM, Sizeland P et al: Quinine-induced disseminated intravascular coagulation. Lancet 336:1535, 1990
42. Chang JC, Gross HM, Jang NS: Disseminated intravascular coagulation due to intravenous administration of hetastarch. Am J Med Sci 300:301, 1990
43. Chistolini A, Mazzucconi MG, Tirindelli MC et al: Disseminated intravascular coagulation and myocardial infarction in a haemophilia B patient during therapy with prothrombin complex concentrates. Acta Haematol (Basel) 83:163, 1990
44. Light RW, Bell WR: LDH and fibrinogen-fibrin degradation products in pulmonary embolism. Arch Intern Med 133:372, 1974
45. Schwartzman RJ, Hill JB: Neurologic complications of disseminated intravascular coagulation. Neurology 32:791, 1982
46. Bell WR, Starksen NF, Tong S, Porterfield JK: Trousseau's syndrome. Devastating coagulopathy in the absence of heparin. Am J Med 79:423, 1985
47. Sotto MN, Langer B, Hoshino-Shimizu S, deBrito T: Pathogenesis of cutaneous lesions in acute meningococcemia in humans: light, immunofluorescent and electron microscopy of skin biopsy specimens. J Infect Dis 133:506, 1976

48. Carr JM, McKinney M, McDonagh J: Diagnosis of disseminated intravascular coagulation. Role of D-dimer. Am J Clin Pathol 91:280, 1989
49. Wilde JT, Kitchen S, Kinsey S et al: Plasma-D-dimer levels and their relationship to serum fibrinogen/fibrin degradation products in hypercoagulable states. Br J Haematol 71:65, 1988
50. Boisclair MD, Lane DA, Wilde JT et al: A comparative evaluation of assays for markers of activated coagulation and/or fibrinolysis: thrombin-antithrombin complex, D-dimer and fibrinogen/fibrin fragment E antigen. Br J Haematol 74:471, 1989
51. Connaghan DG, Francis CW, Ryan DH, Marder VJ: Prevalence and clinical implications of heparin-associated false positive tests for serum fibrin(ogen) degradation products. Am J Clin Pathol 86:304, 1986
52. Gaffney PJ, Creighton LJ, Perry MJ et al: Monoclonal antibodies to crosslinked fibrin degradation products (XL-FDP). Br J Haematol 68:83, 1987
53. Takahashi H, Hanano M, Takizawa S et al: Plasmin-a2-plasmin inhibitor complex in plasma of patients with disseminated intravascular coagulation. Am J Hematol 28:162, 1988
54. Takahashi H, Hanano M, Takizawa S et al: Thrombin vs. plasmin generation in disseminated intravascular coagulation associated with various underlying disorders. Am J Hematol 33:90, 1990
55. Williams EC: Plasma alpha 2-antiplasmin activity: role in the evaluation and management of fibrinolytic states and other bleeding disorders. Arch Intern Med 149:1769, 1989
56. Warrel RP, Kempin SJ: Treatment of severe coagulopathy in the Kasabach-Merritt syndrome with aminocaproic acid and cryoprecipitate. N Engl J Med 313:309, 1985
57. Bell AJ, Chisholm M, Hickton M: Reversal of coagulopathy in Kasabach-Merritt syndrome with tranexamic acid. Scand J Haematol 37:249, 1986
58. Larsen EC, Zinkham WH, Eggleston JC, Zitelli BJ: Kasabach-Merritt syndrome: therapeutic considerations. Pediatrics 79:971, 1987
59. Ortel TL, Onorato JJ, Bedrosian CL, Kaufman RE: Antifibrinolytic therapy in the management of the Kasabach-Merritt syndrome. Am J Hematol 29:44, 1988
60. Shulkin BL, Argenta LC, Cho KJ, Castle VP: Kasabach-Merritt syndrome: treatment with epsilon-aminocaproic acid and assessment by indium-111 platelet scintigraphy. J Pediatr 117: 746, 1990
61. Goldberg MA, Ginsburg D, Mayer RJ et al: Is heparin administration necessary during induction chemotherapy for patients with acute promylelocytic leukemia? Blood 69:187, 1987
62. Rodeghiero F, Avvisati G, Castaman G et al: Early deaths and anti-hemorrhagic treatments in acute promyelocytic leukemia. A GIMEMA retrospective study in 268 consecutive patients. Blood 75:2112, 1990
63. Feldman EJ, Arlin ZAA, Ahmed T et al: Acute promyelocytic leukemia: a 5 year experience with new antileukemic agents and a new approach to preventing fatal hemorrhage. Acta Haematol (Basel) 82:117, 1989
64. Cunningham I, Gee TS, Reich LM et al: Acute promyelocytic leukemia: treatment results during a decade at Memorial Hospital. Blood 73:1116, 1989
65. Blauhut B, Necek S, Vinazzer H, Bergmann H: Substitution therapy with antithrombin III concentrate in shock and DIC. Thromb Res 27:271, 1984
66. Fourrier F, Lestavel P, Chopin C et al: Meningococcemia and purpura fulminans: acute deficiencies of proteins C and S and early treatment with antithrombin III concentrates. Intensive Care Med 16:121, 1990
67. Okajima K, Imamura H, Koga S et al: Treatment of patients with disseminated intravascular coagulation by protein C. Am J Hematol 33:277, 1990
68. Umeki S, Adachi M, Watanabe M et al: Gabexate as a therapy for disseminated intravascular coagulation. Arch Intern Med 148:1409, 1988
69. Hoffmann H, Seibeck M, Spannagl M et al: Effect of recombinant hirudin, a specific inhibitor of thrombin, on endotoxin induced intravascular coagulation and acute lung injury in pigs. Am Rev Respir Dis 142:782, 1990
70. Salem HH, Dudley FJ, Merrett A et al: Coagulopathy of peritoneovenous shunts: studies on the pathogenic role of ascitic fluid collagen and value of antiplatelet therapy. Gut 24:412, 1983
71. Litt MR, Bell WR, Lepor HA: Disseminated intravascular coagulation in prostatic carcinoma reversed by ketoconazole. JAMA 258:1361, 1987
72. Andoh K, Sadakata H, Uchiyama T et al: One stage assay of tissue factor activity of leukemic cells with special reference to disseminated intravascular coagulation. Am J Clin Pathol 93:679, 1990

6

BLOOD COMPONENT THERAPY

THOMAS S. KICKLER
PAUL M. NESS

In order to use blood products safely and effectively, one must know what products are available and their respective therapeutic advantages. In addition, a basic understanding of blood group serology is necessary so that the correct blood type can be transfused. Although there are multiple red cell alloantigens, an understanding of the ABO and D blood groups is of preeminent importance for the average practitioner.

BASIC IMMUNOHEMATOLOGY

ABO System

Providing compatible blood starts with ensuring that the patient is given correct ABO group.

Providing compatible blood starts with ensuring that the correct ABO group is given to a patient. Administration of ABO-incompatible red cells is associated with intravascular hemolysis, leading to renal insufficiency, disseminated intravascular coagulopathy, and possibly death. The fact that patients routinely have anti-A or anti-B or both antibodies in their serum when they lack the corresponding blood groups on their red cells explains the clinical importance of ABO blood group system recognition. The high density of ABO antigen sites on the red cell provides ready targets for the immunoglobulin M anti-A or anti-B isoagglutinin.

This reciprocal relationship is the basis of routine serologic practice in the blood bank. Two antisera, anti-A and anti-B, are used to test the patient's red cells, a practice known as *front-typing* or *forward grouping*. The patient's serum is also tested with cells of known ABO group, known as *back-typing* or *reverse grouping*. These results are compared and are typically confirmatory; discrepant results can be an important clue to hematologic difficulties and require further investigation in all cases. For example, ABO discrepancies commonly occur in patients with warm or cold autoimmune hemolytic anemia.

Patients who are of the uncommon AB red cell type have been considered universal recipients in the past because they lack anti-A and anti-B; likewise, group O red cells (from universal donors) are considered safe to administer to all patients. Blood supplies are generally adequate to avoid using universal donor blood except in cases of major trauma in which transfusion is mandated before blood grouping can be completed. Group O blood is administered as red cells on these occasions to avoid the potential problem of anti-A and anti-B in the donor plasma. Despite this precaution, some donor plasma may contain sufficient levels of isoagglutinins to cause problems. If one wishes to switch such a patient to group specific blood, it is necessary to confirm that no detectable passively administered anti-A or anti-B is present in the patient's plasma to cause hemolysis of the transfused red cells. ABO-incompatible plasma products should be avoided if large volumes are to be administered to small blood volume recipients.

In emergency situations in which the patient's blood type is unknown and there is no time for blood typing or compatibility testing, giving group O red cells is a safe and well accepted policy.

The concept of universal donors (group O) or universal recipients (group AB) is of relevance only to extreme emergencies or when technical support is unavailable (mass casualties or battlefield situations). For elective transfusions it is preferable to provide group-specific blood so that group O blood is not wasted. In an emergency situations in which the patient's blood type is unknown and there is no time to perform type or compatibility testing, giving group O red cells is a safe and well accepted policy.[1]

The Rh System

Although the Rh blood group system has now been shown to include at least 40 specific antigens, the original antigen identified, Rho(D), remains the most important. Unlike ABO system antibodies, antibodies to the D antigen arise only after stimulation from incompatible pregnancies or transfusions. The Rh blood system plays an important role in transfusion practice. Because the Rho(D) antigen is highly immunogenic and because the 85 percent of donors who possess the antigen can readily immunize the 15 percent of patients who lack the antigen, Rh-positive blood components should be administered only to Rh-positive recipients. In extreme emergency situations in which there is a shortage of Rh-negative blood, it may be necessary to transfuse Rh-positive red cells into Rh-negative individuals. This alternative can be chosen without immediate risk although the patient may become immunized. In general, Rh alloimmunization is only a major concern for women who may give birth to children with hemolytic disease of the newborn. Even though the D antigen is limited to red cells and not known to be present in plasma, white cells, or platelets, many of these blood components are contaminated with red cells; therefore, Rh-positive platelets or granulocytes should be avoided in Rh-negative recipients. Frozen plasma products do not contain enough red cells for this to be a clinical problem.[2]

COMPATIBILITY TESTING

Compatibility testing begins with ABO typing of the donor unit and patient, followed by screening of the patient's serum for red cell alloantibodies. If no alloantibodies resulting from alloimmunization by previous transfusions or pregnancies, ABO compatibility between the patient and recipient must be ensured by performing a major cross-match. If the antibody screen is negative and the donor and recipient are ABO-compatible, there is an extremely low probability that the donor red cells will be incompatible. For this reason in emergency situations in which the antibody screen is negative, it is relatively safe to eliminate the major cross-match for ABO-compatible transfusions.

If red cell alloantibodies are detected, they are characterized to ensure that red cells selected for transfusion will lack the offending alloantigen. Since patients can produce several antibodies, antibody identification and subsequent procurement of compatible units may require a great deal of time and effort. For this reason, in the care of patients alloimmunized to red cell antigens and in need of intensive red cell support, close cooperation with the blood bank is required to ensure that blood is available in a timely fashion.

TRANSFUSION WHEN COMPATIBLE BLOOD IS UNAVAILABLE

Patients are occasionally encountered who require blood transfusions because of symptomatic anemia but for whom compatible blood cannot be found. These patients may have been alloimmunized by previous transfusions or pregnancies to high-incidence antigen or to a combination of antigens, which has made compatible blood difficult to find. The obvious first step is communication with the blood bank to convey the urgency of the clinical situation and the complexity of the immunohematologic problem. The blood bank can attempt to find compatible blood from rare donor registries or family members who may have similar phenotypes. An experienced serologist may be able to distinguish clinically significant antibodies from blood group antibodies not known to cause immune hemolysis; a more focused search for blood lacking fewer clinically significant antigens can then be pursued. As a final result of blood bank investigation, the least incompatible blood can be selected in the event that compatible blood cannot be found. This blood can be anticipated to have shortened red cell survival, although an acute hemolytic reaction would be considered unlikely.

When the decision is reached that transfusion must be performed, several additional steps can enhance patient safety. It may be possible to perform a radiolabeled in vivo cross-match to assure the clinician that major hemolysis will not ensue. In some cases transfusions of small aliquots of blood may be sufficient to provide relief of symptoms while avoiding the complications of fluid overload. The use of leukocyte-poor red cells is useful to avoid febrile, nonhemolytic transfusion reactions whose initial presentation can suggest a hemolytic transfusion of more serious consequence. In the final analysis, however, the decision to proceed with incompatible blood requires a risk versus benefit assessment by the physician; in life-threatening emergencies, incompatible blood may be the only means to sustain life until compatible blood can be found or red cell production restores homeostasis.

TRANSFUSION THERAPY IN AUTOIMMUNE HEMOLYTIC ANEMIA

Blood transfusion may be required for patients with autoimmune hemolytic anemia who present with fulminant hemolysis or patients with chronic hemolysis who become symptomatic while awaiting response to primary modes of therapy. The presence of red cell autoantibody coating the patient's red cells or appearing as a panagglutinin in the serum adds additional blood transfusion risks to the general risks of infectious disease transmission or transfusion reaction from alloantibodies to red cells, white cells, platelets, or serum proteins. The autoantibody can make it difficult to detect coexisting red cell alloantibodies, which can cause severe hemolytic transfusion reactions; in addition, the red cell autoantibody will cause increased destruction of the donor red cells. Despite these concerns, transfusion may be required in autoimmune hemolytic anemia and may be life-saving.[3] A 1980 report documented a series of five patients with autoimmune hemolytic anemia and reticulocytopenia despite intense erythroid hyperplasia in the bone marrow. All five patients required transfusion as a life-sustaining measure for profound anemia; these patients had been transferred from other hospitals where transfusions had been withheld because of serologic incompatibilities. Reticulocytopenia persisted for 4 to 160 days before adequate erythropoiesis or control of the hemolytic process with corticosteroids or splenectomy was achieved. These cases emphasize that transfusion should not be avoided in autoimmune hemolytic anemia despite old dogma to the contrary.[4]

The transfusion management of patients with autoimmune hemolytic anemia requires careful communication between the clinician and the transfusion service. It is critical for the clinician to assess the patient's history of pregnancies and previous transfusions with great care; it is unlikely that a previously untransfused male will have masked alloantibodies.

The transfusion management of patients with autoimmune hemolytic anemia requires careful communication between the clinician and the transfusion service.

Since the panagglutinin in the patient's serum typically reacts with all donor red cells, cross-matching blood may be a difficult and time-consuming process. In an emergency or if ABO results are not clear-cut, group O donor blood may be used. Since patients with autoimmune hemolytic anemia are often candidates for chronic transfusion programs, it may be useful to know the red cell phenotype for Rh antigens and common antigens of the Kell, Duffy, or Kidd blood groups. The most pressing problem in a patient with previous pregnancies or transfusions is detecting or identifying alloantibody, which may be hidden by the autoantibody. Sophisticated immunohematology laboratories can use a combination of procedures, including differential absorption, warm autoabsorption, or elution of antibodies with various reagents.

In view of the complications that can arise in patients with autoimmune hemolytic anemia who may require transfusion, measures can be taken during remissions to enhance patient safety. One reasonable approach is autologous transfusion of predeposited frozen storage blood for patients who are likely to relapse in the future or who may require transfusions in the event that splenectomy is required. Another measure to be considered is extended red cell phenotype analysis while the patient remains in remission. Finally, patients who require drugs that often produce immunohematologic problems (e.g., α-methyl dopa) should be evaluated in advance of their transfusion needs to reduce delays.

GENERAL PRINCIPLES OF TRANSFUSION THERAPY

Clinicians can reduce the risk of transfusion by following two basic principles. First, patients should receive only the specific blood components needed to correct the deficiency without unnecessary cells or plasma products. Second, it is unnecessary to correct a cytopenia or a clotting protein deficiency to normal levels.

Every transfusion carries a risk of alloimmunization and incompatibility as well as a risk of viral transmission. When a transfusion is needed, there is much the blood bank can do to ensure its safety. However, clinicians can also reduce the risk by following two basic principles. First, patients should receive only the specific blood components needed to correct the deficiency without unnecessary cells or plasma products. Second, it is unnecessary to correct a cytopenia or a clotting protein deficiency to normal levels. Rather, physiologic levels should be restored, allowing the patient's own homeostatic mechanisms to make any additional correction to normal levels following acute treatment.

INDICATIONS FOR RED CELL TRANSFUSIONS

Until about the early 1980s there was little debate as to when red cell transfusions should be administered. If a patient's hemoglobin fell below 10.0 g/dl, red cells would almost routinely be given. The realization that the human immunodeficiency virus (HIV) and other viruses can be transmitted by transfusion has led to much closer scrutiny of the indications for transfusion. Clinical observations of patients with chronic anemic conditions such as those associated with renal failure or sickle cell anemia suggest that hemoglobin values of 7 to 8 g/dl do not commonly lead to clinical impairment.

The main function of red cells is to deliver oxygen to the tissues. It follows therefore that the purpose of red cell transfusion is to improve the oxygen-carrying capacity of blood, not to treat hypovolemia. Numerous mechanisms exist to maintain oxygen delivery. These mechanisms include control of pulmonary ventilation/perfusion ratio, diffusion of oxygen into the blood, characteristics of red cells and hemoglobin (including the effect of plasma pH), cardiac function, perfusion of tissue, oxygen consumption by tissue, and perhaps the pattern of oxygen utilization within the tissue. No currently available experimental model or single parameter measures these homeostatic mechanisms. Sole reliance on the hemoglobin concentration has grown out of its ease of measurement. Obviously this reliance oversimplifies a complex phenomenon.

In deciding when to transfuse, the physician must decide if the anemia is chronic or acute. Generally in the former situation the clinician must rely upon clinical judgment in deciding whether oxygen delivery needs improvement. If the anemia cannot be corrected by iron or folate replacement and the patient is showing signs or symptoms of decompensation (such as fatigue, dyspnea, tachycardia, or tachypnea), red cell transfusions are justified. In these chronic situations unaccompanied by volume loss, hemoglobin values as low as 7 g/dl or less may be tolerated.

When managing anemias of more acute onset, such as are seen in intensive care units, invasive hemodynamic monitoring may provide a more comprehensive physiologic measure of oxygen delivery. These physiologic measurements include mixed venous oxygen content, extraction ratio, and oxygen consumption along with cardiac output. Agreement is needed concerning what constitutes impaired oxygen delivery and which measurements best reflect this derangement.

RED BLOOD CELL COMPONENTS

Currently, a variety of red blood cell products are available for transfusion, each of which has particular characteristics that determine its effectiveness in a given clinical situation.[1]

Whole Blood

Massive hemorrhage is best treated with whole blood because red cells and plasma are replaced simultaneously. Prompt correction of intravascular volume depletion is important to prevent the sequelae of prolonged hypotension (e.g., acidosis, disseminated intravascular coagulation [DIC], or renal failure). Other red cell components may be used instead of whole blood in combination with volume expanders (e.g., crystalloid, plasma, or plasma derivatives such as albumin or plasma protein fraction).

Red Cell Concentrates

Red cells are the component of choice when restoration of oxygen-carrying capacity alone is required. If the patient has chronic anemia or congestive heart failure or is elderly, transfusion with red cells minimizes volume expansion and maximally improves oxygen delivery. Packed red cells are obtained from a unit of whole blood by removing the plasma and are preserved for 35 to 42 days. The resultant unit of red cells has a volume of approximately 300 ml and a hematocrit ranging between 65 and 80 percent. Some red cell concentrates are collected in an extended preservative solution, which allows storage up to 42 days. These red cells have virtually all the plasma removed and have a volume of 350 ml because of the additive solution used.

Frozen Red Cells

Red cells can effectively be frozen with a cryoprotective agent such as glycerol and stored for several years. The indications for this product are limited. Freezing red cells can provide an inventory of phenotyped red cells for transfusion to patients with complex antibody problems or to patients requiring rare blood types. Freezing also provides a mechanism for storing autologous units, which may be used for future surgery or for patients who are unlikely to have compatible blood available. The freezing and subsequent deglycerolization procedure removes IgA protein and leukocyte antigens; frozen cells are therefore useful in reducing immunologic reactions.

Leukocyte-Poor Blood

Patients receiving multiple transfusions or multiparous women may develop antibodies to leukocytes. When they are transfused with incompatible leukocytes contained in red cells units, febrile reactions may occur. To prevent these reactions use of leukocyte-poor red cells prepared by differential centrifugation, filtration, or cell washing is recommended. These processes remove at least 70 percent of leukocytes, thus preventing most reactions.[6] However, in order to prevent alloimmunization to HLA antigens, more efficient leukocyte removal is necessary. Patients with aplastic anemia who are awaiting bone marrow transplantation should receive transfusions of red cells that have been filtered to reduce the residual leukocyte count to less than 5×10^6 in each blood product transfused.

Washed Red Cells

Washing red cells with isotonic saline solution removes almost all plasma and non-red cell constituents. This preparation is indicated for those patients with severe allergic reactions to plasma constituents. In particular, patients who lack IgA and have been alloimmunized to it and are therefore at risk for anaphylactic transfusion reactions should receive washed cells.[7] Patients with paroxysmal nocturnal hemoglobinuria have traditionally received washed red cells.

PLATELET TRANSFUSION THERAPY

Platelet Transfusion Preparation

Platelets may be prepared from whole blood or by apheresis from a single donor and stored for up to 5 days. When preparing platelets from whole blood, platelet-rich plasma is prepared by centrifugation and subjected to a second concentrating centrifugation step, which results in a unit of platelet concentrate with a volume of approximately 50 to 60 ml. This type of platelet unit contains at least 5.5×10^{10} platelets with approximately 10^8 or more of contaminating leukocytes. For an adult patient 6 to 8 units of platelets are pooled for a single transfusion. If the resulting volume of platelets is too great for the patient, the platelets may be concentrated. This practice is especially useful for patients in precarious fluid balance receiving multiple platelet transfusions. On the other hand, the 400 ml of plasma administered contains good levels of clotting factors, which can reduce the need for plasma components in patients deficient in platelets and coagulation factors.

Platelets may also be prepared by apheresis. A variety of equipment exists to harvest platelets from donors. Depending on the duration of the apheresis procedure, the platelet content of the product will vary. Blood centers generally perform platelet counts on each apheresis collection and label the unit so that the clinical staff can calculate the expected post-transfusion platelet count increment. With improved collection technology, the leukocyte content of an entire pheresis platelet unit may be less than 10^7. This may help prevent alloimmunization to HLA antigens. Use of pheresis platelets also has the advantage of reducing the risk of viral disease transmission, since recipients are exposed to fewer donors than with platelet concentrates.[8]

Platelet Transfusion Practices

It is preferable to use ABO-compatible platelets whenever possible to prevent the passive administration of ABO-incompatible plasma. Some recipients, especially if they are small, may experience hemolytic transfusion reactions with ABO-incompatible platelets. For example, if pooled platelets from eight group O donors are given to a patient who is group A, the 400 ml of plasma contains anti-A isoagglutinin, which may bind to the recipient's group A red cells, leading to intravascular hemolysis. Although renal failure is uncommon, uncomfortable systemic symptoms are not. Platelet shortages may prevent transfusion of ABO-compatible platelets. In these situations platelet washing or removing as much plasma as possible in selected patients may prevent transfusion reactions caused by ABO-incompatible plasma.

Indications for Platelet Transfusions

Generally spontaneous bleeding associated with thrombocytopenia does not occur until the platelet count drops below 20,000/mm^3.[9] (The platelet count of at least 20,000/mm^3 is based upon a large group of patients studied in the early 1960s. It is not clear whether the risk of bleeding may have been influenced by such factors as administration of aspirin, commonly used at that time as an antipyretic. Other clinical problems such as uremia, administration of drugs that affect platelet function (e.g., semisynthetic penicillins), anticoagulation with heparin, and certain paraproteins may impair platelet function or increase the risk of spontaneous hemorrhage, so that patients with platelet

Generally spontaneous bleeding associated with thrombocytopenia does not occur until the platelet count drops below 20,000/mm^3.

counts greater than 20,000/mm^3 may be at risk for bleeding. Other factors that lead to bleeding in thrombocytopenic patients are fever, DIC, and mucositis. Patients with hyperleukocytosis prior to or during cytoreductive chemotherapy and patients with acute progranulocytic leukemia may have an increased risk of hemorrhage and are generally given transfusions to maintain their platelet counts substantially above 20,000/mm^3. There are two approaches to platelet transfusion, prophylactic transfusions and therapeutic transfusions (given only when there is clinical evidence of bleeding). There have been no large-scale randomized studies showing which approach is superior. One small study comparing prophylactic transfusions with therapeutic transfusions showed that morbidity and mortality were not increased by limiting transfusions to episodes of bleeding.[10] Furthermore, the number of platelet transfusions could be decreased although red cell transfusions were not significantly different in the two groups. Since the first bleed may be a life-threatening one (e.g., into the brain), prophylactic platelet transfusions remain a standard transfusion practice. Previously, it was argued that prophylactic transfusions would increase the total number of transfusions, resulting in increased alloimmunization. However, at least in leukemic patients, there is no convincing relationship between the number of platelet concentrates transfused and the rate of alloimmunization.

There are two approaches to platelet transfusion, prophylactic transfusions and therapeutic transfusions (given only when there is clinical evidence of bleeding).

If procedures such as removal or insertion of Hickman catheters, lumbar punctures, or surgery are performed, platelet transfusions may be given to yield a platelet count of at least 50,000/mm^3. If a patient has experienced an intracranial hemorrhage or some other life-threatening bleeding as a result of thrombocytopenia, correction of the platelet count to at least 50,000/mm^3 is also recommended. Platelet transfusions in thrombotic thrombocytopenic purpura have been associated with acute clinical deterioration, however, and should be used with caution.

Refractoriness to Platelet Transfusions

A consistent lack of response to platelet transfusions is termed *platelet refractoriness*. There are two broad causes of refractoriness, nonimmune and immune. Clinically one can assess the response of a platelet transfusion by measuring the platelet count over time. The post-transfusion platelet response should be calculated on the basis of the patient's body surface area and corrected for the number of platelets transfused. The following formula is used to calculate the corrected count increment:

Clinically one can assess the response of a platelet transfusion by measuring the platelet count over time.

Corrected count increment

$$= \frac{(\text{posttransfusion} - \text{pretransfusion increment}) \times \text{body surface area } (\text{m}^2)}{\text{number of platelets} \times 10^{11}}$$

In general, a successful corrected count increment should be greater than 7,500 within 1 hour of transfusion and greater than 4,500 if measured 18 to 24 hours after transfusion. One important variable in this calculation is the timing of the pretransfusion platelet count; this is not obtained immediately before the transfusion, the value used in the calculation may be misleading.

Nonimmune Platelet Refractoriness

The most frequent nonimmune causes of reduced platelet survival are hypersplenism, fever, infection, and DIC. Little is known about the mechanisms of platelet refractoriness in infected patients. Fever alone, immune complexes, platelet sequestration, antibodies to antimicrobial drugs, adverse side effects, and activation of platelets may all contribute to decreased survival of platelet transfusions in patients with infections. Veno-occlusive disease of the liver is a newly reported cause of platelet refractoriness, particularly in patients undergoing marrow transplantation. This condition is characterized by acute onset of painful hepatomegaly, with postsinusoidal intrahepatic portal hypertension and refractoriness to platelet transfusions.

HLA Antigen Alloimmunization

Alloimmunization to human leukocyte antigens is one of the most important complications of platelet transfusion therapy. This response may contribute to failure to achieve adequate hemostasis, increasing the risk of hemorrhagic death. Alloimmunization may develop in 25 to 50 percent of leukemia patients or patients with solid tumors receiving intensive chemotherapy and multiple transfusions. As many as 80 percent of patients with aplastic anemia may become alloimmunized. Leukemia patients who are undergoing induction chemotherapy and become alloimmunized usually do so by the third week of transfusion support.

Selecting Platelets for the Alloimmunized Patient. If a patient becomes refractory to platelet concentrates and has detectable HLA antibodies, a transfusion of HLA-matched platelets should be given. Since the HLA system is highly polymorphic and platelet donor pools are limited in size, it is not always possible to provide identical HLA matches. As a result, a variety of guidelines to provide potentially

If a patient becomes refractory to platelet concentrates and has detectable HLA antibodies, a transfusion of HLA-matched platelets should be given.

compatible platelets have been developed.[11] Traditional selection guidelines have been as follows:

1. If HLA-identical platelets are unavailable, platelets from donors whose HLA types are serologically cross-reactive with those of the recipient may be substituted.
2. Matching for antigens of the HLA-C locus is not necessary.
3. Mismatching for some HLA-B locus antigens that are weakly expressed on platelets is acceptable for some donor-recipient pairs.
4. If cross-reactive platelets are ineffective for some patients, attention to linked HLA specificities may be important (e.g., BW4/BW6).
5. Although expressed on platelets, ABO matching is less critical than HLA matching.
6. Platelet cross-matching is a valuable adjunct to HLA matching for alloimmune refractory patients.

Other Immune Causes of Platelet Transfusion Refractoriness

Autoimmune Thrombocytopenia. In general, platelet transfusions are not considered of benefit in autoimmune thrombocytopenia. There is little evidence that administration of platelets at the time of splenectomy serves any useful purpose. In the case of life-threatening hemorrhage, platelet transfusions should not be withheld. In many cases good 1-hour platelet recoveries may be achieved and in some patients the transfused platelets even survive until the day after transfusion.[12] Administration of high-dose intravenous γ-globulin may serve to increase the efficacy of platelet transfusions in situations in which there is serious bleeding.

Post-Transfusion Purpura. Patients who are negative for platelet-specific antigens may become alloimmunized to these antigens following transfusion or pregnancy. Following blood transfusions these patients may become profoundly thrombocytopenic and be at risk for life-threatening hemorrhage.[13] Post-transfusion purpura was first described in patients who are P1A1-negative and occurs overwhelmingly in females. Platelet counts characteristically drop abruptly about 1 week after transfusion to levels of less than 10,000/mm^3. If the patient has had invasive procedures, management or prevention of severe bleeding may be required. Platelet transfusions are ineffective even if they lack the offending antigen. A variety of therapeutic approaches, including corticosteroids and plasma exchange, have been tried. It is not clear that either therapy shortens the duration of thrombocytopenia. More recently high-dose intravenous γ-globulin has been used. It appears that with infusion of γ-globulin, platelet counts may increase to more than 50,000/mm^3 within 48 hours.[14]

PLASMA PRODUCTS

A variety of plasma products are available for replacing clotting factors. These include fresh-frozen plasma (FFP), cryoprecipitate, serum immunoglobulin, albumin, and plasma protein fraction. In addition, a variety of purified plasma concentrates are available for the treatment of congenital coagulation deficiency states. These specialized plasma products are covered elsewhere in this text.

Fresh-Frozen Plasma

A unit of FFP has a volume of 200 to 250 ml and contains all the labile and stable plasma constituents if maintained frozen. One unit contains approximately 400 mg of fibrinogen and one unit of other clotting factors per milliliter. Appropriate uses of FFP include massive transfusion with hemorrhage; liver disease with bleeding and multiple coagulation defects uncorrected by vitamin K; emergency reversal of warfarin treatment; DIC and bleeding; and thrombotic thrombocytopenic purpura. FFP is not recommended as a volume expander or as a nutritional source, for correction of coagulation abnormalities in an otherwise stable patient, or for prophylactic administration in routinely transfused patients without documented coagulation abnormalities.

Cryoprecipitate

Cryoprecipitate is prepared from a cold insoluble precipitate of plasma. It contains therapeutic levels of clotting factor VIII (contains both the procoagulant activity and von Willebrand factor), fibrinogen, and clotting factor XIII. Insufficient amounts of the other clotting factors are present to be of therapeutic value. Cryoprecipitate can be used to treat hemophilia A and von Willebrand disease (specific recommendations for its use in these disorders is found in Chapter 1). The amount of fibrinogen present in a bag of cryoprecipitate is approximately 200 mg. For hypofibrinogenemic states, cryoprecipitate can be used for replacement therapy in amounts depending upon the severity of the hypofibrinogemia, with the goal of increasing the fibrinogen concentration to 100 to 150 mg/dl. Fibronectin, an opsonic protein important in promoting phagocytosis, is also present in cryoprecipitate. In some patients with multiple organ failure, fibronectin levels may be low, leading to in creased risk of sepsis. Some investigators have suggested that cryoprecipitate may be of benefit in these patients, but efficiency has not been demonstrated in large-scale clinical studies. Uremic platelet dysfunction may be temporarily corrected by cryoprecipitate infusions. However, the efficacy of cryoprecipitate in uremic bleeding should be considered variable.

Coagulation Factor Concentrates

Factor VIII concentrate is the therapy of choice for hemophilia A patients, since large doses can be delivered in small volumes.

The therapy of patients who require coagulation factor support often requires use of coagulation factor concentrates.[15] Factor VIII concentrate is the therapy of choice for hemophilia A patients, since large doses can be delivered in small volumes. These concentrates were associated with a high risk of hepatitis or transmission of the acquired immunodeficiency syndrome (AIDS) in the past, but recent improvements in the facilitation process, including monoclonal antibody purification or heat inactivation treatment, have substantially reduced these problems. The availability of recombinant factor VIII is expected imminently.

Patients with hemophilia B can be treated with two different concentrates. Factor IX complex concentrate contains high levels of factor IX, factor II, and factor X, with variable levels of factor VII. Since it usually contain therapeutic levels of activated factor VII and factor X, which can bypass the factor VIII requirement in hemophilia A patients, it is often used to treat patients with factor VIII inhibitors. This bypassing activity, however, may also increase the thrombogenic potential of the complex, so factor IX concentrate (devoid of other factors) has recently become available to avoid this complication. Two commercial concentrates are also available, which are intentionally activated during the manufacturing process to attain hemostatic efficiency in patients with factor VIII inhibitors. These concentrates (Autoplex and FEIBA) have been shown to be somewhat better than factor IX complex for patients with these inhibitors. Antithrombin III is available as a concentrate to treat patients with clinical deficiency to prevent thrombosis in surgical procedures. Other concentrates that are currently under investigation include factor XI, von Willebrand factor, protein C, and fibrin glue.

TRANSFUSION REACTIONS TO BLOOD PRODUCTS

Acute reactions may occur on an immune or nonimmune basis. Volume overload may occur in patients who have poor cardiac function or who are in renal failure. These episodes may be prevented by limiting the administration rate and the number of transfusions. Septic transfusion reactions, although relatively uncommon, are seen most commonly with platelet transfusions, since a variety of bacteria may contaminate platelets stored at room temperature. Immunologically mediated transfusion reactions are by far the most frequent type of transfusion reaction. Among patients who have received multiple transfusions, as many as 20 percent may experience a transfusion reaction. The most frequent cause of these transfusion reactions is leukocyte antibodies.

Acute Hemolytic Transfusion Reactions

Most immunologically mediated hemolytic episodes are caused by clerical errors. When a hemolytic reaction is suspected, the transfusion should be stopped and a blood sample sent with the offending unit. If the direct Coombs test and visual inspection of the plasma are negative for hemoglobin, an immune hemolytic transfusion reaction is unlikely. Repeat ABO grouping of the patient and donor blood along with a repeat cross-match should also be performed. If an ABO hemolytic reaction occurs, the patient should be well hydrated to maintain urine output. If the patient becomes hypotensive and is unresponsive to fluids, a vasopressor agent such as dopamine should be given. Nonimmunologic causes of hemolysis can occur with transfusion if the red cells are excessively warmed or if hypotonic solutions are added to the unit of red cells.[16,17]

Leukocyte-Mediated Transfusion Reactions

A transfusion recipient who is immunized to leukocyte antigens may experience fever, chills, and dyspnea. These reactions are frequently more uncomfortable than life-threatening. Since fever may be a manifestation of a hemolytic reaction or a septic transfusion, the transfusion should be stopped and the appropriate samples sent to the laboratory for evaluation. Since a patient experiencing one febrile reaction may not have a second reaction, subsequent transfusions need not be modified until the patient has a second febrile reaction. Leukocyte removal by centrifugation, washing, or filtration may prevent further febrile transfusion reactions.[6]

A more serious leukocyte transfusion reaction may occur if the blood product contains an antileukocyte antibody that reacts with the recipient's leukocytes. In these cases acute noncardiogenic pulmonary edema may develop and may progress rapidly to respiratory failure, requiring aggressive management, including intubation. Tests for antileukocyte antibodies should be made to ensure that the blood donor does not precipitate a similar event in another patient.

Allergic Reactions

Urticarial reactions may occur as a result of hypersensitivity to plasma proteins. Antihistamines may alleviate the symptoms and prevent future allergic reactions. If a patient cannot tolerate antihistamines, washed red cells may prevent these reactions. Anaphylactic reactions may occur, sometimes with the first transfusion, in susceptible patients, usually those who are IgA-deficient and have antibodies to IgA. These patients should receive deglycerolized or repeatedly washed red cells. If plasma products are required, a national IgA deficiency registry, such as that maintained by the American Red Cross should be consulted to obtain plasma products collected from IgA-deficient donors.

References

1. Widmann FK (ed): Technical Manual of the American Association of Blood Banks. 8th Ed. American Association of Blood Banks, Washington, 1981
2. Issitt PD, Issitt CH: Applied Blood Group Serology, 2nd Ed. Spectra Biologicals, Oxnard, CA, 1975
3. Petz LD, Garraty G: Acquired Immune Hemolytic Anemias. Churchill-Livingstone, New York, 1980
4. Conley CL, Lippman SM, Ness PM: Autoimmune hemolytic anemia with reticulocytopenia: a medical emergency. JAMA 244:168, 1980
5. Perioperative red cell transfusion. Natl Inst Health Consensus Dev Conf Consensus Statement 7(4):1, 1988
6. Perkins HA, Payne R, Ferguson J, Wood M: Non-hemolytic febrile transfusion reactions. Quantitative effects of blood components with emphasis on isoantigenic incompatibility of leukocytes. Vox Sang 11:578, 1966
7. Vyas GN, Perkins HA, Fudenberg HH: Anaphylactoid transfusion reaction associated with anti-IgA. Lancet 2:312, 1968
8. Dutcher JP: Platelet transfusion therapy in patients with malignancy. p. 26. In Modern Transfusion Therapy. Vol. 2. CRC Press, Boca Raton, 1990
9. Gaydos LA, Freireich EJ, Mantel N: The quantitative relation between platelet count and hemorrhage in patients with acute leukemia. N Engl J Med 266:905, 1962
10. Solomon J, Bokefkamp T, Fahey J et al: Platelet prophylaxis in acute non-lymphocytic leukemia. Lancet 1:267, 1978
11. Slichter SJ: Platelet transfusions a constantly evolving therapy. Thromb Haemost 66:178, 1991
12. Carr JM, Kruskall MS, Kaye JA, Robinson SH: Efficacy of platelet transfusions in immune thrombocytopenia. Am J Med 80:1051, 1986
13. Shulman NR, Jordan JV: Platelet Immunology. p. 274. In Colman HR, Hirsh J, Marder VJ, Salzman E (eds): Hemostasis and Thrombosis. 1st Ed. JB Lippincott, Philadelphia, 1982
14. Vogelsang G, Kickler TS, Bell WR: Post-transfusion purpura. Am J Hematol 21:259, 1986
15. Bloom A: Progress in the clinical management of hemophilia. Thromb Haemost 66:166, 1991
16. Goldfinger D: Acute hemolytic transfusion reactions—a fresh look at pathogenesis and considerations regarding therapy. Transfusion 17:85, 1977
17. Pineda AA, Brzica SM, Taswell H: Hemolytic transfusion reaction. Mayo Clin Proc 53:378, 1978

7

MASSIVE TRANSFUSION

ALEXANDER P. REINER
WILLIAM R. BELL

Massive transfusion is usually defined as the administration of an amount of blood equal to or greater than the patient's blood volume (about 10 units in an adult) within a 24-hour period. Massive blood transfusion generally occurs in critically ill patients; common clinical settings include trauma, gastrointestinal bleeding, cardiovascular surgery, liver failure, and oncologic and obstetric emergencies.[1] In the setting of trauma, abdominal and pelvic injuries are most commonly associated with massive bleeding.[2] Overall survival in massively transfused patients is in the range of 50 percent and correlates with the presence of pre-existing illness, duration of hypotension, and number of units transfused.[1–5] Survival of patients transfused with over 100 units of blood, however, has been reported.[6,7]

The decision to transfuse a given patient should always reflect the relative benefits and risks of transfusion. In the case of massive hemorrhage, the benefits of blood transfusion are obvious. Prolonged hypotension and tissue hypoxia can result in acidosis, disseminated intravascular coagulation (DIC), organ failure, and death. Since tissue oxygen delivery depends in part on both circulating blood volume and red cell mass, prompt administration of appropriate volume-expanding solutions and red cell components is imperative for restoration of tissue perfusion and oxygenation. Furthermore, since components of the coagulation system may become depleted during massive transfusion, administration of platelet and/or plasma products may be required to maintain adequate hemostasis. Even in the massively bleeding patient, however, the risks associated with the transfusion of homologous blood should not be overlooked. In addition to the generally recognized risks of infectious disease transmission and alloimmunization, massively transfused patients may potentially develop several unique complications. Thus, blood components should be used appropriately and discriminately, and alternatives to homologous blood transfusion should be employed when appropriate.

VOLUME-EXPANDING SOLUTIONS

The initial resuscitation of patients with massive hemorrhage involves infusion of isotonic noncellular volume-expanding solutions; this begins repletion of intravascular volume and electrolytes and also allows time for preparation and transportation of blood products. Either crystalloid or colloid solutions may be used for initial volume replacement. Crystalloid or electrolyte solutions such as normal saline or lactated Ringer's solution are generally preferred because they are less expensive and usually more readily available. Colloid or protein-containing solutions, on the other hand, have higher oncotic activity, produce greater volume expansion, and thus require less volume administration than crystalloid solutions. Despite this theoretical advantage, whether the use of colloid solutions results in a lower frequency of fluid overload and pulmonary edema as compared with crystalloid solutions in massively transfused patients remains controversial (reviewed by Kruskall et al.[8]). When using crystalloid, isotonic solutions are preferred: hypertonic saline may exhibit anticoagulant effects and exacerbate bleeding[9] and hypotonic solutions such as 5 percent dextrose provide inadequate volume expansion and simultaneously hemolyze infused red blood cells and thus should not be administered during massive blood transfusion. If a colloid solution is used, 5 percent albumin is preferred, since rapid administration of plasma protein fraction can produce transient hypotension.[10] Dextran[11] and hydroxyethyl starch[12] may impair hemostasis and thus should be avoided.

As volume replacement therapy is initiated, baseline values of serum electrolytes, arterial blood gases, hematocrit, and coagulation laboratory measurements should be obtained. The patient's blood should be typed and cross-matched, and hemodynamic measurements, including urinary output and central venous pressure, should be determined. These values should be followed closely throughout the course of massive transfusion and the rate and composition of the infused fluid adjusted accordingly.

RED CELL PRODUCTS

Although infusion of isotonic noncellular solutions initiates restoration of intravascular volume, red cell mass must also be replaced to maintain adequate tissue oxygenation. Two types of red cell-containing blood products are generally available: (1) whole blood, which contains about 200 ml of red cells and 250 ml of plasma, and (2) packed red cells, containing about 200 ml of red cells and about 70 ml of residual plasma. Whole blood is preferred in the setting of massive transfusion because repletion of red cells, plasma volume, and clotting factors occurs simultaneously. Packed red blood cells should be used initially during massive transfusion therapy only if whole blood is unavailable or if type O blood is released emergently before the recipient's blood type has been established (see below).

Whole blood is the preferred component in the setting of massive transfusion because repletion of red cells, plasma volume, and clotting factors occurs simultaneously. Packed red blood cells should be used initially during massive transfusion therapy only if whole blood is unavailable or if type O blood is released emergently before the recipient's blood type has been established.

In the setting of elective red cell transfusion, routine serologic testing is performed before blood is released from the blood bank. Ideally, ABO and Rh typing of the patient's red cells, screening the patient's serum for atypical non-ABO red cell antibodies, and cross-match between the donor's red cells and recipient's serum are performed to minimize the risk of hemolytic transfusion reaction. During massive hemorrhage, however, depending on the urgency of the situation, blood may be released before routine pretransfusion testing has been completed. In the case of severe trauma associated with massive blood loss, for example, non-cross-matched group O packed red cells may be released for transfusion even before the recipient's ABO and Rh type have been determined.[13] In this situation group O blood *must* be administered as packed red cells since group O plasma contains anti-A and anti-B isoantibodies, which may cause intravascular hemolysis in group A, B, or AB recipients. In emergency situations in which the patient's Rh type is unknown, group O Rh-negative packed red cells are generally administered. The Rh antibody, anti-D, develops in 50 to 70 percent of Rh-negative individuals who receive Rh-positive blood, and in women of childbearing age, it has the potential to cause hemolytic disease of the newborn in future pregnancies. The development of anti-D in men and older women is of less consequence, and these individuals may require transfusion with group O Rh-positive red cells if the supply of O Rh-negative blood is limited.[14]

In emergency situations, a blood sample should be drawn from the patient before the transfusion of group O red cells so that the patient's blood type and antibody screen can be accurately determined retrospectively. Once the patient's blood type has been determined, the decision to switch the recipient to type-specific blood can be made after a new blood sample is obtained and cross-matched. The decision to switch to a different blood type during or after massive transfusion is based on several factors, including the amount of blood already transfused, the total estimated transfusion requirement, the availability of the particular blood type, and the age and sex of the recipient.

In urgent cases in which the patient's blood type has already been determined, ABO type-specific red cell components may be released before completion of cross-match testing. If a clinically significant non-ABO red cell incompatibility (e.g., Rh, Kell, or Duffy) is subsequently identified upon completion of the cross-match, the patient should be monitored for signs of a hemolytic transfusion reaction, which are generally less severe than ABO hemolytic reactions (see below).

Large amounts of blood can be rapidly infused by using multiple infusion sites, using large-bore (14- to 16-gauge) intravenous catheters, and administration under pressure.[15,16] If necessary, a unit of blood can be administered in less than 5 minutes by using a pressure-cuffed bag. The volume of whole blood or packed red cells transfused should be determined by careful hemodynamic monitoring as well as frequent determinations of the patient's hematocrit value. Once the bleeding source has been controlled, a hematocrit of 25 percent is more than adequate in patients without underlying significant myocardial, vascular, or pulmonary disease.

HEMOSTATIC COMPONENTS

Massively transfused patients may develop platelet and/or coagulation factor abnormalities, which occasionally contribute to bleeding during or after resuscitation.[17–19] Theoretically, the coagulopathy associated with massive transfusion may result from a number of factors. First, infusing large amounts of crystalloid or nonplasma colloid solutions will dilute the patient's own coagulation proteins. Second, stored blood is deficient in certain coagulation components. Blood stored for more than 24 hours at 4°C lacks viable platelets.[20] While the majority of clotting factors are stable during blood storage, coagulation factors V and VIII levels decline during storage. Thus, theoretically a dilutional effect may result from the massive transfusion of whole blood or packed red cells. Finally, coagulation proteins and platelets may be depleted as a direct result of the acute hemorrhage or its complications. Hypotension, acidosis, and tissue hypoxia can cause release of thromboplastin from damaged tissues and lead to the destruction and/or consumption of clotting factors and platelets or disseminated intravascular coagulopathy (DIC).

The development of hemostatic abnormalities and consequent bleeding in the massively transfused patient appears to be related more to the extent of injury (e.g., duration of hypotension and development of DIC) than to a dilutional effect of massive blood replacement.

In practice, the development of hemostatic abnormalities and consequent bleeding in the massively transfused patient appears to be related more to the extent of injury (e.g., duration of hypotension and development of DIC) than to a dilutional effect of massive blood replacement.[21,22] Although development of thrombocytopenia correlates with the volume of transfused blood (platelet counts $< 100{,}000/mm^3$ generally occur after 15 to 20 units of blood), bleeding risk correlates poorly with the severity of thrombocytopenia.[23,24] Moderate coagulation factor deficiencies and mild prolongation of the prothrombin time (PT) or activated partial thromboplastin time (aPTT) are relatively common during massive transfusion, but clotting factor levels correlate poorly with the number of units of blood transfused.[23,25] In addition, coagulation screening tests or clotting factor levels are associated with clinical bleeding only if markedly abnormal.[26] One reason that the platelet count and clotting factor levels are not predictably lowered during massive transfusion is that patients may be able to compensate for the dilutional effects of red cell products by acutely increasing production and/or release of platelets and clotting factors.

On the basis of the above considerations, a rational approach for transfusion of coagulation components in massively bleeding patients can be recommended. Since the development of coagulopathy in massively transfused patients is not purely dilutional, prophylactic transfusion strategies for platelets and clotting factors based on the number of units of red cells or whole blood transfused are not advised.[26,27] Rather, replacement of platelets and clotting factors should be guided by assessment of the type and severity of bleeding as well as by frequent monitoring of coagulation laboratory tests, including platelet count, PT, aPTT, and fibrinogen level.

Prophylactic transfusion strategies for platelets and clotting factors based on the number of units of red cells or whole blood transfused are not advised. Rather, replacement of platelets and clotting factors should be guided by assessment of the type and severity of bleeding as well as by frequent monitoring of coagulation laboratory tests.

Platelet Concentrates

Transfusion of platelet concentrates may be indicated in massively transfused patients to correct quantitative or qualitative platelet abnormalities. Platelet transfusions are required if the platelet count falls below 50,000 to 100,000/mm^3, depending upon the severity and location of the patient's bleeding. Platelet transfusion may also be necessary if a qualitative platelet defect exists (e.g., due to recent aspirin ingestion or to cardiopulmonary bypass), as determined by a bleeding time greater than 10 minutes. In patients who have ingested aspirin within the preceding 7 days, 25 percent of the circulating platelet mass must be replaced with fresh, functional unaltered platelets. The platelet dysfunction associated with cardiopulmonary bypass may last up to 3 to 4 hours following the procedure and can be rapidly assessed by measurement of the bleeding time. When generalized microvascular bleeding occurs in a massively transfused patient and a recent platelet count is not immediately available, platelets should be administered empirically, since thrombocytopenia is the most common cause of nonsurgical microvascular bleeding in this setting.[23,28]

When generalized microvascular bleeding occurs in a massively transfused patient and a recent platelet count is not immediately available, platelets should be administered, as thrombocytopenia is the most common cause of nonsurgical microvascular bleeding in this setting.

Each unit of platelet concentrate contains at least 5.5×10^{10} platelets and about 50 ml of plasma. Platelets are usually administered to adults as pools of four to six platelet concentrates, and each unit of platelet concentrate should raise the platelet count by 5,000 to 10,000/mm^3. The actual platelet count increment may be influenced by other factors in an actively bleeding patient, such as the patient's temperature, spleen size, consumption due to DIC, or ongoing hemorrhage. When administering platelet concentrates, a platelet count should always be obtained pre- and post-transfusion to determine the in vivo response and to guide further replacement therapy.

Coagulation Factor Components

The administration of FFP during massive transfusion should be guided by laboratory evidence of significant clotting factor deficiency (i.e., PT or aPTT > 1.5 times control).

Fresh-frozen plasma (FFP), which is separated from whole blood and frozen following blood collection, contains normal amounts of all coagulation proteins including factor V and factor VIII. FFP is used to replace deficits of coagulation factors in patients with specific underlying coagulation abnormalities such as liver disease or congenital bleeding disorders such as factor IX or factor XI deficiency.[29] FFP may also be required to emergently reverse the effects of warfarin therapy. The administration of FFP during massive transfusion should be guided by laboratory evidence of significant clotting factor deficiency (i.e., PT or aPTT > 1.5 times the control value). Usually, two to six units of FFP are administered depending on the severity of coagulopathy. During massive transfusion, FFP should not be used solely for volume replacement, as exposure to the plasma of additional blood donors unnecessarily increases the risk of viral transmission (see below). It should also be noted that a pool of six platelet concentrates contains the clotting factor equivalent of one to two units of FFP. Thus if platelets are transfused, benefit is derived from the plasma contained in the platelet pool.

DIC should be suspected if the patient exhibits generalized bleeding, thrombocytopenia, hypofibrinogenemia, and elevated fibrinogen-fibrin degradation product titers. If the plasma fibrinogen level falls below 100 mg/dl, 10 to 20 units of cryoprecipitate should be transfused in an adult.

Cryoprecipitate is a clotting factor concentrate made from plasma that specifically contains factor VIII, von Willebrand factor, and fibrinogen. In the massively bleeding patient, cryoprecipitate transfusion may be required for fibrinogen replacement. Hypofibrinogenemia in massively transfused patients usually occurs secondary to liver disease (decreased production) or DIC (degradation). DIC should be suspected if the patient exhibits generalized bleeding, thrombocytopenia, hypofibrinogenemia, and elevated fibrinogen-fibrin degradation product titers. If the plasma fibrinogen level falls below 100 mg/dl, 10 to 20 units of cryoprecipitate should be transfused in an adult. One unit of cryoprecipitate should raise the plasma fibrinogen level by 5 to 7 mg/dl. In DIC, platelet concentrates and/or FFP may also be required as indicated by the measured PT, aPTT, and platelet count, but primary control should be directed toward restoring normal blood volume and tissue oxygenation with red cell components.

During massive transfusion, coagulation screening tests, platelet count, and hematocrit should be followed closely until hemorrhage is adequately controlled. Diffuse, generalized oozing usually results from coagulation system abnormalities. If localized bleeding persists from a site of injury, especially in spite of apparently adequate platelet and coagulation factor replacement, inadequate surgical hemostasis should be strongly suspected as the cause.

ADVERSE EFFECTS OF MASSIVE TRANSFUSION

Several complications are unique to massive transfusion and are due to the biochemical differences between stored blood and circulating blood as well as to the rate and volume of blood transfused. Transfused blood differs from circulating blood in two ways: (1) transfused blood is stored at 4°C in an anticoagulant-preservative solution containing citrate, phosphate, dextrose, and adenine; and (2) biochemical changes occur during storage. These biochemical changes are generally corrected by the recipient during "routine" blood transfusion to correct a chronic anemia. In the massively transfused patient, however, such compensatory mechanisms may be overwhelmed, depending on the rate and volume of transfusion. Massive transfusion-related complications are often attributed solely to abnormalities in the transfused blood. The ultimate effect on a patient, however, depends on the complex interaction of many variables related to the patient's underlying medical condition as well as to the acute problem and its associated complications. Since the adverse effects of massive transfusion cannot be accurately predicted for an individual patient, treatment and prevention of these complications should be guided by frequent monitoring of the patient's hemodynamic and biochemical status.

Transfused blood differs from circulating blood in two ways: (1) transfused blood is stored at 4°C in an anticoagulant-preservative solution containing citrate, phosphate, dextrose, and adenine; and (2) biochemical changes occur during storage.

Potassium Abnormalities

Serum potassium abnormalities commonly occur in massively transfused patients. Stored blood accumulates potassium that is released from red cells into the plasma and can reach levels of approximately 40 mEq/L. Because of this potassium load, a transient hyperkalemia can occur during the rapid administration of stored blood[30,31] but is generally clinically insignificant. For massively transfused patients who may not be able to handle this exogenous potassium (e.g., infants or adults with significant pre-existing renal disease), either relatively fresh blood or washed red cells (which are devoid of plasma) can be used. Rare instances of death due to severe hyperkalemia in massively transfused patients have been reported.[32] Hypokalemia, however, occurs more commonly in the massively transfused patient and may require potassium supplementation. Postulated mechanisms for massive transfusion-related hypokalemia include hypotension, alkalosis, and catecholamine release, causing reentry of potassium into the erythrocytes.[33,34] Since the development of hyperkalemia or hypokalemia is not predictable, serum potassium levels should be carefully monitored in massively transfused patients.

Citrate Toxicity

Blood is stored in citrate, which acts as an anticoagulant by binding calcium and inhibiting the calcium-dependent steps of the coagulation system. Once stored blood is transfused, the citrate is rapidly metabolized by the liver, but citrate-induced hypocalcemia has been considered a potential complication of massive transfusion.[35] Despite extremely low levels of serum calcium in massively transfused patients, however, myocardial and hemostatic function are preserved.[36] In fact, administration of supplemental calcium may produce lethal hypercalcemia.[35,37] Thus, supplemental calcium administration is generally unnecessary in massively transfused adults with normal liver function. For neonates or patients with known liver disease or those undergoing liver transplantation who have impaired citrate metabolism and clotting factor synthesis, administration of supplemental calcium should be guided by serum ionized calcium levels.

Citrate also binds ionized magnesium, and hypomagnesemia has been reported during massive blood transfusion.[38] Magnesium chloride administration may be required as determined by serum magnesium measurements.

Acid-Base Disturbances

Massively transfused patients can exhibit a range of acid-base abnormalities. Initially, metabolic acidosis may occur owing to the acid load of stored blood, as well as to lactic acid produced as a result of tissue injury.[39,40] Metabolic alkalosis can subsequently develop, however, as the citrate and lactate are metabolized to bicarbonate.[30,40] Patients undergoing liver transplantation may be particularly prone to massive transfusion-related acid-base disturbances because of the inability of the newly transplanted liver to metabolize the exogenous citrate.[41]

Restoration of adequate blood volume and tissue perfusion is the most critical factor in correcting metabolic acidosis in massively bleeding patients. Sodium bicarbonate administration should be reserved only for those patients who exhibit profound acidosis by arterial pH determination (i.e., pH < 7.00), which is unresponsive to improved tissue perfusion. Alkalosis increases hemoglobin oxygen affinity and reduces tissue oxygen delivery and thus should be avoided.

Restoration of adequate blood volume and tissue perfusion is the most critical factor in correcting metabolic acidosis in massively bleeding patients. Sodium bicarbonate administration should be reserved only for those patients who exhibit profound acidosis by arterial pH determination (i.e., pH < 7.00), which is unresponsive to improved tissue perfusion.

Hemoglobin Function

Storage of blood reduces the red cell intracellular concentration of 2,3-diphosphoglycerate (2,3-DPG). Like alkalosis, low levels of 2,3-DPG increase hemoglobin oxygen affinity and reduce tissue oxygen delivery. Once blood is transfused, however, 2,3-DPG is rapidly regenerated within about 24 hours.[42] Evidence of an adverse effect from the transfusion of 2,3-DPG-depleted stored blood is equivocal. Maintaining a normal red cell mass is much more important for providing adequate tissue oxygen delivery during massive transfusion than concern about 2,3-DPG levels. The only patients for whom it is desirable to use relatively fresh blood containing normal 2,3-DPG levels are those with severe cardiopulmonary disease, who cannot compensate hemodynamically to increase tissue perfusion and thereby improve oxygen delivery.

Hypothermia

Packed red cells and whole blood are stored at 4°C to decrease erythrocyte metabolism and prevent bacterial growth. The hypothermia resulting from rapid transfusion of large volumes of blood stored at 4°C can produce adverse effects on myocardial function, hemoglobin-oxygen affinity, and citrate and lactate metabolism.[43] In addition, hypothermia can worsen the coagulopathy associated with massive transfusion.[44] The use of blood warming devices can reduce these complications in recipients of massive transfusion.[45] Several mechanical devices are available to warm transfused blood to 37°C[46]; when these devices are used, however, the temperature of the blood must be carefully controlled, because hemolysis can result if blood is warmed much higher than 37°C.

Microembolization

Blood stored at 4°C for over 1 week accumulates microaggregates composed of fragments of platelets, white cells, and fibrin that are too small to be removed by standard 170-μm blood filters. Microembolization of these aggregates may contribute to the development of pulmonary insufficiency in some massively transfused patients. Although 40-μm filters are commonly used to remove these microaggregates, a beneficial effect on pulmonary function has not been conclusively demonstrated in recipients of massive transfusions.[47] Filters of even smaller pore size (10 to 20 μm) are available, but these become obstructed more easily and thus may slow transfusion.

Transfusion Reactions

ABO isoantibodies often cause intravascular hemolysis and complement fixation and can be associated with the life-threatening complications of acute renal failure and DIC; these reactions are therefore the most common cause of acute transfusion-related fatalities.

Homologous blood transfusion can result in a number of immune reactions caused by antigen incompatibility between donor and recipient, the most common of which are febrile nonhemolytic reactions and mild allergic reactions (i.e., hives, pruritis). These relatively benign reactions are caused by antibodies to white blood cells and plasma proteins, respectively, and occur with a frequency of about 1 in 100 transfused units. Much less common but potentially more serious are acute hemolytic transfusion reactions, caused by recipient antibodies to donor red cell antigens. Acute hemolytic reactions are usually caused by ABO isoantibodies and less frequently by atypical red cell antibodies such as anti-D, anti-K, or anti-Jk^{a}. ABO isoantibodies in particular often cause intravascular hemolysis and complement fixation and can be associated with the life-threatening complications of acute renal failure and DIC; these reactions are therefore the most common cause of acute transfusion-related fatalities.[48]

Several aspects of massive transfusion increase the likelihood of an acute hemolytic reaction. Since most ABO incompatibility-related transfusion deaths are caused by errors of patient/donor misidentification,[48] they are more likely to occur in an emergency setting. Furthermore, when group O packed red cells are transfused emergently before the patient's blood type has been determined, there is a slight chance of a high-titer ABO isoantibody in the group O plasma, which may cause significant hemolysis of recipient red cells if the patient is not group O.[49] Finally, in the situation in which ABO type-specific blood is released emergently before the cross-match has been completed, a clinically significant non-ABO antibody may be missed. Fortunately, the likelihood of such non-ABO acute hemolytic reactions is relatively small, since the frequency of clinically significant non-ABO red cell alloantibodies in the general population is about 0.3 percent.[50] In addition, such antibodies (e.g., anti-D, anti-K) usually cause predominantly extravascular hemolysis and do not activate complement, and thus are rarely life-threatening.

Typical signs and symptoms of an acute hemolytic transfusion reaction include fever, chills, flank pain, hypotension, falling hematocrit, hemoglobinemia, and hemoglobinuria. In a critically ill, massively transfused patient, however, these signs may be overlooked or attributed to intercurrent complications of resuscitation or the patient's underlying illness or injury. Thus, if a red cell incompatibility is retrospectively identified upon completion of compatibility testing, the patient's physician should be notified and the patient monitored for signs of an acute hemolytic reaction (i.e., falling hematocrit, renal failure, DIC). The diagnosis may be confirmed by laboratory evidence of hemolysis (hyperbilirubinuria, reduced serum haptoglobin) and/or a positive direct Coombs test.

Transfusion-Transmitted Diseases

The transmission of infectious diseases by blood products is a well recognized complication of transfusion. While viral infections represent the most common complication, transmission of bacteria and parasites can also occur. Although the viral safety of homologous blood components has been improved by a combination of more stringent exclusion criteria for blood donors and improved screening of donor blood for viral markers, a small but finite risk of infectious disease transmission remains. The current risk per unit of blood transfused is conservatively estimated to be approximately 1:200 for hepatitis C, 1:2,000 for hepatitis B, 1:50,000 for human immunodeficiency virus (HIV) and human T-cell leukemia/lymphoma virus I, (HTLVI), and 1:1,000,000 for syphilis.[51] Since the risk of disease transmission is related to the number of units (i.e., number of donors) to which a patient is exposed, proper use of blood components is essential for minimizing these infectious complications in massively transfused patients.

ALTERNATIVE APPROACHES

The complications associated with conventional transfusion therapy and the refusal of some patients to receive homologous blood products on religious grounds have led to the study and development of supplemental or alternative means of repleting intravascular volume and oxygen-carrying capacity in acutely bleeding patients. These alternative approaches include autotransfusion and blood substitutes.

Autotransfusion

Autotransfusion devices are increasingly being used to salvage and reinfuse blood that is lost from the surgical or traumatic bleeding site.[52] These devices have been used primarily during cardiovascular surgery but can be useful in orthopedic surgical patients and massively bleeding trauma patients as well. Transfusion of autologous blood contaminated with bacteria or malignant cells, on the other hand, is contraindicated. Autotransfusion can reduce patient exposure to homologous blood[53,54] and thus presumably reduce the problems of infectious disease transmission and alloimmunization. Devices such as the Haemonetics Cell Saver (Haemonetics Corp., Braintree, MA) wash and remove the plasma from the patient's blood before reinfusion; thus, the potential problem of coagulation factor dilution exists. Other types of autotransfusion devices such as the Autotransfusor (Abbott Laboratories, Chicago), which collect blood by gravity from the surgical site, return red cells, platelets, and all coagulation proteins except fibrinogen to the patient. No anticoagulant is employed with this device. For these reasons coagulation factor depletion is less of a problem than with devices that need to wash cells before infusion into the patient.

Blood Substitutes

Substances that either indirectly increase red cell mass by stimulating erythropoiesis or act as substitute oxygen carriers are potentially useful in patients with massive blood loss who refuse homologous transfusion. Iron dextran, which stimulates erythrocyte production by the bone marrow, can be effective in restoring red cell volume in patients with acute, severe blood loss.[55] A stable, synthetic, nonantigenic blood substitute would be highly desirable in the setting of massive transfusion. One such class of compounds, perfluorocarbons (e.g., Fluosol-DA), has been evaluated in bleeding patients who refuse blood transfusion on religious grounds but was not effective as a substitute oxygen carrier in these patients.[56] Numerous studies in this area to identify a suitable hemoglobin- or nonhemoglobin-based oxygen-carrying substitute are in progress.[57,58]

SUMMARY

The principal objective of massive transfusion therapy is restoration of circulatory volume and red cell mass. This is accomplished by immediate administration of acellular volume-expanding solutions and subsequent administration of red cell products, preferably whole blood. Because depletion of coagulation elements may occur in massively transfused patients, supplemental replacement of platelets and/or coagulation factors may occasionally be necessary. The adverse effects unique to massive transfusion result from the biochemical abnormalities of stored blood but are also influenced by the rate and volume of transfusion as well as the physiologic status of the individual recipient. Thus, the administration of all fluids and blood components in the massively transfused patient should be guided by careful monitoring of laboratory and hemodynamic values. Autotransfusion devices should be used whenever possible to reduce the patient's exposure to homologous blood.

References

1. Sawyer PR, Harrison CR: Massive transfusion in adults: diagnoses, survival and blood bank support. Vox Sang 58:199, 1990
2. Kivioja A, Myllynen P, Rokkanen P: Survival after massive transfusions exceeding four blood volumes in patients with blunt injuries. Am Surg 57:398, 1991
3. Phillips TF, Soulier G, Wilson RF: Outcome of massive transfusion exceeding two blood volumes in trauma and emergency surgery. J Trauma 27:903, 1987
4. Wilson RF, Dulchavsky SA, Soullier G, Beckman B: Problems with 20 or more blood transfusions in 24 hours. Am Surg 53:410, 1987
5. Wudel JH, Morris JA Jr, Yates K et al: Massive transfusion: outcome in blunt trauma patients. J Trauma 31:1, 1991
6. Brotman S, Lamonica C, Cowley RA: Massive transfusion without major complications after trauma. Am J Emerg Med 4:514, 1986
7. Michelsen T, Salmela L, Tigerstedt I et al: Massive blood transfusion: is there a limit? Crit Care Med 17:699, 1989
8. Kruskall MS, Mintz PD, Bergin JJ et al: Transfusion therapy in emergency medicine. Ann Emerg Med 17:327, 1988
9. Reed RL, Johnston TD, Chen Y, Fischer RP: Hypertonic saline alters plasma clotting times and platelet aggregation. J Trauma 31:8, 1991
10. Alving BM, Hojima Y, Pisano JJ et al: Hypotension associated with prekallikrein activator (Hageman-factor fragments) in plasma protein fraction. N Engl J Med 299:66, 1978
11. Strauss RG: Review of the effects of hydroxyethyl starch on the blood coagulation system. Transfusion 21:299, 1981
12. Aberg M, Hedner U, Bergentz SE: Effect of dextran on factor VIII (antihemophilic factor) and platelet function. Ann Surg 189:243, 1979
13. Schwab CW, Shayne JP, Turner J: Immediate trauma resuscitation with type O uncrossmatched blood: a two-year prospective experience. J Trauma 26:897, 1986
14. Schmidt PJ, Leparc GF, Samia CT: Use of Rh positive blood in emergency situations. Surg Gynecol Obstet 167:229, 1988
15. Millikan JS, Cain TL, Hansbrough J: Rapid volume replacement for hypovolemic shock: a comparison of techniques and equipment. J Trauma 24:428, 1984
16. Floccare DJ, Kelen GD, Altman RS et al: Rapid infusion of additive red blood cells: alternative techniques for massive hemorrhage. Ann Emerg Med 19:129, 1990
17. Simmons RL, Collins JA, Heisterkamp CA et al: Coagulation disorders in combat casualties: I. Acute changes after wounding. II. Effects of massive transfusion. III. Post-resuscitative changes. Ann Surg 169:455, 1969
18. Lim RC, Olcott IV C, Robinson AJ, Blaisdell FW: Platelet response and coagulation changes following massive blood replacement. J Trauma 13:577, 1973
19. Mannucci PM, Federici AB, Sirchia G: Hemostasis testing during massive blood replacement: a study of 172 cases. Vox Sang 42:113, 1982
20. Murphy S, Gardner FH: Platelet preservation: effect of storage temperature on maintenance of platelet viability—deleterious effect of refrigerated storage. N Engl J Med 280:1094, 1969
21. Harke H, Rahman S: Haemostatic disorders in massive transfusion. Bibliothca Haematol 46: 179, 1980

22. Hewson JR, Neame PB, Kumar N et al: Coagulopathy related to dilution and hypotension during massive transfusion. Crit Care Med 13:387, 1985
23. Counts RB, Haisch C, Simon TL et al: Hemostasis in massively transfused trauma patients. Ann Surg 190:91, 1979
24. Harrigan C, Lucas CE, Ledgerwood AM et al: Serial changes in primary hemostasis after massive transfusion. Surgery 98:836, 1985
25. Murray DJ, Olson J, Strauss R, Tinker JH: Coagulation changes during packed red cell replacement of major blood loss. Anesthesiology 69:839, 1988
26. Ciavarella D, Reed RL, Counts RB et al: Clotting factor levels and the risk of diffuse microvascular bleeding in the massively transfused patient. Br J Haematol 67:365, 1987
27. Reed RL II, Ciavarella D, Heimbach DM et al: Prophylactic platelet administration during massive transfusion: a prospective, randomized, double-blind clinical study. Ann Surg 203:40, 1986
28. Miller RD, Robbins TO, Tong MJ, Barton SL: Coagulation defects associated with massive blood transfusions. Ann Surg 174:794, 1971
29. Consensus Conference: Fresh-frozen plasma: indications and risks. JAMA 253:551, 1985
30. Linko K, Saxelin I: Electrolyte and acid-base disturbances caused by blood transfusions. Acta Anaesthesiol Scand 30:139, 1986
31. Brown KA, Bissonnette B, MacDonald M, Poon AO: Hyperkalaemia during massive blood transfusion in paediatric craniofacial surgery. Can J Anaesth 37:401, 1990
32. Jameson LC, Popic PM, Harms BA: Hyperkalemic death during use of a high-capacity fluid warmer for massive transfusion. Anesthesiology 73:1050, 1990
33. Carmichael D, Hosty T, Kastl D, Beckman D: Hypokalemia and massive transfusion. South Med J 77:315, 1984
34. Reddy SVG, Sein K: Potassium and massive blood transfusion. Singapore Med J 32:29, 1991
35. Dzik WH, Kirkley SA: Citrate toxicity during massive blood transfusion. Transfusion Med Rev 2:76, 1988
36. Howland WS, Schweizer O, Carlon GC, Goldiner PL: The cardiovascular effects of low levels of ionized calcium during massive transfusion. Surg Gynecol Obstet 145:581, 1977
37. Wolf PL, McCarthy LJ, Hafleigh B: Extreme hypercalcemia following blood transfusion combined with intravenous calcium. Vox Sang 19:544, 1970
38. McLellan BA, Reid SR, Lane PL: Massive blood transfusion causing hypomagnesemia. Crit Care Med 12:146, 1984
39. Howland WS, Schweizer O, Boyan CP: The effect of buffering on the mortality of massive blood replacement. Surg Gynecol Obstet 121:777, 1965
40. Collins JA, Simmons RL, James PM et al: Acid-base status of seriously wounded combat casualties: II. Resuscitation with stored blood. Ann Surg 173:6, 1971
41. Driscoll DF, Bistrian BR, Jenkins RL et al: Development of metabolic alkalosis after massive transfusion during orthotopic liver transplantation. Crit Care Med 15:905, 1987
42. Kopriva CJ, Ratliff JL, Fletcher JR et al: Biochemical and hematological changes associated with massive transfusion of ACD-stored blood in severely injured combat casualties. Ann Surg 176:585, 1972
43. Collins JA: Problems associated with the massive transfusion of stored blood. Surgery 75:274, 1974
44. Ferrara A, MacArthur JD, Wright HK et al: Hypothermia and acidosis worsen coagulopathy in the patient requiring massive transfusion. Am J Surg 160:515, 1990
45. Boyan CP: Cold or warmed blood for massive transfusions. Ann Surg 160:282, 1964
46. Iserson KV, Huestis DW: Blood warming: current applications and techniques. Transfusion 31:558, 1991
47. Durtschi MB, Haisch CE, Reynolds L et al: Effect of micropore filtration on pulmonary function after massive transfusion. Am J Surg 138:8, 1979
48. Sazama K: Reports of 355 transfusion associated deaths: 1976 through 1985. Transfusion 30:583, 1990
49. Inwood MJ, Zuliani B: Anti-A hemolytic transfusion with packed O cells. Ann Intern Med 89:515, 1978
50. Giblett ER: Blood group alloantibodies: an assessment of some laboratory practices. Transfusion 17:299, 1977
51. Sandler SG, Popovsky MA: New technologies for a safer blood supply. Technol Rev p. 23, July 1990

52. Popovsky MA, Devine PA, Taswell HF: Intraoperative autologous transfusion. Mayo Clin Proc 60:125, 1985
53. Giordano GF, Goldman DS, Mammana RB et al: Intraoperative autotransfusion in cardiac operations: effect of intraoperative and postoperative transfusion requirements. J Thorac Cardiovasc Surg 96:382, 1988
54. Bovill DF, Norris TR: The efficacy of intraoperative autologous transfusion in major shoulder surgery. Clin Orthop 240:137, 1989
55. Dudrick SJ, O'Donnell JJ, Raleigh DP et al: Rapid restoration of red blood cell mass in severely anemic surgical patients who refuse transfusion. Arch Surg 120:721, 1985
56. Gould SA, Rosen AL, Sehgal LR et al: Fluosol-DA as a red-cell substitute in acute anemia. N Engl J Med 314:1653, 1986
57. Chang TMS: The use of modified hemoglobin as an oxygen carrying blood substitute. Transfusion Med Rev 3:213, 1989
58. Lowe KC: Synthetic oxygen transport fluids based on perfluorochemicals: applications in medicine and biology. Vox Sang 60:129, 1991

8

COMPLICATIONS OF NEOPLASIA AND THEIR THERAPY

MAURIE MARKMAN

As the incidence of cancer in our population increases and the therapy of a number of malignancies intensifies, the number of patients potentially at risk for the major complications of cancer and its therapy will also increase. It is important that all physicians caring for patients with malignant disease recognize these clinical situations when they develop, as appropriate medical management can result in improved quality of life and survival for the affected individuals.

SUPERIOR VENA CAVA SYNDROME

Pathology and Diagnosis

The superior vena cava (SVC) syndrome is characterized by a number of clinical features, which are outlined in Table 8-1. The syndrome is caused by obstruction to venous return from the upper part of the thorax. The SVC is particularly vulnerable to obstruction, as it is surrounded by the mediastinum, sternum, right mainstem bronchus, and lymph nodes. Tumor involving the lung or lymph nodes in this region can cause increased pressure on the thin-walled SVC and consequent obstruction to blood flow back to the heart. Depending on the rate at which the obstruction develops, collateral circulation may or may not be a prominent feature of the syndrome.

Actual thrombosis of the SVC is observed at autopsy in 30 to 50 percent of patients experiencing the SVC syndrome during life.[1] The presence of a large clot may be a cause of failure of specific antineoplastic therapy to successfully treat the disease process, and this feature should be considered in any patient who does not rapidly improve following the institution of such treatment (see below).

More than 95 percent of cases of the SVC syndrome are

TABLE 8-1. Clinical Features of the Superior Vena Cava Syndrome

Symptom	Incidence (%)
Shortness of breath	50
Chest pain	20
Cough	20
Dysphagia	20
Neck vein distension	60
Thorax vein distension	70
Facial swelling	45
Upper extremity/trunk swelling	40
Cyanosis	15

Malignancy is responsible for 95 percent of cases of the SVC syndrome.

secondary to malignant disease. It should be noted that as recently as the 1950s to the early 1960s, 40 percent of patients presenting with this syndrome were found to have either tuberculosis or syphilis, so it should not immediately be assumed that all cases of the SVC syndrome are due to malignancy. Other rare benign causes of this disease process include fibrosing mediastinitis, granulomatosis infections, goiter, and aortic aneurysms. With the increasing use of semipermanent indwelling central venous catheters to provide venous access in cancer patients (e.g., Hickman, Broviac, subcutaneous portal devices), the incidence of nonmalignant etiologies for the SVC syndrome has increased substantially, and catheter-associated caval thrombosis is currently a frequent cause of the signs and symptoms of the SVC syndrome.

Carcinoma of the lung and lymphomas account for approximately 80 and 15 percent, respectively, of cases of the SVC syndrome. Small cell lung cancer accounts for approximately 50 percent of the SVC syndrome cases due to lung cancer, compared with only 25 percent for lung cancers of the epidermoid type. A possible explanation for the high incidence of small cell lung cancer in patients with SVC syndrome is the fact that the malignancy usually involves the central or perihilar areas of the lung.

In patients with the SVC syndrome the chest radiograph will almost always reveal a mass lesion.

The diagnosis of SVC syndrome is usually suspected on the basis of clinical signs and symptoms. The chest radiograph in a patient with this disease process will almost always reveal the presence of a mass, usually in the mediastinum and most frequently on the right side. Hilar adenopathy and pleural effusions are observed in 50 and 25 percent, respectively, of patients. Further diagnostic evaluation to confirm the presence of the SVC syndrome is usually not necessary. While venograms can demonstrate the precise location of the obstruction, they are relatively contraindicated because of the high venous pressure and the risk of excessive bleeding. This is particularly relevant in a patient with a malignancy-related or treatment-related coagulopathy.

There remains considerable controversy as to how rapidly treatment of a cancer-associated SVC syndrome must be initiated. In the past this condition was considered to be a medical emergency and it was believed treatment had to be initiated as soon as the clinical syndrome was recognized. Unfortunately, as patients with lung cancer or lymphoma frequently experience an SVC syndrome as part of the initial manifestations of their malignancy, such individuals may not actually have a histologic diagnosis of cancer when therapy is contemplated.

In addition, as with the performance of a venogram, risk is associated with biopsy of tissue in the upper chest area in the presence of the SVC syndrome because of significantly increased central venous pressure. In general, in such patients the least invasive method available to confirm the presence of malignancy should be attempted initially. This might include sputum cytology and bronchoscopy with washings and limited biopsies. In approximately 60 percent of patients these procedures lead to the correct diagnosis. If it is necessary to obtain more tissue from a patient with the SVC syndrome, the more superficial lymph nodes (where bleeding can be more easily controlled) should be biopsied initially if they are suspected to be abnormal. Unfortunately, in some cases it may be necessary to perform a mediastinoscopy or thoracotomy to confirm the diagnosis of cancer.

The risk of bleeding following biopsy in a patient with the SVC syndrome is increased because of elevated venous pressure.

Treatment

In specific clinical situations it may be necessary to institute therapy of the SVC syndrome *without* histologic confirmation of the presence of malignancy. In patients with severe respiratory compromise or evidence of central nervous system dysfunction believed to be secondary to this disease process, treatment may be initiated immediately and tissue confirmation sought only when the patient's condition has stabilized.

Therapy of the SVC syndrome is directed at the underlying malignancy. In general, radiation therapy is the standard treatment approach unless the tumor is known to be very sensitive to chemotherapy (e.g., small cell lung cancer). The initial radiation treatment usually involves several large fractions (300 to 400 rads), followed by additional daily treatments at lower doses. The total dose of radiation will depend on the tumor being treated, lymphomas (2,000 to 4,000 rads) being much more sensitive to this form of therapy than lung cancers (5,000 to 6,000 rads). Symptom-

Symptomatic improvement is usually rapid following institution of antineoplastic therapy in patients with the SVC syndrome.

atic improvement following the initiation of therapy is usually fairly rapid, 75 percent of patients noting decreased symptoms within 3 to 4 days of starting treatment and 90 percent experiencing improvement by the end of the first week.[2]

As noted above, in the small patient population (10 percent) who do not exhibit improvement in symptoms within the first week of therapy, a clot should be suspected, and initiation of anticoagulants or fibrinolytic drugs should be considered. Anticoagulation should not be routinely used in all patients with the SVC syndrome, as most patients will respond to antineoplastic therapy and in patients with a friable tumor mass under increased venous pressure, the risk of bleeding may be substantially increased when such treatment is given.

Additional adjunctive therapy in this clinical setting includes diuretics and steroids. In a patient with severe respiratory compromise, diuretics may provide temporary relief of symptoms before the effects of the antineoplastic therapy can be observed. Steroids may be helpful in patients with lymphomas, as they are known to be effective agents against this group of neoplasms, but they are of limited usefulness in individuals with lung cancer except perhaps to reduce any tumor-associated edema that may be contributing to the respiratory compromise.

MALIGNANT PERICARDIAL EFFUSIONS

Pathology and Diagnosis

A number of malignancies may metastasize to the pericardium, including cancers of the lung, breast, and gastrointestinal tract and lymphomas, leukemia, and melanoma. Involvement of the pericardium may occur through hematogenous spread or as a result of direct extension from an adjacent structure (e.g., lung, lymph nodes).

While the development of a malignant pericardial effusion may be gradual and cause few symptoms, patients may present with the sudden onset of dyspnea, orthopnea, cyanosis, and venous distension. Additional signs and symptoms of pericardial involvement with cancer include cough, pain, and hepatic engorgement from venous congestion.

The differential diagnosis of a pericardial effusion in a patient with malignancy includes infection and radiation injury.

The differential diagnosis of a pericardial effusion developing in a patient with known or suspected malignancy includes infection (bacterial, viral, and tuberculosis), uremia, trauma, collagen vascular disease, and radiation-induced injury. If the diagnosis is in doubt, particularly in a patient without prior documentation of the presence of metastatic cancer, pericardiocentesis should be performed and the fluid should be sent for cytologic analysis and culture, as well as being stained for acid-fast organisms.

In a patient who has previously received mediastinal radiation it is often difficult to distinguish radiation pericarditis from pericardial involvement with cancer. While cytology will be helpful if found to be positive, a negative result does not rule out the presence of cancer. Other evidence of cancer involving the lung may provide supplementary information to assist in the differential diagnosis, and a detailed knowledge of the radiation history (i.e., volume radiated and dose delivered) may allow an assessment of whether radiation injury is a likely or unlikely possibility in a particular patient.

Cardiac tamponade results when the amount of fluid in the pericardium is sufficient to cause a decrease in the volume of blood reaching the ventricles. This leads to a decrease in cardiac output, tachycardia, and peripheral vasoconstriction. Thus, the signs and symptoms of this condition resemble those of heart failure. One characteristic feature of cardiac tamponade is the greater than normal (> 10 mmHg) fall in systolic pressure with respiration (pulsus paradoxus). While this physical finding is not unique for tamponade and can be observed in patients with severe myocardial failure, asthma, and hemorrhagic shock, in the patient with cancer it is highly suggestive of cancer-associated cardiac tamponade.

Pulsus paradoxus is a classic feature of cardiac tamponade.

The chest x-ray in patients with cardiac tamponade usually demonstrates cardiomegaly, with the heart often appearing globular in contour. The electrocardiogram (ECG) usually demonstrates only nonspecific changes, although the presence of electrical alternans (alternating high and low voltages of both the P waves and QRS complexes) is felt to be almost pathognomonic for tamponade. Echocardiography can be very helpful in determining if a pericardial effusion and cardiac tamponade are present.

Electrical alternans, although uncommon, is almost pathognomonic for cardiac tamponade.

Treatment

Immediate pericardiocentesis of a volume of only 50 to 100 ml may be life-saving in a patient with a pericardial effusion and evidence of severe cardiac compromise. Unfortunately, the fluid will usually rapidly return unless additional measures are employed to prevent reaccumulation. Several methods have been employed in clinical practice to deal with this problem including the instillation of radioactive compounds (e.g., colloidal gold or colloidal chromic phosphate), talc, antineoplastic agents (e.g., cisplatin, thiotepa, nitrogen mustard), quinacrine, and tetracycline.[3]

It is possible to surgically create a "window" in the pericardium to permit the fluid to leak out of the cavity, but scarring in the region often prevents adequate drainage. More extensive surgery, including pericardiectomy, has been shown to be highly effective in preventing fluid recurrence, but it can rarely be recommended in patients with advanced malignancies.[4,5]

Local external-beam radiation to the heart can be effective in patients who have not previously received radiation to this region and whose tumors are anticipated to be responsive to the relatively low doses of cardiac radiation (maximum doses 2,500 to 3,500 rads) that can be safely administered.

SYNDROME OF INAPPROPRIATE ANTIDIURETIC HORMONE SECRETION

As the name syndrome of inappropriate antidiuretic hormone secretion (SIADH) suggests, malignancy-associated SIADH results when there is an abnormal production of arginine vasopressin, either secondary to secretion from the normal posterior pituitary gland or from the tumor itself. The hallmark of SIADH is hyponatremia, which can be severe. The hyponatremia is caused both by loss of sodium in the urine and by renal water retention.

Pathology and Diagnosis

Small cell carcinoma of the lung is the malignancy most frequently associated with SIADH.

While a number of possible etiologies should be considered when a patient presents with the signs and symptoms of (SIADH), including infection (abscess, tuberculosis, pneumonia) and central nervous system dysfunction (infection, hemorrhage, tumor), malignancy is one of the most common causes. Small cell lung cancer is the tumor type most often implicated as the etiology of malignancy-associated SIADH, as many as 10 percent of patients with this disease being found to have SIADH during the course of their illness.[6] In fact, if water loading tests are performed in small cell lung cancer patients, the incidence of inducible abnormalities in water handling is far greater than the 10 percent incidence of symptomatic disease.[7]

The symptoms of SIADH are due to the low serum sodium and the resulting hypo-osmolar state. Early signs include fatigue, emesis, loss of appetite, and muscle aches. However, when serum sodium levels fall below 100 to 115 mEq/L, more serious effects may develop, including seizures, altered mentation, coma, and death. The severity of symptoms is influenced by the rate of fall in the serum sodium content as well as its absolute value.

The differential diagnosis of a low serum sodium in a cancer patient can be quite complex. Possible etiologies in addition to malignancy-associated SIADH include heart, liver, thyroid, kidney, or adrenal dysfunction; severe emesis or diarrhea leading to excessive loss of sodium, which cannot be compensated by renal retention; and dilutional hyponatremia secondary to excessive water intake without sodium. In addition, several chemotherapeutic agents, including vincristine and cyclophosphamide, commonly used in patients with small cell lung cancer, can cause a SIADH-like clinical picture.

Treatment

Treatment of tumor-associated SIADH should be directed at the underlying malignancy if therapy is available. For example, patients with small cell lung cancer and SIADH can experience rapid resolution of their electrolyte abnormalities after institution of systemic chemotherapy.[6] Patients with serum sodium levels below 128 to 130 mEq/L and mild symptoms (e.g., fatigue, anorexia) may demonstrate significant improvement following moderate restriction in fluid intake (to approximately 500 ml/day).

Patients with more severe symptoms of SIADH, including seizures and significant changes in mental status, should be treated with either normal saline or a 3 percent hypertonic saline infusion to raise the serum sodium level. However, despite the fact the hyponatremia may be responsible for a particular constellation of serious symptoms, the serum sodium level should *not* be permitted to increase more rapidly than 1 mEq/L/h, as more rapid rises have been associated with the development of central pontine myelinolysis.

In patients with severe symptoms of SIADH, serum sodium levels should not be increased more rapidly than 1 mEq/L/h.

Demeclocycline is an additional modality available to treat SIADH that is not responsive to chemotherapy. In a dose-dependent manner the agent causes a reversible nephrogenic diabetes insipidus, which counteracts the effect of vasopressin on the kidney. The recommended dose of demeclocycline when used as treatment of SIADH is 200 mg tid or 300 mg bid; high doses have been shown to be toxic to the kidney.

HYPERCALCEMIA

It has been estimated that as many as 10 percent of all patients with metastatic cancer will develop hypercalcemia during their clinical course. In certain advanced malignancies, including breast and lung cancer, more than 20 percent of patients will experience this complication of their disease.

Pathology and Diagnosis

While a number of pathogenic processes have been documented or hypothesized to be responsible for the development of hypercalcemia in patients with cancer, all mechanisms ultimately result in an increase in bone resorption. Direct infiltration of tumor into bone or secretion of humoral factors resulting in increased calcium egress from bone have been shown to be the most important mechanisms of hypercalcemia in this patient population.

Hypercalcemia can result in dysfunction of a number of organs, the severity of which will be greatly influenced by the absolute level and rate of rise of the serum calcium, the extent of the patient's underlying debility from the malignancy, and the presence of other metabolic abnormalities. Neurologic symptoms can progress from mild lethargy to confusion, stupor, or frank psychosis. Patients can develop polydipsia and polyuria secondary to the effect of calcium on the concentrating function of the renal tubules. Additional symptoms include emesis, anorexia, obstipation, ileus, and abdominal pain.

Treatment

Initial therapy of hypercalcemia requires vigorous saline hydration.

Treatment of hypercalcemia of malignancy begins with the institution of vigorous saline hydration, which results in a decrease in proximal tubular reabsorption of calcium. In general, patients with severe hypercalcemia should receive a minimum of 5 to 7 L of saline over the first 24 hours. Once the patient has been adequately hydrated, furosemide is usually added to the treatment regimen, as this agent increases urinary calcium secretion by blocking reabsorption in the ascending loop of Henle. It is important that the furosemide not be administered until any calcium-induced dehydration is corrected by the saline infusion, as any additional dehydration may further exacerbate symptoms of hypercalcemia.

Hypercalcemia will generally recur rapidly when hydration is discontinued.

In general, saline diuresis is quite successful in lowering the serum calcium level in most patients, but the hypercalcemia will usually recur rapidly once the infusion is discontinued. Thus, addition of an agent which can block bone reabsorption is standard practice in this clinical setting.

Unfortunately, the optimal drug for this purpose has yet to be defined. Drugs that have been demonstrated to be successful in controlling malignancy-associated hypercalcemia include gallium nitrate, mithramycin, and the diphosphonates. Gallium nitrate is delivered by the intravenous route at a dose of 200 mg/m^2/day for 5 days,[8,9] and mithramycin is administered intravenously at a dose of 10 to 25 μg/kg. Therapy can be repeated in less than 1 week if no effect on the serum calcium level is noted. The drug is limited by renal toxicity and bone marrow suppressive effects, particularly thrombocytopenia.

Etidronate disodium can be administered by the intravenous route (7.5 mg/kg/day for up to 7 days).[10] The drug can then be taken orally (20 mg/kg/day) to prevent recurrence of the hypercalcemia. Recently, pamidronate disodium was approved for use in the United States in patients with moderate or severe hypercalcemia of malignancy. The recommended dose is 60 or 90 mg as a single intravenous infusion over 24 hours. It is suggested that patients with severe hypercalcemia receive the 90-mg dose level.

Glucocorticoids can be helpful in patients with hypercalcemia associated with myeloma, lymphoma and breast cancer, but is generally of little value in other malignancies. While salmon calcitonin has been shown to rapidly reduce serum calcium levels, its effect is generally very short-lived, which seriously limits the drug's usefulness.

Effective antineoplastic therapy is the most successful method of maintaining normal serum calcium levels in patients who present with hypercalcemia. Therefore in patients with a tumor that may be responsive to a systemic treatment program, such therapy should be instituted as rapidly as possible. It should be noted that women with breast cancer starting hormonal therapy may actually experience an initial worsening of their hypercalcemia before they demonstrate an antitumor response and subsequent lowering of the serum calcium levels. Thus, breast cancer patients must be carefully observed when hormonal therapy is instituted.

TUMOR LYSIS SYNDROME

Pathology and Diagnosis

The tumor lysis syndrome can present as one of the most emergent events in medicine. While this syndrome can develop spontaneously in patients with bulky tumors, it is usually observed in individuals with large tumor masses who have received chemotherapeutic agents to which their tumor is highly responsive. The rapid tumor lysis overcomes the kidney's ability to handle the intracellular material released from the dying cancer cells. The process is most frequently observed in patients with lymphoma (particularly Burkitt's lymphoma) or leukemia,[11] although it has been seen in patients with small cell lung cancer and metastatic breast cancer.

The syndrome is characterized by hyperkalemia, hyperuricemia, and hyperphosphatemia with hypocalemia, which can lead to renal failure, cardiac arrythmias, and death. It is particularly unfortunate to have a patient die from the tumor lysis syndrome, as the process is the direct result of highly successful initial tumor cell kill.

Management

Prevention of the tumor lysis syndrome is far more successful than treatment of an established process.

The goal of management of the tumor lysis syndrome is prevention, rather than treatment of an established process. Individuals who are at risk for the development of this syndrome (i.e., patients with bulky tumors in whom a rapid response to systemic antineoplastic therapy is anticipated) should undergo vigorous hydration prior to initiation of chemotherapy. The urine should be alkalized, which increases the solubility of uric acid, and allopurinol should be added to the treatment regimen to decrease formation of uric acid. Finally, patients at risk for the development of the tumor lysis syndrome must be carefully monitored for 1 to 2 days following the institution of therapy and must have frequent serum electrolyte determinations (at least twice per day) to find and correct any metabolic abnormalities before they become life-threatening.

NEW SEIZURE DISORDER

Pathology and Diagnosis

The development of a new seizure disorder in a patient with malignancy is a cause of great concern. It has been estimated that as many as 30 percent of patients with cancer metastatic to the brain will experience a seizure as the initial manifestation of the spread of cancer to the central nervous system.[12] However, not all seizures developing in cancer patients will be found to be caused by metastatic disease. As previously noted, patients with metabolic abnormalities, including SIADH, may present with seizures, and it is important to exclude these possibilities when considering an evaluation to find a structural lesion in the brain.

The differential diagnosis of seizures in the patient with malignancy includes metabolic abnormalities as well as structural lesions.

While seizures developing in this clinical setting are initially usually self-limited, they will recur if the abnormality causing the seizure is not rapidly corrected. In such a patient with a known or suspected metastatic or primary malignant lesion in the central nervous system, anticonvulsant therapy should be rapidly initiated. Phenytoin is generally started along with dexamethasone, used to reduce any brain swelling from the cancer.

Unless the patient with cancer is previously known to have a primary brain tumor or cancer metastatic to the brain, a computed tomography (CT) or magnetic resonance imaging (MRI) scan should be obtained on an urgent basis. If structural lesions are documented, local radiation therapy should be initiated as soon as possible to prevent additional seizures or further neurologic deterioration. Such therapy can be of great palliative benefit, although the overall impact on survival duration is limited in most patients with cancer metastatic to the brain.

SPINAL CORD COMPRESSION

Spinal cord compression is one of the most devastating complications of malignancy. This is due to the fact that the process can rapidly convert a highly functional individual with known metastatic cancer into a patient who is bedridden and totally dependent on others for all normal daily activities. Thus, the impact of this disease process on quality of life can be dramatic even if its influence on duration of survival is limited.

Pathology and Diagnosis

As many as 5 percent of patients with metastatic cancer will develop epidural metastasis, the principal mechanism of malignancy-associated spinal cord compression.[13] Cancers of the lung, breast, and prostate are particularly likely to metastasize to the vertebral bodies. Spinal cord compression results when tumor growth impinges on the limited space available to the cord within the spinal column. The thoracic spine is the site of 60 percent of epidural metastases, the remaining cases being equally divided between the lumbar and the cervical spine and sacrum.[13] It should be noted that in approximately 10 percent of documented cases of spinal cord compression, which is most frequent with lymphomas, there is no evidence of vertebral body involvement with tumor. In this clinical situation the mechanism of compression is usually discovered to be growth of tumor present in the paravertebral space through the intravertebral foramen.

Localized back pain is the initial symptom in over 90 percent of patients ultimately found to develop spinal cord compression.[13,14] As the disease process worsens, the pain often becomes radicular in nature, spreading down into the muscle groups and cutaneous regions supplied by the compressed nerves. The importance of documenting the spinal cord compression at the time that patients have back pain as their *only* symptom cannot be overemphasized. Treatment of spinal cord compression at this stage has an excellent (approximately 90 percent) chance of preserving ambulatory function. In contrast, once a serious neurologic defect has become established, fewer than 10 percent of patients will regain significant function despite institution of appropriate therapy.[15]

Early recognition that back pain in a patient with cancer may represent spinal cord compression is a most important factor in preserving ambulatory function.

Thus, a high index of suspicion that back pain in the cancer patient may represent the initial sign of spinal cord compression is the essential first step in the diagnosis of spinal cord compression. Plain bone films can be helpful in the differential diagnosis of back pain in cancer patients. In one series 60 percent of cancer patients with localized back pain and radiographic evidence of vertebral body metastatic disease were found to have myelographic evidence of spinal cord compression.[14] Cord compression was subsequently found in 90 percent of patients with abnormal bone radiographs and symptoms of radiculopathy.

The gold standard for confirming the presence of spinal cord compression is the myelogram, although in many centers it has been replaced by the MRI scan as the diagnostic procedure of choice. When a complete cord block is found on a lumbar myelogram, it is critical that a cervical myelogram be obtained to demonstrate the upper level of the block. This is important in defining the upper limit of the radiation therapy portals.

Treatment

In a patient suspected of having spinal cord compression, high-dose corticosteroid therapy (dexamethasone 100 mg, followed by 4 mg every 6 hours) is initiated. If subsequent evaluation fails to confirm the presence of cord block, the steroids can be tapered rapidly. While somewhat controversial, this high-dose steroid regimen has the advantage of optimizing the rate of reduction of any tumor-induced edema that may be contributing to spinal cord dysfunction and injury. Once the patient's condition has stabilized and definitive treatment (radiation or surgery) has been undertaken, the steroids can be tapered fairly rapidly.

In most circumstances local external-beam radiation therapy is preferred to surgery for initial management of spinal cord compression.

The issue of the optimal method of treating spinal cord compression remains unsettled. However, retrospective reviews have suggested that for most patients the results of local external-beam radiation therapy are equivalent to those of surgery (laminectomy) with less morbidity.[13,15] However, there are several circumstances in which immediate surgery should be the treatment of choice for spinal cord compression. These include the cases of patients who have previously received radiation therapy to the area of block or whose neurologic status deteriorates during or immediately following radiation; patients with tumors that are known to be relatively radioresistant (e.g., renal cell carcinoma); patients without a confirmed diagnosis of metastatic cancer; and patients with either an unstable spine or compression due to radiographically demonstrated compressed bone in the epidural space.

OBSTRUCTIVE UROPATHY

Pathology and Diagnosis

An obstructive uropathy developing in a patient with malignancy can be due to bilateral ureteral obstruction (or unilateral obstruction in a patient with only one functioning kidney) by the cancer or can be secondary to obstruction of the bladder outlet. The most common neoplasms associated with this clinical condition are those involving pelvic organs, including cancers of the cervix, prostate, bladder, ovary, uterus, and colon. In addition, obstruction can be caused by extrinsic compression of the ureters by enlarged retroperitoneal lymph nodes, radiation fibrosis, and hemorrhage.

The simplest and least costly test for diagnosing an obstructive uropathy is renal ultrasound, which will demonstrate a hydronephrotic kidney in the presence of obstruction. The size of the kidney, the extent of hydronephrosis, and the amount of residual renal cortex will be helpful in assessing the potential reversibility of the renal dysfunction. However, renal ultrasound is often not successful in determining the actual site of obstruction. A CT scan or retrograde pyelogram may be required to address this important question. In general, a radionuclide scan of the kidneys provides limited information, but it may be helpful in determining the extent of residual function of an obstructed kidney.

Treatment

When obstructive uropathy is demonstrated, efforts to relieve the obstruction are indicated to preserve renal function.

In the patient with symptoms (e.g., pain) due to renal obstruction or in whom infection is present behind an obstructed ureter or bladder, immediate relief of the obstruction is indicated. Even in the patient with minimal or no symptoms it is important to relieve the obstruction to preserve and improve renal function. It is firmly documented in the medical literature that kidneys that have been completely obstructed for 30 to 60 days can regain function when the obstruction is relieved. Thus, it is inappropriate to ignore the presence of an asymptomatic hydronephrotic kidney simply because it is assumed that the obstruction is not acute.

In approximately 50 percent of patients with obstructive uropathies secondary to cancer, a retrograde ureteral stent can successfully relieve the obstruction. Complications of stent placement include infection, migration into the bladder, and obstruction. If necessary, stents can remain in place for considerable periods of time, although various authors have suggested that the catheters be changed on a schedule of every 2 to 6 months. If antineoplastic therapy (e.g., local radiation) is successful in relieving the obstruction, the stents can be removed.

INFECTIONS—FEBRILE NEUTROPENIA

Infections in the cancer patient can be a direct result of the neoplasm itself or may be a consequence of therapy for the malignancy. Patients with certain malignancies, particularly the lymphomas and leukemias, have a compromised immune status and are more susceptible to a variety of both common and uncommon infectious organisms. Patients with the more common solid tumors can develop infection behind an obstructive lesion, and growth of tumor may lead to breakdown of normal tissue barriers responsible for preventing infection.

Pathology and Diagnosis

The most emergent infectious complications of cancer and its therapy are those associated with the neutropenic state. Prior to the introduction of the present powerful armamentarium of broad-spectrum antibiotics, development of fever in the severely granulocytopenia patient was associated with a high mortality rate. In a now classic paper, Bodey et al. noted that 70 percent of neutropenic patients with *Pseudomonas* sepsis died within 48 hours if appropriate antibiotics were not instituted when fever was first noted.[16] This experience and data presented by others have led to the standard practice of *immediately* instituting broad-spectrum antibiotics in a febrile neutropenic (granulocytes $< 1{,}000/mm^3$) cancer patient, even in the absence of any localizing signs of infection on physical or laboratory examination.

Broad-spectrum antibiotics must be started immediately in the febrile neutropenic patient even in the absence of localizing signs of infection.

Fever in the cancer patient is an excellent warning sign of the presence of infection. Thus, neutropenia itself is not generally considered an indication for institution of antibiotics. However, patients receiving cytotoxic chemotherapy, which may result in severe marrow suppression, must always be warned that *any* fever developing during the vulnerable time period after chemotherapy (generally 7 to 15 days after treatment) must be considered a potentially life-threatening event and that immediate medical attention must be sought. It should be noted that patients taking certain medications, such as aspirin or acetaminophen for pain or steroids for spinal cord compression, may not be capable of mounting the same febrile response as individuals not receiving these medication.

Treatment

It is important that appropriate cultures be taken in the febrile neutropenic patient even if broad-spectrum antibiotics are to be administered, as the subsequent finding of a positive culture may lead to important modifications in the antibiotic regimen.

While the choice of antibiotics as empiric therapy in the febrile neutropenic patient remains somewhat controversial, most authorities continue to recommend an aminoglycoside along with a broad-spectrum penicillin. This regimen will cover most important gram-positive and gram-negative organisms that may infect the patient in this clinical setting.

Perhaps the most controversial question today concerning treatment of these patients is the role of vancomycin in the initial antibiotic regimen. As use of indwelling central venous catheters in the cancer patient population has become common as a method to provide convenient venous access, the incidence of staphylococcal infections in these patients has increased substantially. Many of the organisms are methicillin-resistant and susceptible only to vancomycin. For the febrile neutropenic patient with an indwelling central venous catheter it is reasonable to consider addition of this antibiotic to the empiric regimen, pending the results of blood cultures. If cultures fail to reveal any evidence of staphylococcal infection, vancomycin can be discontinued.

Despite the institution of broad-spectrum antibiotics in the neutropenic patient, many individuals remain febrile. In such patients it has become common practice to administer amphotericin B empirically to treat a suspected but undiagnosed fungal infection. Several autopsy series have documented the high incidence of local and disseminated fungal infections in patients who died following a period of prolonged neutropenia. Rarely were these infections diagnosed during life. While amphotericin B administration is associated with considerable side effects (fever, rigors, renal dysfunction, thrombocytopenia), its value in treating serious fungal infections is well documented; therefore until a less toxic alternative with equal efficacy is available, empiric use of the drug in the persistently febrile neutropenic patient should be strongly considered.[17]

The empiric use of amphotericin B has reduced the mortality from fungal infections in the febrile neutropenic patient.

Granulocyte transfusions have been demonstrated to have a limited role in the management of the neutropenic patient, as it is difficult to deliver an adequate number of cells for a sufficiently long time to affect the course of patients with severe, prolonged neutropenia. However, in the patient with severe granulocytopenia and persistent bacteremia despite administration of appropriate antibiotics, granulocyte transfusions may be life-saving by controlling the infection until the patient's own granulocytes recover.

The granulocyte colony-stimulating factors can reduce the severity of chemotherapy-induced neutropenia.

The bone marrow granulocyte colony-stimulating factor (G-CSF) and granulocyte-macrophage colony-stimulating factor (GM-CSF) appear to have far greater clinical utility than granulocyte transfusions in both treating and preventing chemotherapy-induced neutropenia.[18,19] While experience with these two factors remains limited, it is possible to make several important generalizations concerning their use in this patient population. First, the two agents appear to produce equivalent bone marrow stimulatory effects when used at the recommended doses. Second, both GM-CSF and G-CSF can effectively shorten the duration of chemotherapy-induced neutropenia but cannot prevent it. Thus, patients treated with chemotherapeutic agents known to be associated with severe marrow suppression will continue to be at risk for this side effect of therapy but for fewer days.

As the severity of neutropenia for most standard chemotherapeutic regimens used in clinical practice cannot be predicted in individuals patient, the initial course of treatment should probably be delivered without a stimulating factor. However, if the patient experiences an unacceptable degree of marrow suppression with this first course (e.g., nadir fever, granulocytes $< 1,000/\mu l$), subsequent courses may be delivered with the colony-stimulating factor. An alternative and less costly approach would be to use lower doses of the chemotherapeutic drugs without the bone marrow-stimulating agents.

BLEEDING, THROMBOCYTOPENIA, AND COAGULOPATHIES

Bleeding

Patients with cancer may develop abnormal bleeding secondary to a number of etiologies. Bleeding is common in patients with structural lesions (e.g., hematuria from renal or bladder cancers, melena or guaiac-positive stools from gastrointestinal malignancies). Patients with leukemias may present with bleeding secondary to severe thrombocytopenia or disseminated intravascular coagulopathy (DIC). Treatment of these conditions must focus on therapy of the underlying malignancy, although transfusion support (with packed red cells or platelets) is frequently required.

Thrombocytopenia

Thrombocytopenia is a common side effect of chemotherapeutic agents, particularly combination chemotherapy regimens. Fortunately, severe thrombocytopenia (platelets

< 10,000 to 20,000/μl) is uncommon except with the more intensive treatment programs (e.g., for therapy of acute leukemia or in bone marrow transplantation). However, individual patients may experience unanticipated severe marrow suppression and thrombocytopenia, leading to petechiae and the risk of more serious bleeding, including bleeding from and into vital organs. Prophylactic platelet transfusions are generally reserved for patients whose platelets fall below 10,000 to 20,000/μl. Patients with evidence of bleeding, including those with structural lesions due to the cancer, may need transfusion at a higher absolute peripheral platelet count.

Prophylactic platelet transfusions are generally not administered unless the platelet count falls below 10,000 to 20,000/mm³.

It had been hoped that the bone marrow colony-stimulating factors might prevent cancer- or treatment-induced thrombocytopenia. Unfortunately, as predicted by their activity in experimental systems, neither G-CSF nor GM-CSF has any significant effect on the development of chemotherapy-induced thrombocytopenia.[18,19] Thus, although the severity of neutropenia can be decreased by use of these agents, chemotherapy doses may have to be reduced owing to the potential risk to the patient associated with severe thrombocytopenia. It may be hoped that several of the newer colony-stimulating factors entering clinical trials (e.g., interleukin 3, interleukin 6) or a combination of the factors may effectively stimulate platelet recovery.

It should be noted that several groups have found that *peripheral precursor cells* administered to patients after treatment with high doses of chemotherapy drugs can greatly accelerate platelet recovery as compared with administration of the same drugs without these additional cells. The peripheral precursor cells are harvested from the peripheral blood of the same patient at the time of marrow recovery from a previous high-dose chemotherapy regimen. The yield of these precursor cells with thrombopoietic activity can be further enhanced by administration of one of the colony-stimulating factors. The use of peripheral stem cells, while quite appealing, has limited applicability, as it requires leukapheresis and is very costly and labor-intensive. Thus, this treatment should only be given where there is convincing evidence that an intensive chemotherapy regimen can be more efficacious than an alternative program that does not cause severe thrombocytopenia.

Coagulopathy

Abnormal coagulation is a relatively common complication associated with several malignancies, including cancers of the stomach, prostate, pancreas, lung, and breast.[20] A common feature of a number of these neoplasms is their potential to produce mucin, which presumably may enter the vascular compartment to initiate the coagulation cascade.

The coagulopathy associated with acute promyelocytic leukemia may initially worsen following institution of chemotherapy.

Patients with acute leukemia, particularly acute promyelocytic leukemia, can also present with a coagulopathy, which may initially worsen when treatment is initiated owing to the release of procoagulant material into the systemic compartment. Patients with solid tumors may present with abnormal clot formation (e.g., lower extremity deep venous thrombosis, pulmonary emboli, arterial thrombosis) as an initial or later manifestation of their disease process.

The best treatment for all forms of coagulopathy in the cancer patient is successful therapy of the underlying malignancy. Careful attention must be directed to the difficulties associated with such treatment (e.g., the risk of chemotherapy-induced thrombocytopenia) in a patient with a malignancy-associated coagulopathy. For example, prior to the recognition that DIC is common in patients with acute promyelocytic leukemia, this hematologic malignancy was associated with a particularly poor prognosis. However, with meticulous attention to the short-term bleeding risks in this patient population, long-term survival for patients with acute promyelocytic leukemia now exceeds that of patients with other leukemia subtypes.

References

1. Lokich JJ, Goodman RL: Superior vena cava syndrome. JAMA 231:58, 1975
2. Davenport D, Ferree C, Blade D et al: Radiation therapy in the treatment of superior vena cava obstruction. Cancer 42:2600, 1978
3. Shepherd FA, Morgan C, Evans WK et al: Medical management of malignant pericardial effusion by tetracycline sclerosis. Am J Cardiol 60:1161, 1987
4. Gregory JR, McMurtrey MJ, Mountain CF: A surgical approach to the treatment of pericardial effusion in cancer patients. Am J Clin Oncol 8:319, 1985
5. Alcan KE, Zabetakis PM, Marino ND et al: Management of acute cardiac tamponade by subxiphoid pericardiotomy. JAMA 247:1143, 1982
6. Hainsworth JD, Workman R, Greco FA: Management of the syndrome of inappropriate antidiuretic hormone secretion in small cell lung cancer. Cancer 50:161, 1983
7. Comis RL, Miller M, Ginsberg SJ: Abnormalities in water homeostasis in small cell anaplastic lung cancer. Cancer 45:2414, 1980
8. Warrell RP Jr, Israel R, Frisone M et al: Gallium nitrate for acute treatment of cancer-related hypercalcemia: a randomized, double-blind comparison to calcitonin. Ann Intern Med 108: 669, 1988
9. Warrell RP Jr, Murphy WP, Schulman R et al: A randomized double-blind study of gallium nitrate compared to etidronate for acute control of cancer-related hypercalcemia. J Clin Oncol 9:1467, 1991
10. Jacobs TP, Gordon AC, Silverberg SJ et al: Neoplastic hypercalcemia: physiologic response to intravenous etidronate disodium. Am J Med 82:suppl. 2A, 42, 1987
11. Cohen LF, Balow JE, Magrath IT et al: Acute tumor lysis syndrome: a review of 37 patients with Burkitt's lymphoma. Am J Med 68:486, 1980
12. Posner JB: Management of central nervous system metastases. Semin Oncol 4:81, 1977
13. Posner JB: Back pain and epidural spinal cord compression. Med Clin North Am 71:185, 1987
14. Rodichok LD, Harper GR, Ruckdeschel JC et al: Early diagnosis of spinal epidural metastases. Am J Med 70:1181, 1981

15. Gilbert RW, Kim JH, Posner JB: Epidural spinal cord compression from metastatic tumor: diagnosis and treatment. Ann Neurol 3:40, 1978
16. Bodey GP, Jadeja L, Elting L: Pseudomonas bacteremia: retrospective analysis of 410 episodes. Arch Intern Med 145:1621, 1985
17. The European Organization for the Research and Treatment of Cancer, International Antimicrobial Therapy Cooperative Group: Empiric antifungal therapy in febrile granulocytopenic patients. Am J Med 86:668, 1989
18. Gabrilove JL, Jakubowski A, Scher H et al: Effect of granulocyte colony-stimulating factor on neutropenia and associated morbidity due to chemotherapy for transitional-cell carcinoma of the urothelium. N Engl J Med 381:1414, 1988
19. Antman KS, Griffin JD, Elias A et al: Effect of recombinant human granulocyte-macrophage colony-stimulating factor on chemotherapy-induced myelosuppression. N Engl J Med 319:593, 1988
20. Sack GH Jr, Levin J, Bell WR: Trousseau's syndrome and other manifestations of chronic disseminated coagulopathy in patients with neoplasms. Clinical, pathophysiologic and therapeutic features. Medicine (Baltimore) 56:1, 1977

9

THROMBOTIC THROMBOCYTOPENIC PURPURA–HEMOLYTIC UREMIC SYNDROME

WILLIAM R. BELL

The onset of thrombotic thrombocytopenic purpura (TTP) is unexpected and sudden, arriving in a thunderbolt or avalanche manner, and is unrelentingly devastating in character. During the years immediately following its original description in 1924 by Moschcowitz, [1,2] it was established that this disease process had a 100 percent mortality. In 1955 Gasser[3] sequentially observed five children with the same tetrad of features (severe hemolytic anemia, thrombocytopenic hemorrhage, central nervous system changes, and renal failure) described by Moschcowitz but was seriously impressed by the degree of renal failure. Gasser designated this *hemolytic uremic syndrome* (HUS). Since the mid-1980s as the features of these two disease states have been sufficiently studied in detail, it has been established that the two disorders are the same pathogenetic process, each with slightly different spectra.[4,5]

The diagnosis of TTP-HUS is particularly difficult. The pentad of diagnostic features (thrombocytopenia, hemolytic anemia, central nervous system abnormalities, renal disease, and pyrexia), singly or together, are nonspecific findings. Only when this pentad occurs and no cause can be identified can the diagnosis of TTP-HUS be made. Characteristically and as initially described, this devastatingly destructive disease process suddenly appears in a completely healthy normal person. Within hours to 1 to 2 days, the patient is commonly transformed from a person in excellent health to one who is near death. TTP-HUS is a primary disease entity and is not a malady superimposed on an underlying disease process. Until the etiologic agent(s)

TTP-HUS appears abruptly in previously completely normal healthy individuals as a result of an unidentifiable cause and etiology.

are identified, the diagnosis of this problem remains one of exclusion.

PATHOLOGIC FEATURES

The target organ that is extensively damaged in TTP-HUS is the vascular endothelium and this damage results in thrombi in the microcirculation.

Pathologically, the classic feature associated with TTP-HUS is the presence of hyaline microthrombi, which occlude small arteries and arterioles throughout the body. Moschcowitz believed these lesions to arise from agglutinated red cells[2]; however, Baehr and associates[6] have disputed this theory and suggested that the lesions are formed by fibrin, platelets, and extensive endothelial proliferation. Gore[7] suggested that a subintimal deposit of hyaline material results in damage in the overlying endothelium. He believed that this is the initiating factor leading to vascular occlusion and can result in platelet accumulation, thrombosis, and endothelial proliferation. Orbison[8] noted that involved arterioles frequently demonstrate marked vascular dilation, taking the form of small aneurysms. This observation supported the concept and universally recognized finding that the vascular endothelium is the target organ and the primary pathologic lesion in TTP-HUS.

Hyaline microthrombi are known to consist of fibrin and platelets[6,9,10] and account for the clinical findings and symptoms associated with TTP-HUS. These formations are seen in various stages of organization and generally do not cause complete vascular occlusion of involved vessels. Venules are normally spared.

The two organs relatively spared by the vascular occlusive thrombi are the lungs and liver.

Although TTP-HUS is reported to involve virtually every organ system examined histologically, the lungs[11,12] and liver are often relatively unaffected.[11,13] The pancreas, adrenal glands, myocardium, brain, and kidneys are the most frequently affected organs.[11–14]

Hyaline microthrombi are not pathognomonic for TTP-HUS. Similar lesions have been described in mercury, abrin (phytoxin from *Abrus precatorius* leguminosae) and phenol poisoning, pneumonia, diphtheria and other infectious processes, burns,[2] as well as disseminated intravascular coagulopathy (DIC),[15] leukemia,[16] and malignancies.[17]

DISEASE ENTITIES ASSOCIATED WITH TTP-HUS

Although the precise cause and complete pathogenesis of TTP-HUS remain unknown, a number of widely different diseases have been described as immediately preceding or being concomitantly associated with TTP-HUS.

Obstetric and Gynecologic Disorders

A number of cases reported in the literature identify an association between TTP-HUS and pregnancy or the postpartum period.[11,18–29] As many as 9 percent of TTP-HUS cases may be associated with these conditions,[11] and most cases occur during the third trimester. Some authors believe that this association has been overemphasized because TTP-HUS is known to occur more frequently in young women who coincidentally are in their childbearing years.[23] In addition, this disorder can be confused with immune thrombocytopenic purpura, pre-eclampsia, eclampsia, and HELLP (hemolysis, elevated liver enzymes, low platelet count) syndrome, all evident during pregnancy and with postpartum renal failure.[11,24] Recently my colleagues and I observed an 18-year-old woman who experienced fulminant TTP-HUS during the third to fourth week of pregnancy and who during treatment had a spontaneous abortion. After 14½ months (with normal hematologic studies during the interval) while in the fourth to fifth week of pregnancy she experienced her second bout of fulminant TTP-HUS, and during the remission that followed treatment she again had a spontaneous abortion. This is the only patient in whom we have observed TTP-HUS in the early days of pregnancy.

Some authors believe that in pregnancy the placenta protects the fetus from TTP-HUS because histologic evidence has not been reported in the infant.[23,26,29] Others note that the fetus may have a plasma factor that is missing in the mother with TTP-HUS and is thereby protected. The fetal mortality rate is high,[27] and TTP-HUS remains a serious disorder during pregnancy. Treatment and survival rates are similar to those of nonpregnant individuals.[11,25] More recently immediate evacuation of the uterus has been advocated if other therapies fail.[28]

Infectious Diseases

TTP-HUS is commonly preceded by a prodromal illness often characterized by nonspecific abdominal complaints and has been reported to follow a wide variety of infections. The frequency has been reported to vary between 9 and 40 percent,[11,13] and among the infections implicated are those caused by coxsackie virus B,[30] mycoplasmas,[31] Microtatobiotes,[32] and *Legionella pneumophila,* [33] as well as influenza,[34] herpes simplex,[35] meningococcemia,[36] measles,[37] and nonspecific viral-type upper respiratory tract syndromes.[11]

TTP-HUS is also frequently associated with a preceding infection.[18] Recently, it has been shown that TTP-HUS may be associated with *Campylobacter jejuni*,[38,39] bacillary dysentery,[40] and *Escherichia coli* 0157:H7, an enteric verotoxin-producing pathogen.[41] Although the frequency of this last agent has been high in several reports of patients with this illness,[42] this microbe could not be identified in 71 consecutive patients recently reported.[43] Whether the association between infectious agents and TTP-HUS is more than incidental remains to be determined.

Drugs and Toxins

There has been speculation that TTP-HUS may be induced by drugs, and in a few reports a temporal relation has been observed. Drugs that have been implicated include oral contraceptives,[44–46] sulfa compounds,[47,48] penicillamine,[49–51] procaine and chlorpropamide,[52] iodine,[52] oxophenarsine,[53] and a combination of chloramphenicol and penicillin.[54] Phenytoin has been implicated as causing a syndrome similar to TTP-HUS but not involving microangiopathic hemolytic anemia.[55] These associations with a few different medications have been particularly suggestive when the same medication that was initially associated with the TTP-HUS has been inadvertently reintroduced after an interval of 1 to 2 years and has resulted in another bout of TTP-HUS.

Implicated toxins include chloronapthalene in varnish,[56] carbon monoxide,[57] and poliomyelitis and influenza vaccinations.[58,59] Dog bites and bee stings have also been mentioned as possible toxins.[60,61] In 1991 five patients were reported to have experienced TTP-HUS following treatment with the antiplatelet agent ticlopidine.[62]

Neoplastic Diseases Receiving Cytotoxic Therapy

Microangiopathic red cell hemolysis and thrombosis have been reported in some patients with neoplastic diseases following treatment with cytotoxic agents.[63–69] Following mitomycin therapy, fulminant microangiopathic red cell hemolysis, thrombocytopenia, and pronounced renal failure have been observed in some of these patients. In others slow but progressive renal failure has been noted, with modest abnormalities in red cells, white cells, and platelets.[63,66,67] Similar observations have been reported following chemotherapy with cisplatin in combination with vinblastine, bleomycin, or vindesine.[64,65,69] Small vessel thrombosis has been observed during treatment of acute lymphoblastic leukemia in children with the combination vincristine–prednisone–L-asparaginase.[68]

In the majority of patients with TTP-HUS or TTP-HUS-like illness following chemotherapy, the outcome has been fatal. Plasmapheresis has been helpful in a few such patients.

At our present state of knowledge it would appear reasonable to be cautious in labeling as TTP-HUS victims those patients with devastating neoplasms who are terminally ill and receiving systemic nonspecific cytotoxic drugs. The physician must be aware that TTP-HUS, as originally and subsequently defined, is a severe illness that abruptly occurs in apparently healthy people in whom there is no apparent cause. Patients with systemic neoplastic diseases are frequently seriously ill with high fevers, severe malnutrition, and almost always septic from one—or more frequently multiple—bacterial, fungal, and protozoal organisms. These patients who receive systemic nonspecific cytotoxic therapy superimposed on severe derangement in many if not all metabolic pathways that are catabolically overburdened, later experience several nonspecific features of TTP-HUS. The results of such a complex multitude of problems may give rise to abnormalities that suggest a TTP-HUS-like illness. However, the original and subsequent definitions of TTP-HUS would have to undergo considerable alteration to categorically include these problems, which are directly related to and result from the combination of neoplasms and chemotherapy, as bona fide TTP-HUS. It is instructive to note that when these same cytotoxic drugs are used to treat non-neoplastic disease, TTP-HUS-like illness has not been reported.

Immune-Mediated Diseases

TTP-HUS has been described in association with systemic lupus erythematosus (SLE),[11,13,14,70–73] Sjögren's syndrome,[74] rheumatoid arthritis,[75–77] ankylosing spondylitis,[11] polymyositis,[78] immune thrombocytopenic purpura,[79] polyarteritis,[80] and Graves' disease.[35] Although many authors advance an immunologic basis for TTP-HUS, most of the above-mentioned disorders are only rarely associated with it. SLE is most commonly cited as occurring in patients with TTP-HUS, but in the extensive review by Ridolfi and Bell[11] only three cases of associated SLE were reported. In other series the frequency has been less than 10 percent.[19] Those who support the concept of an immune-related disturbance in TTP-HUS believe that it is probably due to either an immune-mediated vasculopathy or the presence of circulating immune complexes.[18,19]

Miscellaneous Disease Processes

Additional associations between TTP-HUS and other underlying disease processes are noted throughout the literature. Neoplastic disorders,[81,82] including cholangiocarcinoma,[83] giant lymph node hyperplasia,[84] acute myelogenous leukemia,[17] and gastric[17,74,85] and colon[85] adenocarcinoma, have been described.

Infective endocarditis[86] and genetic[87] and congenital[88] factor deficiencies have also been reported. Reports of TTP-HUS occurring in siblings, twins,[89–91] and husbands and wives[92] have been documented. Despite numerous patient reports, it appears that most of these cases are coincidental. Over 90 percent of TTP-HUS cases develop without either an apparent causal event or an underlying disease process.[11]

PATHOGENESIS

Microthrombi observed widely disseminated in the small arterioles and capillaries of patients with TTP-HUS account for most of its clinical manifestations. It has been speculated that platelet consumption during thrombus formation may lead to thrombocytopenia (which, however, is not true) and that the passage of red blood cells through partially occluded vessels with irregular endothelium leads to the microangiopathic hemolytic anemia.[13] Fever may be due to ischemic events in the hypothalamus, and renal and neurologic dysfunction is believed to result from thrombotic occlusions in the kidney and brain.

A number of theories have been advanced to explain the cause of TTP-HUS. Most hypotheses center around platelet aggregation or endothelial injury, but the pathogenesis of TTP-HUS probably involves many different mechanisms.

Byrnes and Lian,[93] Lian and colleagues,[94] and Lian[95] reported finding a platelet aggregating factor (PAF) in the plasma of patients with active TTP-HUS and suggested this as a possible cause. These authors demonstrated that plasma from TTP-HUS patients induced aggregation of autologous and homologous platelets and noted that agglutination was neutralized by preincubation with normal plasma.[93]

The source of the PAF or PAFs remains unknown, but it is probably heterogenous in nature and might represent a normal plasma component[94] or an infectious agent.[96] A platelet agglutinating protein that might contribute to the development of microthrombi has recently been isolated.[97]

Byrnes and Lian[93] earlier speculated that there is a deficiency of a PAF inhibitor in a TTP-HUS patient's plasma. This inhibitor, if present, would normally prevent the platelet aggregation that occurs in TTP-HUS. An inhibitor has been isolated from normal plasma.[98]

Moake and colleagues[99,100] studied patients with chronic relapsing TTP-HUS and found von Willebrand factor multimers larger than those present in normal plasma. These unusually large multimers normally support platelet-related function in hemostasis. In TTP-HUS, however, it is speculated that they decrease or disappear during relapses of the illness and attach to platelets in vivo in the presence of an inciting event such as tissue necrosis, inflammation, or pregnancy.[99–101]

Kelton and associates[12] detected a PAF in the plasma of some patients with known TTP-HUS. They believed that either more than one aggregating factor may be responsible for this disorder or the primary defect could be due to the absence of an inhibitor. In addition, they speculated that platelet agglutination is due to an interaction between the unusually large von Willebrand factor multimers and a platelet agglutinating factor.

Some investigators concluded that the synthesis or activity of prostacyclin, a potent inhibitor of platelet aggregation, may be defective in patients with TTP-HUS.[102–104] Others detected a severe deficiency in circulating prostacyclin by measuring plasma levels of prostaglandin $F_1\alpha$, a metabolite of prostacyclin; following plasma exchange therapy, these levels returned to normal.[105] This is not particularly surprising because the vascular endothelium, the site of prostacyclin synthesis, is the major site of extensive damage in TTP-HUS.

According to Remuzzi and co-workers,[102,103] there may be a missing plasma factor that would normally stimulate vascular prostacyclin activity. If this factor is missing, platelet aggregation may result. Whether this factor deficiency is congenital or acquired is unknown.

Cocchetto et al.[104] indicated that there is a deficiency of prostacyclin, either systemically or at the level of the vascular endothelium. They speculated that this might lead to increased production of thromboxane A_2 (a potent vasoconstrictor responsible for intense vascular spasm) or β-thromboglobulin (which is capable of reducing or inhibiting endogenous prostacyclin production), thereby increasing platelet aggregation or consumption.

Wu and colleagues[106] found abnormal prostacyclin binding in the plasma of patients with TTP-HUS and believed that this could predispose patients to recurrent microangiopathy. Kwaan[107,108] noted that the widely disseminated TTP-HUS lesions are composed mainly of platelets. In TTP-HUS there is an absence of local vascular fibrinolytic activity and a resultant lack of lysis of these microthrombi.

Evidence for immune-mediated vascular injury has included the finding of complement-dependent cytotoxic antibodies (to cultured endothelial cells) in the serum of seven of nine patients with TTP-HUS.[109] Some reports have supported this hypothesis[110,111] although other authors have failed to document the presence of immune complexes.[19,112]

The increased platelet levels of immunoglobulin G[113–115] noted in some reports suggest that the immune system is involved in TTP-HUS, although in other studies none were found.[115] Most recently (in a 1991 report) a cathepsin-like cysteine proteinase has been identified in 11 patients with TTP-HUS.[116] The role of this agent may be very important in this disease process, but additional confirmation is needed.

There is apparently no overwhelming proof that TTP-HUS is immune-mediated. The most compelling argument against an immune-mediated process is the total failure of acute plasma taken from patients in the original hours of illness to initiate or induce any abnormality when transfused into normal recipients.[117–119]

The identification of abnormal substances in the circulating blood or a deficiency of normal components from the blood in patients with TTP-HUS are most likely secondary phenomena.

With respect to the pathogenesis of TTP-HUS, there have been some new observations. Each of these observations is intriguing, instructive, and potentially of considerable importance. However, one must seriously and intellectually discuss whether these observations represent primary events or rather secondary happenings induced by a primary trigger, the precise nature of which remains unidentified and without definition. The information that is currently available supports the idea that these observations—the presence of an aggregating factor, the absence of an inhibitor, unusually large von Willebrand factor molecular multimers, prostacyclin deficiency, complement-dependent cytotoxic antibodies, etc.—are secondary effects which result from the primary devastating insult that represents the key to initiation of the TTP-HUS process. At present this is the great unknown in this disease. It is hoped that further investigation and delineation of these recent observations will lead to identification of the primary initiator in this serious illness.

FREQUENCY AND CLINICAL FEATURES

TTP-HUS is a rare disorder. Ridolfi and Bell[11] noted only one new patient per year over a 25-year interval in a hospital averaging nearly 50,000 admissions annually, whereas Evans and associates[120] noted one patient for as few as 5,000 admissions. Petitt[121] thought the frequency approached one case per 1 million population, whereas others have noted regional outbreaks.[122] In a series of 3,300 consecutive autopsies, only three cases of TTP-HUS were found.[123]

TTP-HUS is seen more frequently in females, who account for as many as 60 to 70 percent of patients.[11,13,124] It is found more often in whites than in blacks,[11] although the survival rate may be lower in the latter.[125] Most cases of TTP-HUS occur between the ages of 10 and 40 years,[11,13] but it has been seen in infants[126] as well as in elderly people.[75] TTP-HUS appears to peak during the third decade of life.[11,13]

The age range of peak frequency for TTP-HUS is the third decade.

The clinical features of TTP-HUS are classically thought of as a pentad, including fever, renal manifestations, neurologic symptoms, thrombocytopenia, and hemolytic anemia.[12,18,127,128] The actual symptoms, however, may be markedly variable, and most patients will have vague, nonspecific complaints, including malaise, fatigue, severe abdominal discomfort, and weakness, which may be present for 2 to 5 days before the patient seeks medical attention.[125] The clinical course most frequently recognized, however, is an acute, fulminant illness in a patient with thrombocytopenia, yielding extensive hemorrhage, focal neurologic disturbances, and hemolytic anemia and rapidly progressing to seizures, coma, and death.[129] Up to 70 percent of patients will have relapses, often during their initial hospitalization in the first month after the diagnosis.[43]

Relapse is common within the first month after the initial diagnosis.

Fever

Fever may not be a presenting feature of TTP-HUS, although it is generally seen at some point during the illness. Temperatures generally range between 37.8° and 38.9°C but can approach 40° to 40.6°C.[13,125] The cause of fever is unknown, but it may be due to tissue necrosis,[13] vascular involvement of the thermoregulatory center in the hypothalamus, release of the products of hemolysis, or endogenous pyrogens.[130,131]

Renal Findings

Renal manifestations are frequently seen with TTP-HUS and include gross or microscopic hematuria, pyruia, proteinuria, abnormal urinary sediment, and elevations of serum urea nitrogen or creatinine.[11,13,18] In one series gross or microscopic hematuria was the most frequent renal abnormality.[11] In others, however, gross hematuria was considered unusual but microscopic hematuria was common.[18] Acute renal failure was noted in 11.5 percent of patients,[11] although chronic renal failure is an uncommon complication.[132] Renal failure is more prominent than other renal effects in TTP-HUS, although some form of renal manifestation was present in 76 to 89 percent of patients with established TTP-HUS.[11,13]

Neurologic Manifestations

The neurologic symptoms of TTP-HUS may be varied and include confusion or mental status changes, headaches, aphasia, syncope, dysarthria, paresis, paresthesias, ataxia, organic brain syndromes, seizures, and coma.[11,13,18,124] In one series the most common neurologic finding was an organic brain syndrome, with paresis, headache, and aphasia noted less frequently.[124] Other studies have reported headache to be a frequent symptom, followed by coma, mental status changes, seizures, and aphasia.[18] Neurologic symptoms are seen in up to 92 percent of patients with TTP-HUS and are usually transient and often recurrent.[13] A rare complication is serous retinal detachment.[133]

Thrombocytopenia

Thrombocytopenia may be severe in patients with TTP-HUS, and in one large series platelet counts below 20,000/mm^3 were noted in 56 percent of patients.[11] Hemorrhagic manifestations are common in this disorder, and bleeding into the skin and mucous membranes, producing petechiae, ecchymoses, and purpura, is frequently noted. Major gastrointestinal and genitourinary hemorrhage may occur, as well as retinal hemorrhage, gross or microscopic hematuria, and conjunctival or mucous membrane bleeding. Epistaxis and hemoptysis are seen less frequently. Antiplatelet antibodies have been documented in a few cases,[113,114] and the bone marrow aspirate typically reveals normal to increased number of megakaryocytes. Salkey et al. noted that if the platelet count is below 25,000/mm^3 the prognosis is poor.[134]

Microangiopathic Hemolytic Anemia

The anemia of TTP-HUS may be quite severe, and the peripheral blood smear typically shows burred cells, helmet cells, schistocytes, nucleated red blood cells, polychromatophilia, and fragmented cells of all varieties to an extreme degree. In 38 percent of patients tested, the hemoglobin level was below 6.5 g/dl.[11] The Coombs test is generally negative,[135] and the bone marrow demonstrates erythroid hyperplasia and pallor and jaundice are frequently seen.[113] Fragmented red blood cells are present and are probably due to mechanical trauma.[136] Reticulocyte counts as high as 19 percent may be seen.[18]

Disseminated intravascular coagulopathy, (DIC), when

present, is always a secondary event in TTP-HUS.[137,138] In one series 88 percent of patients had normal prothrombin times, 94 percent had normal partial thromboplastin times, and 79 percent had normal plasma fibrinogen levels. Only 25 percent of patients in this series had a significant elevation of fibrinogen-fibrin degradation products,[11] whereas in another study this was reported to be as high as 70 percent.[138] Jaffe and co-workers[137] studied 12 patients and found no abnormalities in 6, minimal coagulation abnormalities in 3, and major abnormalities compatible with DIC in 3. They concluded that DIC was not a primary factor in the pathogenesis of TTP-HUS.

Other Laboratory Tests

The serum lactate dehydrogenase (LDH) level is elevated in TTP-HUS, reflecting the presence of red cell hemolysis.[138] A number of authors have recommended monitoring the serum level of LDH;[11,18,139,140] the elevated LDH levels are reported to correlate with prognosis. Others recommended following the ratio of the platelet marker proteins β-thromboglobulin and platelet factor 4 in assessing treatment of TTP-HUS. These proteins, localized in the α-granules of platelets, are released during platelet aggregation.[141]

The unconjugated fraction of bilirubin and the plasma hemoglobin levels are elevated in TTP-HUS, whereas the serum haptoglobin and hemopexin levels are decreased.[11,13] An elevated total bilirubin level has been reported to represent an unfavorable prognosis.[134]

DIAGNOSIS

TTP-HUS should be suspected in any patient with neurologic deficits, fever, renal abnormalities, a Coombs-negative microangiopathic hemolytic anemia, and thrombocytopenia. Its presentation is almost always one of an overwhelming illness, with acute onset or less commonly, a more gradual onset over several days, with any combination of the above-mentioned symptoms. Laboratory findings are nonspecific, although thrombocytopenia and microangiopathic hemolytic anemia should be observed.

Tissue biopsies to demonstrate the characteristic hyaline microthrombi may not be rewarding.[11] Various biopsy sites have been recommended, including spleen, liver, pancreas, kidney, gingiva, skin, lymph nodes,[120] and bone marrow.[10,58,121] According to Berkowitz and colleagues[10] and Petitt,[121] bone marrow is the preferred tissue site if blood vessels are obtained, although Berkowitz et al. frequently examined gingival tissue and bone marrow to increase the yield. Machin[142] recommended gingival or skin biopsies and noted that a petechial lesion should be examined to demonstrate the characteristic vascular lesion.

It must be clearly recognized that the sensitivity of tissue biopsy of the various sites mentioned is considerably less than 30 percent. Because extensive hemorrhage may be present, tissue biopsy cannot be simple, easily, and routinely performed. One is frequently limited to a site that visibly can be compressed mechanically to secure hemostasis. A positive biopsy is helpful, but a negative one does not rule against the diagnosis. In most patients with TTP-HUS, a tissue biopsy is not necessary but may be helpful (if positive) in a complex, confusing situation.

The differential diagnosis of TTP-HUS is varied but frequently includes immune thrombocytopenia purpura, Evans syndrome (autoimmune hemolytic anemia and thrombocytopenia), scleroderma, SLE, autoimmune hemolytic anemia, polyarteritis nodosa, paroxysmal nocturnal hemoglobinuria, purpura fulminans, subacute bacterial endocarditis, nonbacterial thrombotic endocarditis, septic abortion, malignant hypertension, postpartum renal failure, and eclampsia.[11,13,138,143]

Immune thrombocytopenic purpura generally lacks anemia and is dominated by petechial lesions and mucosal hemorrhage. The Coombs test is positive in Evans syndrome and is also frequently positive in SLE. In addition, leukopenia is commonly seen with SLE. With septic abortion or eclampsia it may be difficult to exclude TTP-HUS. DIC is a secondary event, whereas malignant hypertension often overlaps with TTP-HUS.

The most helpful test for diagnosis of TTP-HUS is examination of a peripheral blood film prepared by direct finger puncture, with identification of striking red cell fragmentation, polychromatophilia, spherocytes, and nucleated red cells in the absence of platelets.

TTP-HUS as originally defined remains a diagnosis of exclusion; there is no single clinical sign, feature, or laboratory test that is pathognomonic. Cautious, thorough, and detailed analysis of all the clinical features, peripheral blood film, laboratory data, and tissue biopsy, together with the absence of a recognizable cause, will permit accurate identification of TTP-HUS. The diagnostic line between TTP-HUS, toxemia of pregnancy, pre-eclampsia, eclampsia, the HELLP syndrome (hemolysis, elevated liver enzymes, low platelet count), and postpartum renal failure in some patients may be extremely thin and delicately narrow. In some clinical situations even the wisest and most knowledgeable and seasoned clinicians and scientists (at our present state of knowledge) cannot in truth and certitude diagnostically separate these disease entities. Serologic studies are very helpful in identification of SLE when the presentation is central nervous system/SLE, anemia, thrombocytopenia, and renal failure.

TREATMENT

Because TTP-HUS is a relatively rare disorder, evaluation of therapy is a major and difficult problem. The optimum treatment remains controversial, although a number of different approaches have been advocated. To date no controlled studies have been performed to demonstrate the effectiveness of any one form of therapy. In most centers multiple approaches are employed, including any combination of the following: corticosteroids, plasmapheresis and plasma infusion, antiplatelet agents, splenectomy, immunosuppressive agents, and hemodialysis. If TTP-HUS is untreated, mortality is high, and spontaneous remission has never been reported.[143]

Once TTP-HUS is suspected, intense and unrelenting efforts must be made to establish the diagnosis (see above), and to promptly institute therapy. As experience grows, it is now reasonably obvious that the earliest possible treatment provides the best results, and delay in treatment is more commonly associated with failure in the form of fatality or of residual organ damage if the patient survives.

In the current regimen employed by us, a patient who presents with minimal symptoms and is free of central nervous system abnormalities (except for a mild headache) promptly receives 200 mg of oral prednisone per day, or if there is any evidence of hepatic dysfunction (reduced serum albumin in the presence of adequate nutrition, elevation in hepatic enzymes or prolonged prothrombin time), 200 mg of IV methylprednisone is administered per day. However, a more drastic regimen is used if the patient evidences moderate to severe symptoms, with changes in mental status or other neurologic abnormalities or if there is rapid clinical deterioration with the hematocrit value decreasing below 0.20 (20 percent), the platelet count falling below 10×10^9/L, (10,000/mm^3), the serum lactate dehydrogenase level rising above 600 units/L, or the serum creatinine suddenly increasing above 442 μmol/L (5.0 mg/L). These patients should be treated with 200 mg/day of methylprednisone IV plus daily plasmapheresis and plasma exchange (infusion of 65 to 140 ml fresh-frozen plasma per kilogram of body weight per exchange). It is critically important that if the hematocrit value is below 0.30, the patient should receive packed red cells to elevate the hematocrit value to the 0.20 to 0.25 range before plasmapheresis/exchange is instituted.

Plasmapheresis/exchange should not be instituted if the hematocrit value is below 0.20 (20 percent); red cells should be given to raise the hematocrit value to 0.20 to 0.25, and plasmapheresis can then be performed.

If a patient who was initially treated with corticosteroids alone does not show improvement after 48 hours or before that time experiences any central nervous system abnormalities or shows clinical or laboratory evidence of deterioration, plasmapheresis and plasma exchange are promptly instituted, and the corticosteroids are continued at the same dose.

In those patients treated with corticosteroids alone who improve, when laboratory values recorded for three successive days return to near normal or normal range, the dose of corticosteroids is rapidly reduced to 60 mg/day and then more slowly reduced by 5 mg/week to zero. In patients treated with both steroids and plasmapheresis/exchange, the plasma therapy is discontinued when there is improvement in clinical status and the laboratory values are normal or near normal on two successive days. The dose of corticosteroids is tapered as indicated above. If during the tapering of the corticosteroid dose, the clinical or laboratory status deteriorated, plasmapheresis and plasma exchange are reinstituted promptly, and corticosteroids are increased to the starting dose.

If a given patient does not respond to either corticosteroids or the combination treatment, given either initially or following a relapse, consideration should be given to treatment with intravenous vincristine (1.4 mg per square meter of body surface) not to exceed 2.0 mg on days 1, 4, 7, and 10;[143,144] antiplatelet agents (300 mg aspirin PO q8h plus 100 mg dipyridamole PO q8h; splenectomy; or high-dose intravenous immunoglobulin.[145–156]

It must be emphasized that relapse is common with the present modality of therapy. Relapse is defined as the recurrence of any or all of the following: the initial signs and symptoms, microangiopathic hemolytic anemia, thrombocytopenia, abrupt (more commonly) or slowly progressive deterioration in clinical status, and abrupt (more commonly) or insidious deterioration in laboratory values. In a 1991 study, 69 (64 percent) of 108 patients experienced relapse.[43] In this series 84 percent of the relapses occurred within 30 days of the diagnosis, these relapses being more frequent in females. Two months after initial diagnosis an additional 13 percent relapsed. Relapse after 5 years is extremely rare. In the group of patients who experienced relapse, 72 percent had single relapse, and 28 percent relapsed more than once. In view of the fact that this is the first study of a population of TTP-HUS survivors, more accurate information about relapse, prognosis, and survival awaits definition.

Platelet transfusions should not be given to patients with TTP-HUS because of documented CNS and renal deterioration immediately thereafter.

It is apparent that if at all possible, platelet concentrates should not be infused in patients with TTP-HUS. There is a growing recognition of abrupt, striking deterioration in clinical status (immediate seizures and coma) and increase in the frequency of hemorrhage and renal failure when this type of transfusion is administered.

Discontinuation of the initial intensive therapy is guided

by appropriate daily monitoring of the clinical status of the patient, which should include vital signs, central nervous system function every 6 to 8 hours, hematocrit, white cell count, platelet count, reticulocyte count, and serum levels of urea nitrogen, creatinine, and LDH. A smear of peripheral blood obtained by direct finger puncture should be examined at least once every third day.

Initial therapy should not be decreased or discontinued until the LDH is below 500 units/dl and the hematocrit value and platelet count are progressing toward normal.

Since about the early 1980s there has been a dramatic change in the survival of patients afflicted with TTP-HUS which has risen from zero to over 90 percent at present. At least three important factors have contributed to this impressive improvement in survival: (1) earlier recognition and diagnosis; (2) progressive improvement in general medical care and facilities; and (3) plasma therapy. Simpler treatment that is more readily available is needed. Although several valuable and hopefully important clues have emerged, the most critically important need is to promptly discover the etiology of this devastating disease.

References

1. Moschcowitz E: Hyaline thrombosis of the terminal arterioles and capillaries; a hitherto undescribed disease. Proc N Y Pathol Soc 24:21, 1924
2. Moschcowitz E: An acute febrile pleiochromic anemia with hyaline thrombosis of the terminal arterioles and capillaries. An undescribed disease. Arch Intern Med 36:89, 1925
3. Gasser VC, Gautier E, Steck A et al: Hamolytisch-urämische Syndrome: bilaterale Nierenrindennekrosen bei akuten erworbenen hämolytischen Anämien. Schweiz Med Wochenschr 85: 905, 1955
4. Byrnes JJ, Moake JL: Thrombotic thrombocytopenic purpura and the haemolytic-uraemic syndrome; evolving concepts of pathogenesis and therapy. Clin Haematol 15:413, 1986
5. Remuzzi G: HUS and TTP: variable expression of a single entity. Kidney Int 32:292, 1987
6. Baehr G, Klemperer P, Schifrin A: An acute febrile anemia and thrombocytopenic purpura with diffuse platelet thromboses of capillaries and arterioles. Trans Assoc Am Physicians 51: 43, 1936
7. Gore I: Disseminated arteriolar and capillary platelet thrombosis. A morphologic study of its histogenesis. Am J Pathol 26:155, 1950
8. Orbison JL: Morphology of thrombotic thrombocytopenic purpura with demonstration of aneurysms. Am J Pathol 28:129, 1952
9. Feldman JD, Mardiney MR, Unanue E, Cutting H: The vascular pathology of thrombotic thrombocytopenic purpura. Lab Invest 15:927, 1966
10. Berkowitz LR, Dalldorf FG, Blatt PM: Thrombotic thrombocytopenic purpura. A pathology review. JAMA 241:1709, 1979
11. Ridolfi RL, Bell WR: Thrombotic thrombocytopenic purpura: report of 25 cases and review of the literature. Medicine (Baltimore) 60:413, 1981
12. Kelton JG, Moore J, Santos A, Sheridan D: Detection of a platelet-agglutinating factor in thrombotic thrombocytopenic purpura. Ann Intern Med 101:589, 1984
13. Amorosi EL, Ultmann JE: Thrombotic thrombocytopenic purpura: report of 16 cases and review of the literature. Medicine (Baltimore) 45:139, 1966
14. Barondess JA: Thrombotic thrombocytopenic purpura. Review of the literature and report of three cases. Am J Med 13:294, 1952
15. Robboy SJ, Colman RW, Minna JD: Pathology of disseminated intravascular coagulation (DIC). Hum Pathol 3:327, 1972

16. Husebye KO, Stickney J, Bennett WA: Platelet thrombosis in leukemia. Ann Intern Med 44: 975, 1956
17. Komori R: Thrombotic microangiopathy in patients with malignant tumor. Acta Pathol Jpn 12:379, 1962
18. Bukowski RM: Thrombotic thrombocytopenic purpura: a review. Prog Hemost Thromb 6: 287, 1982
19. Neame PB: Immunologic and other factors in thrombotic thrombocytopenic purpura (TTP). Semin Thromb Hemost 6:416, 1980
20. Yang C, Nussbaum M, Park H: Thrombotic thrombocytopenic purpura in early pregnancy. Remission after plasma exchange. Acta Haematol (Basel) 62:112, 1979
21. Vanderkerchove F, Noens L, Colardyn F et al: Thrombotic thrombocytopenic purpura mimicking toxemia of pregnancy. Am J Obstet Gynecol 150:320, 1984
22. Walker BK, Ballas SK, Martinez J: Plasma infusion for thrombotic thrombocytopenic purpura during pregnancy. Arch Intern Med 140:981, 1980
23. Lian ECY, Byrnes JJ, Harkness DR: Two successful pregnancies in a woman with chronic thrombotic thrombocytopenic purpura treated by plasma infusion. Am J Hematol 16:287, 1984
24. Ambrose A, Welham RT, Cefalo RC: Thrombotic thrombocytopenic purpura in early pregnancy. Obstet Gynecol 66:267, 1985
25. May HV, Harbert GM, Thornton WN: Thrombotic thrombocytopenic purpura associated with pregnancy. Am J Obstet Gynecol 105:452, 1976
26. Upshaw JD, Reidy TJ, Groshart K: Thrombotic thrombocytopenic purpura in pregnancy: response to plasma manipulations. South Med J 78:677, 1985
27. Blakowski SA, Zacharski LR, Telfer MC: Pregnancy complicated by thrombotic thrombocytopenic purpura with fetal sparing. Arch Intern Med 143:2207, 1983
28. Natelson EA, White D: Recurrent thrombotic thrombocytopenic purpura in early pregnancy: effect of uterine evacuation. Obstet Gynecol 66:54S, 1985
29. Wurzel JM: TTP lesions in placenta but not fetus. N Engl J Med 301:503, 1979
30. Berberich FR, Chene SA, Chard RL Jr, Hartman JR: Thrombotic thrombocytopenic purpura: three cases with platelet and fibrinogen survival studies. J Pediatr 84:503, 1974
31. Reynolds PM, Jackson JM, Brine JAS, Vivian AB: Thrombotic thrombocytopenic purpura—remission following splenectomy. Am J Med 61:439, 1976
32. Mettler NE: Isolation of a microtatobiote from patients with hemolytic-uremic syndrome and thrombotic thrombocytopenic purpura and from mites in the United States. N Engl J Med 281:1023, 1969
33. Riggs SA, Wray NP, Waddell CC et al: Thrombotic thrombocytopenic purpura complicating legionnaires' disease. Arch Intern Med 142:2275, 1982
34. Wasserstein A, Hill G, Goldfarb S, Goldberg M: Recurrent thrombotic thrombocytopenic purpura after viral infection. Arch Intern Med 141:685, 1981
35. Myers TJ, Waken CJ, Ball ED, Tremont SJ: Thrombotic thrombocytopenic purpura: combined treatment with plasmapheresis and antiplatelet agents. Ann Intern Med 92:149, 1980
36. Nussbaum M, Dameskek W: Transient hemolytic and thrombocytopenic episode (acute thrombohemolytic thrombocytopenic purpura) with probable meningococcemia. N Engl J Med 256:448, 1957
37. Swaiman KM, Schaffhausen M, Krivit W: Thrombotic thrombocytopenic purpura: report of an unusual clinical case and chromium 51 red cell survival studies. J Pediatr 60:823, 1962
38. Chamovitz BN, Hartstein AI, Alexander SR et al: *Campylobacter jejuni*-associated hemolytic-uremic syndrome in a mother and a daughter. Pediatrics 71:253, 1983
39. Denneberg T, Friedberg M, Holmberg L et al: Combined plasmapheresis and hemodialysis treatment for severe hemolytic-uremic syndrome following Campylobacter colitis. Acta Paediatr Scand 71:243, 1982
40. Date A, Raghopathy P, Jadhau M et al: Outcome of the haemolytic-uremic syndrome complicating bacillary dysentery. Ann Trop Paediatr 2:1, 1982
41. Karmali MA, Steele BT, Petric M, Lim C: Sporadic cases of haemolytic-uraemic syndrome associated with faecal cytotoxin and cytotoxin-producing *Escherichia coli* in stools. Lancet 1: 619, 1983
42. Marshall WF, McLimans CA, Yu PKW: Results of a 6-month survey of stool cultures for *Escherichia coli* 0157:H7. Mayo Clin Proc 65:787, 1990
43. Bell WR, Braine HG, Ness PM, Kickler TS: Improved survival in thrombotic thrombocytopenic purpura–hemolytic uremic syndrome. N Engl J Med 325:398, 1991

44. Vesconi S, Langer M, Rossi E et al: Thrombotic thrombocytopenia purpura during oral contraceptive treatment. Thromb Haemost 40:563, 1978
45. McShane PM, Bern MM, Schiff I: Thrombotic thrombocytopenic purpura associated with oral contraceptive: a case report. Am J Obstet Gynecol 145:762, 1983
46. Holdrinet RSG, Depauw BE, Haanen C: Hormonal dependent thrombotic thrombocytopenic purpura (TTP). Scand J Haematol 30:250, 1983
47. Burke HA Jr, Hartman RC: Thrombotic thrombocytopenic purpura: two patients with remission associated with the use of large amounts of steroids. Arch Intern Med 103:105, 1959
48. Symmers WS: Thrombotic microangiopathy: histological diagnosis during life. Lancet 1:592, 1956
49. Speth PAJ, Boerbooms AM, Holdrinet RSG et al: Thrombotic thrombocytopenic purpura associated with D-penicillamine treatment in rheumatoid arthritis. J Rheumatol 9:812, 1982
50. Ahmed F, Sumalnop V, Spain DM, Tobin MS: Thrombohemolytic thrombocytopenic purpura during penicillamine therapy. Arch Intern Med 138:1292, 1978
51. Symmers WStC: So-called 'collagen diseases' as a manifestation of sensitivity to drugs. Symp Boerhaave Courses (Leyden) 123, 1962
52. Ehrich WE, Seifter J: Thrombotic thrombocytopenic purpura caused by iodine. Arch Pathol Lab Med 47:446, 1949
53. Symmers WC: Thrombotic microangiopathy (thrombotic thrombocytopenic purpura) associated with acute haemorrhagic leucoencephalitis and sensitivity to oxophenarsine. Brain 79: 511, 1956
54. Case records of the Massachusetts General Hospital. N Engl J Med 278:36, 1968
55. Zidar BL, Mendelow H, Winklestein A, Shadduck RK: Diphenylhydantoin-induced serum sickness with fibrin-platelet thrombi in lymph node microvasculature. Am J Med 58:704, 1975
56. Pilz P: Moschcowitz syndrome with involvement of the central nervous system. Virchows Arch [A] 366:59, 1975
57. Stonesifer LD, Bone RC, Hiller FC: Thrombotic thrombocytopenic purpura in carbon monoxide poisoning. Arch Intern Med 140:104, 1980
58. Blecher TE, Raper AB: Early diagnosis of thrombotic microangiopathy by paraffin sections of aspirated bone marrow. Arch Dis Child 42:158, 1967
59. Brown RC, Blecher TE, French EA, Toghill PJ: Thrombotic thrombocytopenic purpura after influenza vaccination. Br Med J 2:303, 1973
60. Mars DR, Knochel JP, Cotton JR, Fuller TJ: Thrombotic thrombocytopenic purpura after a dog bite. South Med J 73:676, 1980
61. Jones MB, Armitage JO, Stone DB: Self-limited TTP-like syndrome after bee sting. JAMA 242: 2212, 1979
62. Page Y, Tandy B, Zeni F et al: Thrombotic thrombocytopenic purpura related to ticlopidine. Lancet 337:774, 1991
63. Gulati SC, Sordillo P, Kempin S et al: Microangiopathic hemolytic-anemia observed after treatment of epidermoid carcinoma with mitomycin C and 5-fluorouracil. Cancer 45:2252, 1980
64. Jackson AM, Rose BD, Graph LG et al: Thrombotic microangiopathy and renal failure associated with antineoplastic chemotherapy. Ann Intern Med 110:41, 1984
65. Harrell RM, Sibley R, Vogelzang NJ: Renal vascular lesions after chemotherapy with vinblastine, bleomycin and cisplatin. Am J Med 73:429, 1982
66. Lyman NW, Michaelson R, Viscuso RL et al: Mitomycin-induced hemolytic-uremic syndrome: successful treatment with corticosteroids and intense plasma exchange. Arch Intern Med 143: 1617, 1983
67. Cantrell JE, Philips TM, Schein PS: Carcinoma-associated hemolytic uremic syndrome: a complication of mitomycin C chemotherapy. J Clin Oncol 3:723, 1985
68. Chesney CM, Pui CH, Weed J, Jackson CW: Apparent role of factor VIII complex in thrombosis during asparaginase-prednisone-vincristine therapy for childhood leukemia. Thromb Haemost 54:139, 1985
69. Licciardello JTW, Moake JL, Rudy CK et al: Elevated plasma von Willebrand factor levels and arterial occlusive complications associated with cisplatin-based chemotherapy. Oncology 42: 296, 1985
70. Biegelman PM: Variants of the platelet thrombosis syndrome and their relationship to disseminated lupus. Arch Pathol Lab Med 51:213, 1951
71. Levine S, Shearn MA: Thrombotic thrombocytopenic purpura and systemic lupus erythematosus. Arch Intern Med 113:826, 1964

72. Dekker A, Obrien ME, Cammarata RJ: The association of thrombotic thrombocytopenic purpura with systemic lupus erythematosus. A report of two cases with successful treatment of one. Am J Med Sci 267:243, 1974
73. Laszlo MH, Alvarez A, Feldman F: The association of thrombotic thrombocytopenic purpura and disseminated lupus erythematosus. Report of a case. Ann Intern Med 42:1308, 1955
74. Steinberg AD, Green WT, Talal N: Thrombotic thrombocytopenic purpura complicating Sjögren's syndrome. JAMA 215:757, 1971
75. Dunea G, Muehrcke RC, Nakamato S, Schwartz FD: Thrombotic thrombocytopenic purpura with acute anuric renal failure. Am J Med 41:1000, 1966
76. Fisher WB: Exchange transfusion in acute thrombosis thrombocytopenic purpura. Case report. Milit Med 142:789, 1977
77. Blackman NS, Cohen BM, Watson J: Thrombotic thrombocytopenic purpura. Report of a case. JAMA 148:546, 1952
78. McLeod BC, Wu KK, Knospe WH: Plasmapheresis in thrombotic thrombocytopenic purpura. Arch Intern Med 140:1059, 1980
79. Stein RS, Flexsner JM: Idiopathic thrombocytopenic purpura during remission of thrombotic thrombocytopenic purpura. South Med J 77:1599, 1984
80. Benitez L, Mathews M, Mallory GK: Platelet thrombosis with polyarteritis nodosa. Arch Pathol 77:116, 1964
81. Brook J, Konwaler BE: Thrombotic thrombocytopenic purpura associated with metastatic gastric carcinoma and a possible autoimmune disorder. West J Med 102:222, 1965
82. Case records of the Massachusetts General Hospital. N Engl J Med 278:1336, 1968
83. Caggiano V, Choseny B, Way LW: Thrombotic thrombocytopenia purpura, cholangiocarcinoma, and oral contraceptives. Lancet 2:365, 1980
84. Couch WD: Giant lymph node hyperplasia associated with thrombotic thrombocytopenic purpura. Am J Clin Pathol 74:342, 1980
85. Kressel BR, Ryan KP, Duong AT et al: Microangiopathic hemolytic anemia, thrombocytopenia, and renal failure in patients treated for adenocarcinoma. Cancer 48:1738, 1981
86. Bayer AS, Theofilopoulos AN, Eisenberg R et al: Thrombotic thrombocytopenic purpura-like syndrome associated with infective endocarditis. JAMA 238:408, 1977
87. Hellman RM, Jackson DV, Buss DH: Thrombotic thrombocytopenic purpura and hemolytic-uremic syndrome in HLA-identical siblings. Ann Intern Med 93:283, 1980
88. Upshaw JD: Congenital deficiency of a factor in normal plasma that reverses microangiopathic hemolysis and thrombocytopenia. N Engl J Med 298:1350, 1978
89. Wallace DC, Lovrich A, Clubb JS, Carseldine DB: Thrombotic thrombocytopenic purpura in four siblings. Am J Med 58:724, 1975
90. Paz RA, Elijovich F, Barcat JA, Sanchez Avalos JC: Fatal simultaneous thrombocytopenic purpura in siblings. Br Med J 4:727, 1969
91. Norkin SA, Freedman HH, Evans GW: Thrombotic thrombocytopenic purpura in siblings. Am J Med 43:294, 1967
92. Watson CG, Cooper WM: Thrombotic thrombocytopenic purpura. Concomitant occurrence in husband and wife. JAMA 215:1821, 1971
93. Byrnes JJ, Lian ECY: Recent therapeutic advances in thrombotic thrombocytopenic purpura. Semin Thromb Hemost 5:199, 1979
94. Lian ECY, Harkness DR, Byrnes JJ et al: Presence of a platelet aggregating factor in plasma of patients with thrombotic thrombocytopenic purpura (TTP) and its inhibition by normal plasma. Blood 53:333, 1979
95. Lian ECY: The role of increased platelet aggregation in TTP. Semin Thromb Hemost 4:401, 1980.
96. Tofflemire EB, Clark WF, Cordy PE et al: Plasma exchange in thrombotic thrombocytopenic purpura. Can Med Assoc J 131:1371, 1984
97. Siddiqui FA, Lian ECY: Novel platelet-agglutinating protein from a thrombotic thrombocytopenic purpura plasma. J Clin Invest 76:1330, 1985
98. Lian ECY, Jui P, Siddiqui FA, Chin LLS: Purification and some properties of a protein obtained from normal human plasma which inhibits the platelet aggregation induced by thrombotic thrombocytopenic purpura plasma. Thromb Res 33:69, 1983
99. Moake JL, Rudy CK, Troll JH et al: Unusually large plasma factor VIII: von Willebrand factor multimers in chronic relapsing thrombotic thrombocytopenic purpura. N Engl J Med 307: 1432, 1982
100. Moake JL, Byrnes JJ, Troll JH et al: Effects of fresh frozen plasma and its cryosupernatant

fraction on von Willebrand factor multimeric forms in chronic relapsing thrombotic thrombocytopenic purpura. Blood 65:1232, 1985
101. Marcus AJ: Moschcowitz revisited, editorial. N Engl J Med 307:1447, 1982
102. Remuzzi G, Misiani R, Marchesi D et al: Haemolytic-uraemic syndrome: deficiency of plasma factor(s) regulating prostacyclin activity? Lancet 21:871, 1978
103. Remuzzi G, Rossi EC, Misiani R et al: Prostacyclin and thrombotic microangiopathy. Semin Thromb Hemost 6:391, 1980
104. Cocchetto DM, Cook L, Cato AE, Niedel JE: Rationale and proposal for use of prostacyclin in thrombotic thrombocytopenic purpura therapy. Semin Thromb Hemost 7:43, 1981
105. Machin SJ, Defreyn G, Chamone DAF, Vermylen J: Plasma 6-keto-PGF1 levels after plasma exchange in thrombotic thrombocytopenic purpura, letter. Lancet 1:661, 1980
106. Wu KK, Hall ER, Rossi EC, Papp AC: Serum prostacyclin binding defects in thrombotic thrombocytopenic purpura. J Clin Invest 75:168, 1985
107. Kwaan HC: The pathogenesis of thrombotic thrombocytopenic purpura. Semin Thromb Hemost 5:184, 1979
108. Kwaan HC: Role of fibrinolysis in thrombotic thrombocytopenic purpura. Semin Thromb Hemost 6:395, 1980
109. Wall RT, Harker LA: The endothelium and thrombosis. Annu Rev Med 31:361, 1980
110. Garvey MB, Freedman J: Complement in thrombotic thrombocytopenic purpura. Am J Hematol 15:397, 1983
111. Meister RJ, Sacher RA, Phillips T: Immune complexes in thrombotic thrombocytopenic purpura. Ann Intern Med 90:717, 1979
112. Celada A, Perrin LH: Circulating immune complexes in thrombotic thrombocytopenic purpura (TTP). Blood 52:855, 1978
113. Morrison J, McMillan R: elevated platelet associated IgG In thrombotic thrombocytopenic purpura. JAMA 238:1944, 1977
114. Sims PJ, Boswell EB: Elevated platelet bound IgG associated with an episode of thrombotic thrombocytopenic purpura. Blood 58:682, 1981
115. Cuttner J, Zaroulis CG, Leiderman IZ et al: Normal platelet associated IgG and undetectable circulating platelet antibodies in thrombotic thrombocytopenic purpura, abstracted. Blood 58: suppl. 1, 192a, 1981
116. Falanga A, Consonni R, Ruggenenti P, Barbiro T: A cathepsin-like cysteine proteinase proaggregating activity in thrombotic thrombocytopenic purpura. Br J Haematol 79:474, 1991
117. Adelson E, Heitzman EJ, Fennessey JF: Thrombohemolytic thrombocytopenic purpura. Arch Intern Med 94:42, 1954
118. Brittingham TE, Chaplin H: Attempted passive transfer of thrombotic thrombocytopenic purpura. Blood 12:480, 1957
119. Stemerman MB: Thrombotic thrombocytopenic purpura. Med Grand Rounds 1:48, 1982
120. Evans TL, Winkelstein A, Zeigler ZR et al: Thrombotic thrombocytopenic purpura: clinical course and response to therapy in eight patients. Am J Hematol 17:401, 1984
121. Petitt RM: Thrombotic thrombocytopenic purpura: a thirty year review. Semin Thromb Hemost 6:350, 1980
122. Crowley JP, Zaroulis CG, O'Shea PE, Clark DD: Thrombotic thrombocytopenic purpura in southeastern New England. Arch Intern Med 143:1011, 1983
123. Fossgreen J: Thrombostisk thrombocytopenisk purpura. Nord Med 67:51, 1962
124. Cuttner J: Thrombotic thrombocytopenic purpura: a ten year experience. Blood 56:302, 1980
125. Kennedy SS, Zacharski LR, Beck JR: Thrombotic thrombocytopenic purpura. Analysis of 48 unselected cases. Semin Thromb Hemost 6:341, 1980
126. Monnens LAH, Retera RJM: Thrombotic thrombocytopenic purpura in a neonatal infant. J Pediatr 71:118, 1967
127. Lukes RJ, Rath CE, Steussy CN, Mailliard J: Thrombotic thrombocytopenic purpura—clinical and pathologic findings in 49 cases, abstracted. Blood 17:336, 1961
128. Kulkarni GA, Pellegrini JR, Nathanson L: Thrombotic thrombocytopenic purpura. Am Fam Physician 31:141, 1985
129. Pisciotta AV, Gottschall JL: Clinical features of thrombotic thrombocytopenic purpura. Semin Thromb Hemost 6:330, 1980
130. Clinicopathologic conference: Thrombotic thrombocytopenic purpura. Am J Med 27:115, 1959
131. Snell ES, Goodale F Jr, Wendt F, Cranston WI: Properties of human endogenous pyrogen. Clin Sci 16:615, 1957

132. Rooney JC, Anderson RM, Hopkins IJ: Clinical and pathological aspects of central nervous system involvement in the haemolytic uraemic syndrome. Aust Paediatr J 7:28, 1971
133. Lambert SR, High KA, Cotlier E, Benz EJ Jr: Serous retinal detachments in thrombotic thrombocytopenic purpura. Arch Ophthalmol 103:1172, 1985
134. Salkey BA, Kreel I, Gelernt IM et al: Splenectomy for thrombotic thrombocytopenic purpura. Mt Sinai J Med (NY) 50:56, 1983
135. Deuel T, Gardner F, Peck WA, Avioli LV: Thrombotic thrombocytopenic purpura. Arch Intern Med 140:93, 1980
136. Monroe WM, Strauss AF: Intravascular hemolysis: a morphologic study of schizocytes in thrombotic thrombocytopenic purpura and other diseases. South Med J 46:837, 1953
137. Jaffe EA, Nachman RL, Merskey C: Thrombotic thrombocytopenic purpura—coagulation parameters in twelve patients. Blood 42:499, 1973
138. Nalbandian RM, Henry RL, Bick RL: Thrombotic thrombocytopenic purpura: an extended editorial. Semin Thromb Hemost 5:216, 1979
139. Taft EG: thrombotic thrombocytopenic purpura and dose of plasma exchange. Blood 54:842, 1979
140. Crowley JP, Metzger JB, L'Europa RA: The blood counts and lactate dehydrogenase levels in thrombotic thrombocytopenic purpura (TTP). Am J Clin Pathol 80:700, 1983
141. McRoyan DK, Daniel SJ, Liu PI: Beta-thromboglobulin and platelet factor 4 levels in a case of acute thrombotic thrombocytopenic purpura. South Med J 78:745, 1985
142. Machin SJ: Thrombotic thrombocytopenic purpura. Br J Haematol 56:191, 1984
143. Gutterman LA, Stevenson TD: Treatment of thrombotic thrombocytopenic purpura with vincristine. JAMA 247:1433, 1982
144. Gutterman L: Treatment of thrombotic thrombocytopenic purpura (ITP) with exchange plasmapheresis (EP), vincristine (VCR), and methylprednisolone (MP): a standardized initial treatment in 11 patients, abstracted. Blood 76:suppl. 1, 509a, 1990
145. Gilscher RO: Refractory TTP responding to IV gammaglobulin, abstracted. Blood 64:suppl 1, 237a, 1984
146. Krishnamurthy M, Bellevue R, Lian E et al: Intravenous immunoglobulin in thrombotic thrombocytopenic purpura—a new mode of treatment, abstracted. Blood 66:suppl. 1, 291a, 1985
147. Messmore HL, Yeshwant C, Remlinger K, Seghatchian MJ: Intravenous gamma globulin in refractory thrombotic thrombocytopenic purpura (TTP). Thromb Haemost 54:127, 1985
148. Viero P, Cortelazzo S, Buelli M et al: Thrombotic thrombocytopenic purpura and high-dose immunoglobulin treatment. Ann Intern Med 104:228, 1986
149. Wong P, Itoh K, Yoshida S: Treatment of thrombotic thrombocytopenic purpura with intravenous gamma globulin. N Engl J Med 314:385, 1986
150. Keltin JG, Moore JC, Murphy WG: Studies investigating platelet aggregation and release initiated by sera from patients with thrombotic thrombocytopenic purpura. Blood 69:924, 1987
151. Finn NG, Wang JC, Hong KJ: High-dose intravenous gamma-immunoglobulin infusion in the treatment of thrombotic thrombocytopenic purpura. Arch Intern Med 147:2165, 1987
152. Chin D, Chyczij H, Etches W et al: Treatment of thrombotic thrombocytopenic purpura with intravenous gammaglobulin. Transfusion 27:115, 1987
153. Siddiqui FA, Lian EYC: Platelet-agglutinating protein P37 from a thrombotic thrombocytopenic purpura plasma forms a complex with human immunoglobulin G. Blood 71:299, 1988
154. Schmidt JL: Thrombotic thrombocytopenic purpura: successful treatment unlocks etiologic secrets. Mayo Clin Proc 64:956, 1989
155. Heyman MR, Sweet T: Thrombotic thrombocytopenic purpura treated with high-dose intravenous gamma globulin. South Med J 83:1471, 1990
156. Raniele DP, Opsahl JA, Gensen NJ et al: Treatment of thrombotic thrombocytopenic purpura (TTP) with intravenous immunoglobulin G (IgG): 88% response rate. p. 90. In International Society For Blood Transfusion and American Association of Blood Banks Abstracts. Vol. 1. American Association of Blood Banks, Arlington, VA, 1990

10

PLASMAPHERESIS

HAYDEN G. BRAINE
R. BEN DAWSON

Hemapheresis, the therapeutic process of removing fractions of whole blood, can involve the removal of cellular fractions (cytapheresis) or removal of plasma (plasmapheresis). When the process involves not only the removal of plasma but its replacement with biologically active plasma, the procedure is called *plasma exchange*. These technologies have evolved rapidly since the early 1970s and become an essential part of our management of many hematologic and oncologic problems.

The first organized study of plasmapheresis was published in 1914 by Abel and co-workers.[1] In their classic studies they explored techniques of managing the metabolic abnormalities of experimental anephric dogs. Although they identified dialysis as a superior methodology, their work with plasmapheresis led them to feel that this technology could be used to harvest antisera prepared in horses. With the development of physiologic anticoagulants and biocompatible containers, single-unit manual plasmapheresis became feasible in the late 1940s. To facilitate the collection of larger volumes of plasma, the technologies developed for the continuous separation of cream from milk by the dairy industry were applied by E. J. Cohn to the separation of plasma from whole blood.[2] By the mid-1960s, this technology had evolved to the point that there were two clinically available systems (the Latham bowl and the NCI-IBM Cell Separator)[3,4] capable of fractionating large volumes of whole blood into plasma, leukocyte, platelet, and red cell fractions. Over the next 20 years these technologies were refined and developed.

PHYSIOLOGIC MODELING OF PLASMAPHERESIS AND CYTAPHERESIS

Hemapheresis offers the clinician the possibility of acutely removing large quantities of intravascular components. However, materials in the intravascular compartment are in equilibrium with the extravascular compartment, and their total body concentration is a balance between synthesis and catabolism. Thus the effectiveness of hemapheresis in depleting total body stores of various materials varies with synthetic rate, catabolic rate, intravascular and extravascular distribution, and rate of movement between these two compartments. In making rational decisions with regard to the volume of material removed with each plasmapheresis, the frequency of plasmapheresis procedures, and the overall number of procedures, one must consider not only the physiologic parameters but also the acuteness of the clinical problem. In most hemapheresis procedures the therapeutic aim is to remove immunoglobulins, which are either involved in the hyperviscosity state or are the effector molecules in the disease process being treated. Thus, an understanding of the biology of immunoglobulins allows us to arrive at a logical model for hemapheresis in general.

Biology of Immunoglobulins and Hemapheresis Strategies

Volume of Hemapheresis Procedures

To determine the optimal volume of each plasmapheresis procedure, one must consider the patient's vascular volume. An average patient's plasma volume is usually about half of the patient's 5-L blood volume, or 2 to 3 L, the remainder being blood cells. Thus, one plasma volume would be a 2- to 3-L exchange. This would totally remove circulating factors if plasmapheresis were 100 percent efficient. Unfortunately, it is not. As plasma is removed, replacement solutions are given; soon previously infused replacement solutions are being removed. Thus, when the equivalent of one volume of plasma has been removed, there will only be a 63 percent reduction in circulating intravascular factors; with removal of two plasma volumes this reduction is 86 percent, and with three plasma volumes it is 95 percent.[5]

Removal of one plasma volume reduces intravascular constituents by 63 percent. Doubling the volume and time decreases constituents by only an additional 23 percent.

Frequency of Hemapheresis

Volumes of Distribution of Immunoglobulins. Immunoglobulin M molecules present in IgM macroglobulinemias are large molecules, the size of fibrinogen: 76 percent of them are in the 5-L vascular space, the remaining 24 percent being in the 10-L extravascular space. These and other large plasma proteins are virtually excluded from the 25-L intracellular space, a compartment whose small protein metabolites are not accessible to plasmapheresis but are reached by dialysis. IgM-sized molecules circulate between the vascular and extravascular spaces with a half-life of 3 days. Thus for maximum efficiency, plasmapheresis designed to reduce IgM should be performed at 2- to 3-day intervals. However, in emergency situations in which rapid removal of damaging antibodies is the goal, more frequent procedures may be carried out in spite of some loss of efficiency. For example, a serious, symptomatic hyperviscosity with life-threatening dysfunction may warrant a more frequent plasmapheresis schedule. However, as new IgM molecules are synthesized slowly (1 to 3 weeks), plasmapheresis rarely needs to be carried out longer than 2 to 4 weeks unless synthesis is more rapid, as in Waldenström's macroglobulinemia.

IgG molecules, on the other hand, are distributed with 45 percent in the intravascular and the remaining 55 percent predominant within the 10-L extravascular space. The circulation time of IgG between those two extracellular spaces for IgG is approximate a half-life of 24 hours. Therefore removal efficiency is optimal with an alternate-day schedule.[5]

Metabolism of Plasma Proteins (Table 10-1). A further aid to planning the frequency of plasmapheresis is consideration of the half-life of these proteins, which is 5, 6, and 21 days for IgM, IgA, and IgG, respectively.[6] The half-life of these immunoglobulins defines the time to replace, in equal amounts, one-half of the amount catabolized. The recirculation half-times (in and out of intravascular space) for these proteins are 72 hours for IgM and 24 hours for IgA and IgG. These are matched somewhat by the intravascular protein coefficient 70 to 80 percent for IgM and 40 to 50 percent for IgA and IgG.[7]

The fractional catabolic rate (FCR) for these and other proteins is a function of the intravascular mass (IVM), which is expressed as the product of plasma concentration (PC) by plasma volume; (thus IVM = PC × PV). For IgG FCR is 6.7 percent of the IVM per day; for albumin it is 10 percent, for IgM, 18 percent, for fibrinogen 25 percent, and for the complement component (the third component of C3) 53 percent.

Intravascular/Extravascular Exchange. Exchange between the intra- and extravascular compartments is determined by the relationship of EVM to the product of the transcapil-

TABLE 10-1. Summary of Immunogblobulin Kinetics

Immunoglobulin class	IGM	IGG
% Intravascular	76	45
% Catabolized per day	13	6 (variable)
Plasma half-life	72 h	6 h
Transcapillary escape rate (% of intravascular mass/h)	1	3

lary escape rate (TER), and the return rate (RR); the equation is EVM = K × TER × RR, where K is a constant. TER and RR are 6 percent of the IVM per hour for albumin, 3 percent for IgG, 2 percent for fibrinogen, and 1 percent for IgM. For general reference purposes, the recycling time of these proteins might be compared with the blood volume (5 L) circulation time of once per minute (cardiac output equals 5 L/min). For albumin and IgG, the recycling time (in and out of the vascular space) is once per day, and for fibrinogen and IgM, once per 2 to 3 days.[7]

Fractional catabolic rate varies eight- to ninefold with concentration, from about 2 percent per day with very low IgG levels to a maximum of 16 to 18 percent per day in patients with very high IgG levels (usually multiple myeloma patients). Also, the survival of IgG can be shortened by IgG infusions but not by infusions of other immunoglobulins or albumin.

It is obvious that larger molecules will redistribute much more slowly than smaller ones after a process such as plasma exchange. This is a function of capillary permeability, molecular weight, and to a lesser extent, effective molecular radius. However, for molecules smaller than albumin, capillary permeability is not limiting, and such molecules leave the circulation very rapidly.

Depletion of Clotting Factors. Another consideration in determining the frequency of apheresis is the rate to which clotting factors are replaced. Following a one-plasma volume apheresis, one can detect a prolongation of the prothrombin and partial thromboplastin times to 1.3 to 1.5 times normal, which is caused by depletion of clotting factors. There also is a significant decrease in fibrinogen level. The partial thromboplastin and prothrombin times usually correct within 24 hours, but it may take 48 hours for fibrinogen to return to normal. Thus, following a one-PV pheresis, clotting proteins are not normally completely reconstituted for 24 to 48 hours.[5] This is another reason for an alternate day pheresis schedule in many situations.

One plasma volume exchange every other day usually will not significantly deplete clotting factors. Larger or more frequent exchanges usually require replacement with fresh-frozen plasma.

The reduction in immunoglobulins in patients undergoing multiple plasma exchanges with 3.5 to 5 percent albumin replacement is directly related to the volume of exchange. The change is cumulative and in the order IgG, IgA, IgM, which is in the reverse order of the product of percent IVM by FCR. Replacement with fresh-frozen plasma (FFP) instead of albumin will prevent lowering of all immunoglobulins, except the pathogenic one(s). However, because of the risk of disease transmission with FFP, volumes and frequency of exchanges are usually limited, so that FFP is hardly needed. FFP is used routinely in plasma exchange only in thrombotic thrombocytopenic purpura/

hemolytic uremic syndrome (TTP-HUS), in which a missing normal inhibitor of platelet aggregation is being replaced until some unpredictable time when it is again available. The blood bank product PF 24 (plasma frozen within 24 hours of blood collection) is equivalent to FFP for treating TTP-HUS by either plasmapheresis or infusion.

Plasma and Blood Volume Calculations

Normal Volumes

The volume of each plasmapheresis should be individualized according to the patient's estimated plasma volume. One can roughly estimate the plasma volume by calculating the vascular volume to be approximately 70 ml/kg. By using the patient's hematocrit, the fraction of the vascular volume containing plasma can be calculated. If a more accurate measure of vascular volume is desired, there are several published tables that normalize for sex and frame.

Abnormal Volumes

In estimating vascular volumes, one should also be aware of the effects of various disease states on vascular volumes. Patients with hyperviscosity or severe anemia frequently have vascular volumes that are larger than calculated. This is important to recognize, as these patients may become more susceptible to congestive heart failure with further increases in their vascular volume. In addition, the therapeutic effect of the procedure may appear to be less than expected because vascular volume has been underestimated.

Technique of Plasma Exchange

When starting a hemapheresis procedure, some intravenous fluid is usually given first to expand the vascular volume; for example, 200 ml of 5 percent albumin or saline. When blood drawing starts, a citrate anticoagulant is added to the blood as near the venipuncture as possible. In the most widely used discontinuous device, Haemonetics Model 30 or V-50 (Haemonetics Corp., Braintree, MA), the centrifuge bowl becomes filled with approximately 200 ml of red cells from which the plasma has been separated. This takes 20 to 30 minutes depending on bleeding rate. The red cells are then returned to the donor and another cycle begins. The volume removed with each cycle should be chosen so that no more than 15 percent of the patient's vascular volume or 25 percent of the red cell mass is extracorporeal at any one time. The cycle is repeated, with replacement of the collected plasma with an equal or slightly higher volume of replacement solution, as many times as necessary to collect the desired plasma volume. If 5 percent albumin is used, replacement volumes can be equal to the volume removed. If significant volumes of saline are used to replace plasma, up to 115 percent of the volume removed must be replaced to account for third spacing. All other systems separate plasma from cells on a continuous flow basis, making vascular volume more stable and operation somewhat simpler.

It is the general practice in the United States to exchange one plasma volume at a time and to repeat the procedure every 1 to 3 days to allow equilibration with the extravascular space. If no ongoing synthesis is assumed, the total body amount of γ-globulin can be reduced 88 percent by six one-volume exchanges performed over 2 to 3 weeks.

Anticoagulation

Hematologically oriented services predominantly use anticoagulant citrate dextrose (ACD), familiar from its use as the anticoagulation preservative for blood collection and transfusion. An amount of citrate sufficient to prevent initiation of plasma clotting acts by chelating calcium. Sodium citrate solutions are also used and provide more versatility than ACD with respect to lowering concentration to avoid symptoms of hypocalcemia. Perimoral paresthesias secondary to hypocalcemia can be observed, but severe signs of hypocalcemia (e.g., tetany or cardiac arrhythmia) are rare, and calcium supplementation is not commonly needed. One of us (R.B.D.) has used intravenous calcium perhaps a dozen times for symptoms (e.g., perioral paresthesias) but oral calcium carbonate (Tums) a few hundred times in about 5,000 procedures. In this experience electrocardiographic (ECG) monitoring has been performed for hypocalcemia several times and only one diagnosis made. No death suspected to be due to hypocalcemia has occurred in this 13-year experience.

Most centrifugal cell separators use citrate. This nearly provides extracorporeal anticoagulation, as most of the citrate is retained in the collected plasma. A small amount of citrate returns with cells in plasma exchange and most citrate is returned with the plasma in cytapheresis, but citrate is rapidly metabolized by the liver. When paresthesias develop, slowing down the procedure will allow the metabolism to catch up with citrate infusion. Oral calcium carbonate supplementation (Tums) may be required in some patients who are sensitive to citrate. Systemic anticoagulation with heparin is generally not required for centrifugal cell separation. Most filtration systems, however, require some heparinization and citrate for plasma flow through the membrane pores.

Replacement Fluids

Plasmapheresis replacement fluids usually are albumin-based, usually 5 percent human serum albumin, in the United States. In some centers 4 percent solutions are preferred. As the normal plasma albumin concentration is 3.5 to 5 g/dl, a 4 percent solution is more physiologic. Indeed, volume for volume replacement with 5 percent albumin expands the normal plasma volume, lowering the hematocrit by up to 20 percent over several procedures.[7]

A 5 percent plasma protein fraction (PPF) is equivalent to 5 percent albumin with respect to oncotic activity and is mostly (86 percent) albumin, the remainder being α- and β-globulins of insignificant biologic activity except for oncotic properties. PPF is made for economic reasons, being 20 percent less expensive to manufacture than albumin, although its market price, may be the same. In the past some incompletely processed lots of PPF containing prekallikrein activator were released with resulting cases of morbid hypotension. This has not occurred for over a decade, since the U. S. Food and Drug Administration (FDA) began screening all lots.[11]

Protein replacement solutions nearly one-third the cost of a plasmapheresis. Use of 50 percent saline significantly lowers the cost.

Albumin is preferred to PPF when hyperviscosity or red cell aggregation should be avoided. Whereas even nonspecific globulins may participate in aggregation, albumin in any concentration will not promote red cell agglutination.[9]

Replacement of up to 50 percent of removed plasma with crystalloid, usually normal saline, at an increased volume (15 to 30 percent), is theoretically safe and economical. The procedure cost for 5 percent albumin may thus be cut by 50 percent, and the edema threshold for albumin of 2.5 g/dl is not usually breached. Normal plasma albumin has a concentration of 3.5 to 5 g/dl, or 4.2 g/dl on average. A one plasma volume exchange reduces plasma proteins by about 60 percent, and a 60 percent reduction of 4.2 g/dl yields 2.5 g/dl, just above the edema threshold. Unfortunately, saline, when used to replace plasma, can require a greater volume.[12] Thus, hypotension may be more common when saline replacement for plasma is used.[13]

Decrease in other plasma proteins with albumin replacement has been well studied by Flaun et al.[14] and a useful summary has been provided by Dawson et al.[12] Fortunately, even a 4-L plasmapheresis will lower the critical, labile coagulation factors V and VIII by only 50 percent, and recovery is 75 to 90 percent, respectively at 4 hours. Thus, FFP is usually not required. Other factors are not lowered as much as these.

MECHANISMS OF HEMAPHERESIS

In some disease states the mechanism of hemapheresis seems quite clear (i.e., removal of paraproteins and improvement in blood viscosity) (Table 10-2). In other disease states in which the pathologic agent is well known, such as anti-acetylcholine receptor antibodies in myasthenia gravis, the actual mechanism whereby pheresis interferes with the pathologic molecule may be multifactorial. Removal of plasma may result in reduced antibody levels,[15] reduced antigen levels, alteration in the number of structure of immune complexes,[16] improved reticuloendothelial clearance of immune complexes,[17] reduction in serum complement,[5] or alterations in fibronectin levels.[18]

In addition, replacement solutions may have a role in determining outcome of therapy. When FFP is used as the replacement solution, a broad spectrum of biologically active molecules is infused. In particular, infusion of γ-globulin has been shown to alter disease states through reticuloendothelial blockade.[19] Use of PPF protein fraction has been reported to be associated with infusion of prekallikrein activators,[11] and increased levels of serum aluminum[21,22] been noted with use of albumin solutions. When staphylococcal protein A columns have been used, there has been concern that small amounts of protein A may be infused, with concomitant activation of complement and other bioregulatory systems.[23]

Finally, a number of authors have described significant changes in cellular function following plasmapheresis,

TABLE 10-2. Mechanism of Hemapheresis

Reduction in blood viscosity
Antibody reduction
Antigen reduction
Immune complex reduction
Improved reticuloendothelial function
Hypocalcemia
Increase in trace metals and aluminum
Effect of replacement solutions
Intravenous immunoglobulin G
Fresh frozen plasma
Plasma protein fraction/bradykinin
Activation of complement
Removal of toxins
Altered cellular function
Decreased granulocyte phagocytosis
Decreased suppressor T cells
Increased natural killer cells

These include decreased, nonspecific granulocyte phagocytosis, decreased suppressor cells, and increased natural killer cells.[24,25] Thus, the effects of hemapheresis on biologic systems are manifold, and caution should therefore be used in attributing observed outcomes to any specific mechanisms.

HEMAPHERESIS SYSTEMS

Currently six different hemapheresis systems are in common use in the United States. These include three systems that separate cells on the basis of centrifugal force: the Haemonetics V-50 (Haemonetics Corp., Braintree, MA), the CS3000 (Baxter Healthcare Corp., Evanston, IL), and the COBE Spectra (COBE Laboratories Inc., Lakewood, CA). One membrane filtration system is the COBE TPE (COBE Laboratories, Lakewood, CA), and one staphylococcal protein A adsorption column, Prosorba (Imre Corp., Seattle) are also marketed. In addition, one photopheresis unit is marketed in the United States, but its use will not be discussed here.

Selection of a particular hemapheresis system involves multiple factors. Clinically, the most important factors are efficiency and extracorporeal volume. Membrane separation systems are slightly less efficient than centrifugal systems, but this can be compensated for by high flow rates not possible in centrifuges for physical reasons. Attention to extracorporeal volumes is important, especially if pediatric hemapheresis is planned. The ability to perform single-needle procedures is also of value, as it allows patients with marginal vascular access to be treated. Other factors involved in choosing instrumentation include portability, the cost of software and hardware, and the ability to use the equipment for cell collection. No single system is optimal for all needs. The equipment used will therefore vary from hospital to hospital.

VASCULAR ACCESS

Efficient centrifugal hemapheresis requires a blood flow between 40 and 80 ml/min; higher flow rates may be used with membrane separation systems. If adequate vascular access is not achieved, flow rates can be slow and target plasma volumes may not be achieved. Thus, adequate venous access is mandatory for effective hemapheresis.

Adequate venous access is critical for effective plasmapheresis. "Tinkering" with inadequate peripheral venous access invariably results in failure to remove desired plasma volumes.

Optimally, peripheral venous access should use antecubital or forearm veins. Steel needles (16-gauge) or plastic catheters are employed. In the experience of one of us (H.G.B.), the former has caused less local irritation. If adequate peripheral venous access cannot be achieved, one should not hesitate to catheterize a large central vein. Use of the subclavian, internal and external jugular, and femoral veins and the inferior vena cava has been described. Basically, any catheter that can be used for dialysis can be used for hemapheresis.

Recently many patients have had Hickman catheters placed for semipermanent venous access. These catheters are placed in the superior vena cava via the subclavian vein and tunneled subcutaneously to exit the skin above the breast. Separation of the skin exit port from the vein entrance port has proved effective in preventing infection. However, most of these catheters are long, with narrow lumina. The resulting resistance makes rapid blood flow difficult. Shorter, larger-bore, single-lumen Hickman-like catheters are available.

Arteriovenous shunts and fistulae have also been used for venous access. Whereas these techniques work well for dialysis, they have proved less effective in nonuremic patients. The high cardiac output secondary to the low hematocrit of renal disease and the associated uremic platelet dysfunction both inhibit thrombosis. These protective factors are usually not present in patients requiring hemapheresis. Additionally, one can usually achieve adequate vascular access by using one of the above-describe catheters.

Maintenance of catheters, once they are in place, has been somewhat problematic. Catheter thrombosis has been the greatest problem. Infusion of heparin solutions to fill the catheter seem to be effective; doses of heparin have ranged from 1,000 to 10,000 units/ml. Systemic treatment of patients with antiplatelet agents (aspirin) or low-dose warfarin (1 mg/day) has also been used.

COMPLICATIONS OF PLASMA EXCHANGE

During the 1980s, the period when therapeutic hemapheresis became available not only in research medical centers but also in community hospitals in the United States, complications of plasma exchange were described. The first review, initially published by Huestis in 1983 as a letter,[26] cited 42 deaths, 60 percent of which were cardiovascular or pulmonary and most of which were related to use of FFP. (These are summarized below.[27]) More recently this experience has been updated and the Canadian experience has also been summarized.[28,29] This work was begun by Huestis, who announced his concern at an International Society of Blood Transfusion meeting in Budapest in the early 1980s and requested assistance in collecting, analyzing, and reporting adverse reactions to hemapheresis.

Hypocalcemia and Fluid Overload

Hypocalcemia, the commonest side effect of hemapheresis, usually can be controlled by merely slowing the procedure to allow hepatic metabolism of citrate to catch up or by administration of oral calcium carbonate supplements.[30] Perioral paresthesia is the commonest symptom. Other symptoms and signs include tremor, muscle twitching, chills, nausea and vomiting, tetany, and arrhythmia. ECG changes include bradycardia and a-wave prolongation.

Slowing the rate of return of blood to allow metabolism of citrate by the liver to occur will help dissipate citrate toxicity. If a severe reaction occurs, plasmapheresis can be continued with a lower citrate concentration. Citrate reactions (hypocalcemia) are most common when FFP is used. If symptoms of hypocalcemia persist, calcium gluconate, 1 g in 100 ml of normal saline given at the rate of a few milliliters per minute, is appropriate. It should be noted that respiratory alkalosis will exacerbate hypocalcemia. Diagnosis and effective management of hyperventilation are essential.

Anxiety-related hyperventilation frequently accompanies symptomatic hypocalcemia, and this respiratory alkalosis further lowers the ionized calcium. Attention to hyperventilation is helpful in managing citrate reactions.

Other reactions related to infusion fluids include pulmonary edema, especially when normal saline is used in excess. Failure to provide high enough oncotic pressures to prevent extravasation of fluid sometimes results in pulmonary edema after one or two plasma exchanges in hypoproteinemic syndromes.

Fresh-Frozen Plasma

FFP is a needed replacement fluid in TTP-HUS. Allergic reactions frequently result, hives being the most common. One or two hives may be allowed to resolve spontaneously, but more are an indication for 20 or 50 mg of diphenhydramine PO or IV. If the hives are over a large region, diphenhydramine should be given and steroids should be considered. Usually a dose of 60 mg methylprednisolone or equivalent can be repeated once for extensive hives. Stridor, suggesting the development of laryngeal edema, necessitates epinephrine 3 to 5 mg IV (1:1,000 dilution) up to 1 mg in the dire situation of the unstable patient. For the uncommon febrile reaction, acetaminophen is indicated, as with any transfusion.

Mortality in Therapeutic Hemapheresis

Huestis's 1983 letter to the *Lancet*[26] tabulated 42 deaths, 20 in France, mostly associated with use of FFP. Of the 42 deaths, 12 were cardiovascular, 13 were respiratory, 3 anaphylactic, 2 due to pulmonary thromboembolism, 3 due to vascular perforation, 2 due to hepatitis, and 2 due to sepsis, and for 3 the data were incomplete. Since FFP is now almost exclusively reserved for TTP-HUS, deaths associated with its use have greatly decreased. On the basis of the number of therapeutic procedures done during 1979 to 1983, this gives a case fatality rate for the United Kingdom, the United States, France, and Canada of 3 per 10,000 procedures. The procedure is generally considered reasonably safe, as plasma exchange is performed in seriously ill patients.

Metabolic Alkalosis

Sodium citrate is metabolized to sodium bicarbonate, which results in metabolic alkalosis in patients with renal failure, especially glomerulonephritis. Substituting a 3 percent albumin solution for FFP can reduce potential bicarbonate production by 300 mEq daily, thereby resulting in rapid resolution of metabolic alkalosis. As mentioned above, the amount of citrate administered can be further reduced. Also substitution of heparin anticoagulant or use of half heparin and half citrate has been employed to prevent this complication.[31]

Hypotension in Therapeutic Hemapheresis

Hypotension is invited by substituting replacement fluids that contain oncotic proteins at less than the patient's plasma oncotic pressure (e.g., using 2.5 percent albumin, which corresponds to the edema threshold, or the equivalent in other replacement fluids). In companion papers in 1985, Trandaugh and Lewis[32] and Dawson et al.[33] have discussed crystalloid and colloid fluids.[32,33] As in most reports of crystalloid fluid use, the volume used has been less than half the blood volume, resulting in reduction of plasma oncotic proteins (e.g., albumin to no less than the edema threshold, 2.5 g percent). In spite of this limitation in use of crystalloid fluid, peripheral edema, but rarely pulmonary edema or other compromises, can result.

In a 1989 review from the Canadian Apheresis Study Group, there was a 12 percent rate of side effects, or 612 reactions in 5,235 procedures involving 252 (40 percent) of the 627 patients treated.[29] The common reactions were fever, chills, urticaria, muscle cramps, and paresthesias and these were encountered more frequently with plasma than with other replacement fluids. Most reactions had little to no clinical consequence, but there were 28 severe complications, including one case of cardiac arrest and two of respiratory arrest. Five late deaths occurred, but these were not directly related to plasma exchange. As in most series, neurologic diseases accounted for the greatest number of cases treated, with Guillain-Barré syndrome the most common disease in that group. Hematologic diseases accounted for the next greatest number, with paraproteinemia the most common but with TTP-HUS showing the most reactions and a larger number of cases as well.

Therapeutic hemapheresis is performed for serious illness. It is an invasive procedure involving one or more plasma or blood exchanges. Reaction should be anticipated because of the invasive, exchange nature of the procedure. Moreover, the replacement fluids, especially FFP and citrate, represent hazards. Precautions include listening for breath sounds in both lung bases and cardiac sounds before, during, and after the procedure, as well as checking for edema and urinary output. Monitoring vital signs is crucial as is watching the rate of blood withdrawal and reinfusion. The patients should be asked, when possible, for signs of reaction, such as tingling or numbness in the lips, or any other signs or symptoms. The ready availability of an experienced cardiac arrest and resuscitation team is essential. Additionally, the pheresis physician, if unable to be on site throughout the procedure, must be available by page and phone for advice.

CURRENT CLINICAL APPLICATIONS OF HEMAPHRESIS

Plasmapheresis

Hyperviscosity

Whole blood viscosity is affected by complex interactions between cellular and noncellular elements. Red blood cell mass affects whole blood viscosity even in the normal hematocrit range. Usually, white cells do not affect whole blood viscosity until they are present in pathologic numbers. Plasma proteins, especially large asymmetric molecules, also contribute to the blood viscosity. The important plasma proteins include the immunoglobulins and fibrinogen. In addition to these variables, temperature and blood flow rate also affect whole blood viscosity.

The size and concentration of immunoglobulin molecules both have a profound effect on blood viscosity. IgM or polymeric IgA affect blood viscosity at lower concentrations than does IgG. In high concentration, however, even IgG, either polyclonal or monoclonal, increases blood viscosity. In general there is a logarithmic relationship between immunoglobulin concentration and plasma viscosity (i.e., at higher immunoglobulin concentrations, very small concentration increments can result in profound increases in blood viscosity). This is important to recognize, as at high protein concentrations even small decreases in plasma protein concentrations induced by plasmapheresis may have significant effects on blood viscosity and clinical symptomatology.[34]

Most patients with significant hyperviscosity manifest global symptoms such as fatigue and anorexia. The onset may be chronic, and patients may not be aware of the degree of their fatigue. Headache is a frequent complaint. Epistaxis and upper gastrointestinal bleeding from engorged veins are not uncommon. Specific organ symptomatology varies considerably from patient to patient; presumably this is related to anatomic variations in vascular integrity. Thus, hyperviscosity can result in renal insufficiency, congestive heart failure, angina, or a variety of focal or nonfocal neurologic symptoms.

In general, patients who manifest in vitro evidence of hyperviscosity with associated clinical symptomatology should undergo plasmapheresis. This should be individualized from patient to patient, as individual patient thresholds are quite variable. Furthermore, it may be difficult to evaluate symptomatology because of its chronic nature. In many cases a trial of plasma exchange is undertaken to determine if the clinical symptomatology will respond.

Traditionally, blood viscosity has been evaluated by relative plasma viscosity as measured by an Oswald viscometer. This technique does not account for interactions between red cells and plasma proteins, and therefore measurement of whole blood viscosity at variable shear rates is quite useful. Finally, blood viscosity can be evaluated in vivo by measuring retinal circulation times. Visualization of the clearance of the timed flow of a fluoresceinated dye from the arterial to the venous circulation can be used to evaluate the clinical importance of other in vitro determinations. Protein evaluation with quantitative immunoglobulins is also helpful. Clinical endpoints, then, include symptomatology, plasma viscosity, whole blood viscosity, and immunoglobulin concentration.

Plasmaphresis was first reported to be effective in hyperviscosity,[35–37] and subsequent studies have elaborated on its use.[38,39] Plasmapheresis is usually undertaken with exchange of one to two plasma volumes. Response may be dramatic, as plasma viscosity has a logarithmic relationship to protein concentration. Usually two to three procedures are required on an alternate day basis to return the plasma viscosity to normal. This is more likely to be achieved with IgA or IgG molecules, which undergo significant re-equilibration with the extravascular compartment.

Initially the plasma viscosity may be too high to permit adequate flow in the cell separator. In this situation additional crystalloid can be supplied at the venipuncture site to dilute the blood entering the separation device. As protein depletion takes place, flow usually increases. In addition, it should be noted that patients with paraproteinemia have an expanded vascular volume, which is ostensibly due to the increased oncotic strength of their protein load. Thus, they may be in a state of incipient congestive heart failure, and fluid replacement should be given cautiously. This is also true for red cell transfusion. In many patients epistaxis produces an iron deficiency anemia, which functionally protects the patient from symptomatic whole blood hyperviscosity. Thus, red cell transfusion should usually be delayed until plasma viscosity has been reduced. It should also be noted that in emergent situations, a one- or two-unit whole blood phlebotomy and replacement with normal saline can result in significant improvement in symptoms related to hyperviscosity. Thus, therapy may be instituted even before a full pheresis team can be mobilized.

Cryoglobulinemias

Cryoglobulinemia has been reported in conjunction with a variety of lymphoproliferative diseases, autoimmune disorders, and postinfectious states. The pathologic molecules can be single monoclonal immunoglobulins (type 1), mixed (usually IgG and IgM) monoclonal gammopathic molecules (type 2), or mixed polyclonal immunoglobulins (type 3). Tissue damage can be related to viscosity, cryoprecipitation, vasculitis, or rapidly progressive glomerulonephritis. Indications for plasmapheresis are made on a case by case basis. In general, 25 percent of cryoglobulins are IgM (type 1) monoclonal macroglobulins (e.g., in Waldenström's macroglobulinemia; 25 percent are mixed usually IgM-IgG or IgA (type 2) complexes with a monoclonal component (e.g., in multiple myeloma); and 50 percent are mixed polyclonal (type 3) with low levels of antibodies (e.g., in chronic hepatitis B virus infections with false positive rheumatoid factor). Vascular purpura, often palpable, is usually associated with types 2 and 3. Cryoglobulinemia may be associated with hemolysis (discussed in the section on autoimmune hemolytic anemia).

Blood samples for immunoglobulin testing in cryoglobulinemia should be promptly transported to the laboratory in 37°C water to prevent cryoprecipitation, which can result in falsely low estimates of serum proteins.

There have been no controlled trials of plasma exchange in this complex group of disorders. When symptoms are related to hyperviscosity, plasmapheresis is usually effective. The role of plasmapheresis in rapidly progressive glomerulonephritis or other vasculitic manifestations is poorly defined. However, in small series there have been anecdotal reports of the efficacy of plasmapheresis combined with immunosuppressive therapy in renal disease,[40–43] gangrene,[43] and neutropenia.[44] However, for selected patients who have failed conventional immunosuppressive therapy, a trial of plasmapheresis may be indicated.

Therapy is usually directed at clinical symptomatology. In most cases total protein level and cryocrit are also of assistance. Monitoring of serum complement or immune complexes has not been reported to be helpful. In following patients with cryoglobulinemias, it is important to ensure that cryoprecipitation during specimen procurement or transportation does not give erratic results.

Plasma exchange can be undertaken by either centrifugal or filtration methodologies. Some authors have reported difficulties with membrane clogging in some filtration systems. In isolated cases, extracorporeal precipitation of cryoproteins has also been somewhat problematic. This problem may be solved by performing plasmapheresis in warm atmospheres or including in-line blood warmers.

Thrombocytopenia

Thrombocytopenia can result from deficient platelet production, platelet sequestration, increased platelet consumption, or a combination of these effects. The key to the management of thrombocytopenia is establishing an accurate diagnosis. This may be difficult, as clinical symptomatology is frequently nonspecific and laboratory parameters can overlap. Plasmapheresis has been shown to be effective in a number of thrombocytopenic states.

Thrombotic Thrombocytopenic Purpura. TTP was classically described as a pentad of fever, thrombocytopenia, microangiopathic hemolytic anemia, renal disease, and central nervous system signs.[46] Today, however, we recognize it as one end of a spectrum of illnesses that result in microangiopathic hemolytic anemia secondary to mechanical destruction of red cells in platelet and fibrin thrombi in the microcirculation.[47,48] Other variants of this syndrome include HUS[49] and the HELLP syndrome (hemolysis, Elevated liver enzymes, low platelet count), seen in patients with pre-eclampsia.[50] The cause of these microthrombi, which are common to all these syndromes, is unclear. A variety of studies suggest that both the presence of a toxic material, favoring platelet adhesion to endothelial cells, and depletion of a normal plasma factor are important. This dual etiology is further substantiated by trends in published trials, which seem to imply that both plasmapheresis and plasma infusions are required to obtain the greatest therapeutic benefit. Apparently, a wide variety of factors can initiate this syndrome. In a number of patients a history of an antecedent viral illness is commonly obtained. *Escherichia coli* toxins, pregnancy, an drugs such as mitomycin C have also been implicated. Once initiated, however, the process appears to be self-perpetuating.[47,48] Prior to the institution of effective plasmapheresis and exchange, fewer than 30 percent of TTP patients survived despite therapy with corticosteroids, antiplatelet drugs, and splenectomy. With plasmapheresis and exchange as the center of therapy, survival has increased to more than 90 percent.[51–54]

In approximately 30 percent of patients, this syndrome will resolve spontaneously or after therapy with corticosteroids. This is particularly true of patients with HUS and pregnant patients with the HELLP syndrome who complete delivery. However, the development of severe thrombocytopenia (platelet count $< 10{,}000/mm^3$) or of focal neurologic signs is generally accepted as being a poor prognostic sign and an indication for the initiation of plasmapheresis and exchange.

Clinical assessment of the patient with TTP is quite difficult to quantitate. Neurologic signs can be transient, and hematocrit is dependent upon transfusion. In general, it is recommended that the hemolytic process be followed closely with daily hematocrits, reticulocyte counts, and serum lactic dehydrogenase levels. The platelet count and creatine should also be closely monitored. After a definitive improvement in these variables has been documented, the frequency of plasma exchange can be modified as indicated by these parameters. Red cell transfusions should be given to keep the hematocrit above 20 percent or higher if indicated. Platelet transfusion should be avoided.

TTP and the equivalent syndromes are emergent indications for plasmapheresis with exchange of FFP. Clinical symptoms can develop rapidly, and coma develop within hours. Patients with focal neurologic signs frequently require roentgenographic examination to document that a hemorrhagic space-occupying lesion is not present. Once the diagnosis of severe TTP is established and hemorrhage is excluded, emergency plasmapheresis with exchange should be undertaken. One to two plasma volumes should be removed and replaced with FFP. A central venous catheter is nearly always required, as patients with changing mental status are unable to cooperate adequately in order to use peripheral veins. Patients with delirium frequently require sedation with benzodiazepines. Not uncommonly, patients are being treated with antiseizure medications. As Dilantin is highly protein-bound, levels should be carefully monitored and replacement doses adjusted during and following each procedure. With the infusion of large volumes of fresh plasma from 15 to 30 donors, allergic transfusion reactions are not uncommon. Premedication with diphenhydramine is usually undertaken. Selection of the appropriate pheresis equipment is also indicated; with pre-existing severe thrombocytopenia, a pheresis system that does not require heparinization should be selected.

To maintain Dilantin levels, one-half the maintenance dose should be given at the midpoint of a one plasma volume procedure and one half at the end. Serum Dilantin levels must be monitored.

At our institutions daily plasma exchange is undertaken.

If the clinical status worsens despite daily plasma exchange, the exchange volume is increased to two to three times the patient's estimated plasma volume. When improvement is noted, plasma exchange frequency can be reduced to accommodate weekends and holidays and finally tapered on an alternate day basis. It is not uncommon to have a relapse following cessation of plasmapheresis. For this reason, close on a daily monitoring of indicators of active disease is required for several weeks.

Post-Transfusion Purpura. Post-transfusion purpura (PTP) is a rare syndrome predominantly seen in women. It is characterized by the sudden onset of severe thrombocytopenia 5 to 10 days after a blood transfusion. Nearly all patients investigated have been shown to be homozygously negative for a common platelet-specific antigen system, most commonly the PLA-1 system. Although the exact pathophysiology is unclear, the disease behaves as if transfused PLA-1 antigen is passively attached to the patient's platelets.[55]

By definition, patients with this syndrome are symptomatic (purpura) from their thrombocytopenia. If immediate improvement is clinically required, institution of plasmapheresis would seem logical. Both whole blood exchange[56,57] and automated plasmapheresis have been effective.[58] PTP is the one situation wherein one plasmapheresis procedure is curative. More recently, infusions of intravenous immunoglobulin G (IVIGG) have also proved effective.

Patients reported in the literature have been treated with whole blood exchange or plasmapheresis. Apparently, whole blood exchange is not required, the usual protocol of one to two plasma volumes of plasmapheresis being adequate.

Immune Thrombocytopenic Purpura. Immune thrombocytic purpura (ITP) is a disorder of autoimmune platelet destruction. Apparently this can be mediated by immune complexes passively adhering to platelets, as well as by specific antiplatelet antibodies. The acute syndrome, seen predominantly in children, is usually self-limited. The adult syndrome, seen predominantly in women, can be much more chronic.[59]

Plasmapheresis to remove offending antibodies would seem a logical therapeutic modality. However, despite the initial reports of successful plasmapheresis in this disease in the 1970s, plasmapheresis is not commonly used,[60] possibly because in many cases this is a benign disorder and also because there are multiple alternate therapeutic modalities. Nonetheless, there may be a role for plasma exchange in this disease.

In a 1990 review of this syndrome, Williams et al. compiled the results of 39 cases published to date.[61] Despite the fact that only 17 patients were believed to be adequately treated, 14 out of 19 patients with acute and 11 out of 22 with chronic cases showed a positive response to plasmapheresis. The one large attempt at a prospective study (The Canadian National Study) of this disease[61] has fortunately not accrued an adequate number patients (23 patients to date). Although remissions were commonly seen, all patients subsequently relapsed and frequently required alternate therapy. Plasmapheresis may be an effective adjuvant to conventional therapy in patients who have severe disease refractory to conventional therapy and are demonstrating hemorrhage.

Most investigators have employed one to two plasma volumes every other day for 7 to 10 days. More recently (1988) it was suggested that daily plasmapheresis for three days followed by IVIGG infusions may be efficacious.[62]

Specific immune absorption of IgG has also been attempted. The most commonly used device is the Prosorba column (Imre Corp., Seattle), which employs a staphylococcal protein A fixed to a stable "backbone." Each column typically binds approximately 1 g of IgG. Reports have indicated effectiveness in ITP, particularly ITP occurring in patients with the acquired immunodeficiency syndrome (AIDS).[61,63] Paradoxically, this response has been seen both with large-volume perfusion and with perfusion volumes as small as 250 ml. It is clear that this device is not capable of depleting significant amounts of circulating IgG, and the reported beneficial effects are therefore probably attributable to an alternate mechanism, perhaps an immune modulation.

Refractoriness to Platelet Transfusion Secondary to Alloantibodies. Approximately 60 percent of patients who receive platelet transfusions will develop anti-human leukocyte antigen (HLA) class I antibodies, which result in alloimmune platelet destruction with subsequent transfusions. Post-transfusion alloimmunization has been very difficult to manage. Steroids have had little effect. HLA-matched platelets can be effective, but frequently the gene frequency of the patient's HLA type precludes finding adequate numbers of donors. Consequently there has been great interest in the use of plasma exchange to ameliorate this situation.

Only one group has reported successfully ameliorating post-transfusion alloimmunization with plasma exchange. Bensinger et al. have reported beneficial responses in 11 of 18 patients undergoing bone marrow transplant.[64] Their patients received one to three exchanges, and those having the most exchanges had the best result. The benefit was also reported to be most marked when employed just before bone marrow transplant. Thus, the immunosuppression of the bone marrow transplant may have added to the overall effect of plasmapheresis. Other groups have not been able to duplicate this result.

Plasmapheresis is not itself curative. If the underlying disease is not in remission, some degree of immunosuppression is required. Cyclophosphamide may be more immunosuppressive than azathioprine but carries the risk of secondary leukemia.

Paraneoplastic Neuromuscular Syndromes

Myasthenia Gravis. Myasthenia gravis is a peripheral neuropathy mediated by antibodies to postsynaptic cholinesterase receptors. These antibodies can usually be documented in 80 to 90 percent of cases and result in antigen-antibody-mediated blockade, impaired neuromuscular transmission due to enhanced destruction of the receptor, and/or a complement-mediated effect with lysis of the membrane. Approximately 66 percent of cases are associated with thymic hyperplasia and 10 to 15 percent with thymoma. Management is focused on enhanced neurotransmission with anticholinesterases, immunosuppression to decrease antibody production, thymectomy, and plasmapheresis. To date there have been no large randomized studies of the efficacy of plasmapheresis in this disease, but results of nonrandomized trials have been fairly consistent. Improvement, if it occurs, may be seen 24 to 48 hours after one to two plasmapheresis procedures. Approximately 70 percent of patients appear to respond, but the benefit is short lived, usually of less than 1 month's duration. Neither pretherapy antibody titer nor post-therapy reduction of titer has been correlated with degree of response. In fact, several authors have noted clinical improvement occurs during the first week following exchange, when serum titers were actually increasing. This was believed to reflect some degree of redistribution of antibody from the extravascular to the intravascular compartment.[65–67]

The general strategy for use of plasmapheresis in patients with myasthenia gravis is to manage acute side effects that are unresponsive to conventional therapy. Indications include (1) myasthenic crisis or rapidly progressive myasthenia, with decreasing forced vital capacity or respirator dependence; (2) prethymectomy, to maximize pulmonary toilet in the postoperative period; (3) during institution of high-dose steroid therapy, when there may be a paradoxical weakening; and/or (4) worsening myasthenia during pregnancy when use of antimetabolites may be contraindicated. In addition, several clinicians have used plasmapheresis in a subacute or chronic setting when patients were refractory to conventional therapy or had a specific contraindication to use of effective agents such as steroids.

Clinical evaluation of muscle strength and of forced vital capacity is the most important measure to follow. However, timing observations, with regard to medications and time of day, are important. Measurement of serial titers of antibodies to anticholinesterase receptors has not proved useful.[15] Measurement of total IgG can be useful in indicating that a maximum effect has been achieved. Usually total IgGs can be reduced to less than 500 mg/dl.

Various plasma exchange protocols have been recommended, ranging from weekly plasma exchange for 6 weeks to daily plasma exchange for 5 days. Antozzi et al. have recently reported that an exchange series as short as two procedures, one day apart, can result in a 75 percent response rate.[68] In general, one to two plasma volumes are exchanged with each procedure. The protocol chosen should match the clinical strategy. If one is intervening acutely in a reversible situation, a rapid series of two or three plasmapheresis procedures would seem the best strategy to induce response as soon as possible; if one is attempting to use plasmapheresis to substitute for alternate therapies on a chronic basis, a weekly strategy may be more appropriate. It should be noted, though, that the more intensive strategies will induce deficiencies in clotting protein profiles and require replacement with FFP, which has potential for serious consequences due to infectious disease transmission.

Several authors have been concerned about a postplasmapheresis overshoot of antibody titers. This has been documented in several animal systems and in some patients with myasthenia gravis. Thus, some authors have recommended concomitant immunosuppressive therapy whenever plasmapheresis is undertaken in order to blunt this overshoot. This has usually not been a problem in most series, perhaps because concomitant immunosuppression has generally been employed.

It is of interest that several authors have noted a reduction in normal cholinesterases following plasma exchange. This has been hypothesized to be a potential postoperative complication when anesthetics have included cholinesterase inhibitors. Although this has not been widely reported as a problem, whenever plasmapheresis is used as an adjuvant during thymectomy, patients have generally been given a 48-hour rest period between plasmapheresis and surgery, which allows reconstitution not only of plasma cholinesterases, but also of any clotting proteins that may have been depleted.

Eaton-Lambert Syndrome. Eaton and Lambert in 1957 were the first to describe a syndrome mediated by decreased peripheral neuromuscular transmission.[69] This abnormality is related to a reduced release of presynaptic acetycholine vesicles and can be differentiated from myasthenia gravis by characteristic electromyographic changes. Clinically it tends to involve the large muscles of the trunk and proximal extremities. Although it can occur in the absence of neoplasia, nearly two-thirds of cases are associated with a neoplastic process, especially small cell carcinoma of the lung. Its management relates not only to control of the syndrome but also to control of the primary malignancy. Although there has been no large prospective study, there have been several anecdotal reports. Dau and Denys[70] reported a series of five patients treated with sequential plasmapheresis and immunosuppression and noted that the optimal regimen appeared to be concomitant plasmapheresis and immunosuppression.

The aim of therapy in the Eaton-Lambert syndrome is generally to maintain as much muscle strength as possible in a chronic disorder. Thus, most authors have used plasmapheresis of one to two plasma volumes on a weekly basis. Concomitant immunosuppression has also been suggested.

Acute and Chronic Guillain-Barré Syndrome. The acute Guillain-Barré syndrome is an ascending motor and sensory neuropathy, which over a period for days to weeks can lead to tetraparesis and ultimately to pulmonary failure.[71] The etiology of this syndrome is not clear. In about two-thirds of cases there is an antecedent viral infection. An association with *Campylobacter jejuni* enteritis has been noted. Guillain-Barré syndrome has also been observed as a paraneoplastic syndrome. The acute disorder is usually self-limited, but some cases may progress to either a chronic progressive or a chronic relapsing pattern. Most investigators believe that this syndrome is an autoimmune phenomenon. Antimyelin antibodies have been described in many cases but have not been predictive of response to therapy. More suggestive of an autoimmune origin is the observed response of both acute and chronic Guillain-Barré syndrome to manipulations of the immune system, including plasmapheresis, high-dose γ-globulin infusion, and immunosuppression.[72–76]

Plasmapheresis is usually reserved for patients who have progressed to the stage of difficulty in walking or who have marginal pulmonary vital capacity. Three randomized trials have documented the efficacy of plasmapheresis. In the North American trial it was shown that a series of five plasma exchanges of 50 ml per kilogram of plasma resulted in a 50 percent decrease in the time required to walk unassisted and in the duration of mechanical ventilation.[73] Following a response to plasmapheresis, approximately 10 percent of patients have a brief relapse. Those who develop the chronic form of Guillain-Barré syndrome can be symptomatically relieved by chronic plasmapheresis, but chronic immunosuppression is required to maintain remission.

A recent trial has compared plasma exchange with high-dose intravenous immunoglobulin and shown the latter to be as efficacious as plasma exchange.[72] If confirmed in other studies, this would be a significant advance over plasma exchange, as immunoglobulin infusions can be begun immediately and are easier to administer in small children or cardiovascularly unstable patients.

Peripheral Neuropathy Associated With Paraproteins. It has been recognized that paraproteins associated with malignant and nonmalignant diseases seem to be associated with an increased incidence of peripheral neuropathy. Two distinct syndromes have been noted. One of these comprises a unique combination of polyneuropathy, osteosclerotic lesions, endocrinopathies, monoclonal proteins and skin changes (POEMS syndrome).[77–79] These are usually non-IgM monoclonal proteins, and their association with sclerotic lesions is remarkable as most myeloma patients manifest lytic lesions. Another neuropathic syndrome is shown by patients with IgM monoclonal neuropathies whose paraprotein can be demonstrated to have activity against myelin-associated glycoprotein.[80] This syndrome is usually not associated with Waldenström's macroglobulinemia. Because of the success of plasmapheresis in acute or chronic Guillain-Barré syndrome, another illness with documented antimyelin antibody activity, one might have hoped that plasmapheresis could be more effective than has been documented to date.

At this time there is no absolute indication for plasmapheresis in polyneuropathy. However, selected patients, particularly those with motor weakness that interferes with walking, may be candidates for a therapeutic trial.[78,81]

As the clinical symptoms in this patient population are usually not acutely life-threatening, therapeutic strategies have usually employed periods of weekly plasmapheresis for several months before determining clinical benefit. In this manner reduction in protein concentration can be achieved, and enough time will have elapsed to allow some degree of remyelination.

Renal Failure Associated With Multiple Myeloma

It is recognized that patients with multiple myeloma are susceptible to acute and chronic episodes of renal insufficiency. It has become clear that the paraproteins associated with multiple myeloma, in particular the light chains (Bence-Jones protein), are particularly toxic to the renal tubular epithelium. As long as the glomerular filtration rate remains high, light chains are usually filtered and rapidly

Hydration is the most important factor in preventing nephrotoxicity in patients with Bence-Jones protein.

excreted in the urine. During periods of dehydration, their exposure to the tubular epithelium during low urine flow is believed to result in renal toxicity. There are now more than 16 reports of plasmapheresis for renal failure associated with multiple myeloma. Response rates vary from 0 to 75 percent, with most studies showing approximately half of the patients benefiting.[82–84] This wide spectrum of activity is to be anticipated, since the causes of renal failure were multifactorial and not always reversible. However, patients with adequate pre-existing renal function who experienced an acute insult apparently benefited from the plasma exchange most, possibly because of reduction in the concentration of light chains presented to the injured kidney. Studies have not specifically addressed this mechanism.

Plasma exchange should be considered in patients with oliguric renal failure who have had other causes of renal failure reversed and who show increasing levels of Bence-Jones paraproteinemia. Plasmapheresis for chronic progressive renal failure or renal failure in end-stage diseases would not seem to be indicated.

The major endpoint appears to be to reduce the Bence-Jones circulating paraproteinemia. This should be assessed by serum protein electrophoresis, quantitative immunoglobulin determinations, and 24-hour urine collections to quantitate immunoglobulin excretion. The primary organ function can be measured by creatinine levels and creatinine clearance.

Most studies have employed semi-intensive regimens with 4 to 5 days of pheresis over a 7-day period. Care should be taken during plasmapheresis not to induce periods of hypotension or oliguria, which could further exacerbate the nephrotoxicity of light chains. This requires meticulous attention to fluid balance during plasma exchange.

Circulating Plasma Coagulation Inhibitors

Antibodies to factor VIII, factor IX, and von Willebrand factor have been noted to be formed spontaneously and following replacement therapy. These antibodies are usually of the IgG class and can become life-threatening, as they block effective replacement therapy. Removal of such circulating antibodies in conjunction with subsequent factor replacement would seem to be logical. However, there have been no large clinical trials to document this, and the limited number of anecdotal experiences do not seem to justify its routine use. Further, since very small amounts of factor VIII antibody are associated with clinical interference with factor VIII, plasmapheresis would not be expected to be as effective as a high-dose factor replacement for the treatment of factor VIII antibody.

At this time there are no established indications for plasmapheresis in this disease. In selected situations in which rapid correction of circulating coagulants is required, one could consider plasmapheresis in conjunction with factor replacement.[85] However, one should be aware that in the long run this will exacerbate the situation owing to antibody rebound.

There is no set protocol for removal of circulating anticoagulants. In general, as this is an emergent situation, large-volume exchanges on a daily basis would seem to be indicated. At this time several groups are developing specific immune absorption columns that may be capable of absorbing such factors. One column has been described in which factor IX is fixed to Sepharose columns, making perfusion with whole blood feasible, and rapid specific reduction in anti-factor IX activity has been documented.

Anticancer Therapy

Over the last century there have been numerous attempts to direct the patient's immune system to the destruction of cancer cells. Techniques have ranged from vaccination to removal of toxic or blocking substances.[23,86] 'There have been intermittent reports of responses of various cancers to plasmapheresis (with or without plasma infusion) and most recently to immunoabsorption on protein A columns (Imre Corp., Seattle). One recent study by Messerschmidt et al. reported the results of a large collaborative group study, which indicated an object response in 5 of 22 patients treated for breast cancer, 6 of 17 patients treated for Kaposi's sarcoma, and 1 of 18 patients with colon cancer.[87] If minimal responses are included the response rate in breast cancer increases to 36 percent (eight patients). While these responses are encouraging, it should be noted that no complete responses were observed and that the partial responses were transient. It is doubtful that these responses could have significantly contributed to the patient's survival.

The technology used in these studies involved perfusion of 250 to 2,000 ml of plasma through columns containing 15 to 200 mg of staphylococcal protein A. The treatments were continued three times per week for 12 treatments. In contrast to previous studies with staphylococcal protein A columns, side effects were minimal and related mainly to chills and fever. Despite this promising result, which has been documented in a multi-institution study, a definitive role for the staphylococcal protein A column in the management of cancer has not been established, nor has any other mode of plasma protein depletion.

Hemolytic Anemia

Hemolytic Disease of the Newborn. Plasmapheresis would seem to be a logical therapy for hemolytic disease of the newborn, which results from maternal antibodies being directed against red cell antigens in the fetus. However, attempts to lower maternal antibodies with plasmapheresis have in general been unsuccessful. This probably relates to the large volume of distribution of IgG and its hemolytic effect even at low titers. This subject has been recently reviewed by Rock.[88]

Autoimmune Hemolytic Anemia. In Dacie's extended series,[89] antibodies in 11 of 18 patients with autoimmune hemolytic anemia (AIHA) were more active at 37°C (warm type), while in the other 7 the activity was markedly potentiated by falling temperature. This original observation has been confirmed. Cold-active antibodies are responsible for less than half of all cases and less than 20 percent of severe ones.[9]

Warm AIHA (IgG). Warm-active antibodies causing immunohemolytic anemia are usually IgG, and rarely IgA or IgM. Reactivity is usually pan-specific for antigens of the Rh locus on the red cell but is rarely specific for one or more actual Rh phenotypes.[9]

Of Dacie's 11 patients with warm AIHA, 9 had idiopathic antibodies, causing chronic hemolytic anemia.[89] In the other two, the antibodies were secondary to lymphoblastic lymphoma and chronic lymphocytic leukemia. Hemolysis was more severe than in the idiopathic cases. The cold titers were in the normal range in nine and just above normal in two of the idiopathic cases.

Warm-active antibodies are more chronically troublesome, as their reactivity is greatest at body temperature. Most belong to the IgG1 and IgG3 subclasses, which never cause agglutination and usually do not activate complement.[9] The antibodies are mostly bound as a coating on the red cells, which is confusing to blood bank personnel, who must elute to remove blocking antibody to determine specific Rh type.

Plasma exchange in warm AIHA is not often needed but is probably useful when required for patient management. In a small series, improved red cell survival could not be demonstrated for warm antibodies, probably because they are so tightly bound.[89] However, transfusion requirements were reduced by 75 to 85 percent. Three consecutive daily exchanges removed 80 to 90 percent of warm and cold antibodies.

Cold AIHA (IgM). Cold-active antibodies are mostly directed against the I antigen present on 95 percent of adult red cells. However, they are IgM, are usually circulating free, and easily bind complement. Occasionally they have blood group A specificity, causing violent intravascular hemolysis as well as agglutination promoted by exposure to cold. (Anti-A is perhaps the strongest red cell hemolysin responsible for most fatal hemolytic transfusion reactions.) More rarely, specificity is against the B or P antigens of the red cell.

Virtually all cold agglutinin disease is caused by IgM κ-antibodies, which agglutinate red cells at low tissue temperatures, causing vaso-occlusion in peripheral cutaneous areas. Glove-stocking paresthesias and acrocyanosis are typical. Hemolysis may result from mechanical trauma or from complement activation, but the sequence is interrupted in the cold. Thus, only a brief period of overlap between IgM agglutination (cold) and complement activation (warm) produces an opportunity for dangerous hemolysis. Exchanges in cold AIHA have improved red cell survival threefold and reduced transfusion requirements by 90 to 100 percent.[90]

Individual case reports seem to substantiate the use of plasmapheresis. In cold climates many patients seek relief by spending the winter in warmer locations. In the experience of one of us (R.B.D.) with weekly plasmapheresis, one patient began spending winters at home (Baltimore) without the twice monthly hospitalizations she had required during the previous 4 years. Monthly cryofiltration provided better control of the paresthesias, relieving the hand symptoms and moving the numbness level from the upper calves down into the feet. Cryoglobulins remained negative, but brisk hemolysis recurred. Weekly plasmapheresis was resumed to control hemolysis, and paresthesias returned.[91]

Secondary Cold Agglutinin Disease. Mycoplasm (atypical) pneumonia stimulates low level anti-I IgM antibodies over 1 to 3 weeks in 80 percent of infections. In a minority of patients antibody titers become very high, abruptly causing severe hemolysis. High transfusion requirements may be reduced by plasmapheresis in this self-limiting disease. Cold agglutinin levels return to normal in 1 month. Other infectious agents, from viruses through protozoa, stimulate high-titer cold agglutinins in less than 1 percent of cases.[9]

Lymphoproliferative, usually B cell-derived monoclonal IgM may cause mild hemolytic anemia. However, hemolysis is often overshadowed by the much more troublesome hyperviscosity, as in Waldenström's macroglobulinemia.

Related cryopathic syndromes: Mixed cryoglobulins, like

cold agglutinins, involve interactions between IgM, complement, and the red cell I antigen. In addition, some cold-reactive IgG may be present, especially in chronic Epstein-Barr and hepatitis B viral infections. As in cold agglutinin disease, joint stiffness may reflect immune complex reactions in joints as well as in blood vessels.

Besides skin signs, vascular palpable purpura, and joint symptoms, neurologic involvement occurs in at least 15 percent of cryopathic patients. Central nervous system findings of headache, weakness, blindness, dysarthria, hemapheresis, and paresthesias in three patients were alleviated by 8 to 14 plasmapheresis procedures, which removed 25 to 90 percent of cryoproteins per procedure.[92]

Drug-induced hemolytic anemia, like drug-induced thrombocytopenia,[93] is usually self-limiting. The antibodies are IgG, and production ceases when the drug is stopped. However, clearance of antibody may be hastened when the antibody is not drug-dependent, as in thiazide-induced thrombocytopenic purpura.[12] The Coombs test (direct using patient's red cells with bound antibody, or indirect, using plasma antibodies with reagent red cells) has been positive in the presence of drug plus hapten with all the following drugs: penicillin, aspirin, phenacetin, *p*-aminosalicylic acid (PAS), quinine, quinidine, nitrofurantoin, stibophen, phenylhydantoin, and methyldopa.[94] Penicillin-induced immunohemolytic anemia is the prototype for haptene-dependent drug-induced hemolysis. Classically, high-dose penicillin is implicated. However, after 5 days of prophylactic penicillin one patient had profound hemolysis with a red cell half-life of 9 days, requiring transfusions.[95]

Radiographic contrast media given repeatedly has been shown by the coombs test to be the cause of IgG hemolysis requiring transfusions.[96]

Malaria. Malarial infestation in red cells can be so predominant that rapid death is accurately predictable. In one such case red cell exchange was the crucial therapy, which by reducing parasitemia from 70 percent to less than 1 percent was responsible for the patient's recovery.[97] There have been no large reported series employing plasmapheresis in a controlled manner.

Cytapheresis

Leukostasis and Leukapheresis

In the 1960s an increased incidence of hemorrhagic deaths in patients with acute leukemia and white cell counts greater than 300,000/μl was first recognized. Further, patients with high counts who underwent chemotherapy were also noted to have a high incidence of renal failure and disseminated intravascular coagulopathy. These syndromes have now come to be recognized as leukostasis and tumor lysis syndrome.

In patients with high white counts, the total cytocrit (hematocrit plus leukocrit) is a major determinant of whole blood viscosity. With white counts in the 300,000/μl range, it is not unusual to have a total cytocrit in excess of 50 percent. Usually some degree of anemia is protective in lowering the total value of the cytocrit. With high cytocrits, there is increasing viscosity and sludging in the microcirculation, particularly in patients with acute myelocytic leukemia (AML) and chronic myelocytic leukemia (CML) in blast crisis.[99] Acute lymphocytic leukemia (ALL) cells are more deformable but in high numbers can also contribute to leukostasis. Chronic lymphocytic leukemia (CLL) counts in excess of 1,000,000/μl can be observed without apparent adverse effects.

With decreased blood flow in the microcirculation, there is an opportunity for stasis, agglutination, and proliferation of leukemia cells. This results in obstruction of the vessel by "balls" of proliferating leukemia cells, which eventually violate the arterial wall and result in hemorrhage. These are characteristically seen in the brain and the lungs. Their occurrence is a medical emergency requiring immediate reduction in the total cell count.

In addition to the danger of leukostasis, patients with high white counts are also at risk for the tumor lysis syndrome at the initiation of chemotherapy. Lysis of a large number of cells results in a large metabolic load of nucleic acid material, resulting in hyperuricemia and hyperphosphatemia. Despite hydration and treatment with allopurinol, urates and phosphates can precipitate in the microtubules of the kidney and result in acute renal failure. Similarly, bioactive proteins can apparently trigger disseminated intravascular coagulopathy. In theory, reduction of cell mass in patients with high counts prior to cytotoxic therapy should ameliorate the tumor lysis syndrome.

Because of these risks many centers have recommended leukapheresis for patients with AML, ALL, or CML in blast crisis with white counts in excess of 100,000 to 200,000/μl. While most authors consider leukapheresis of high-count leukemia patients of definite benefit, there have been no randomized control studies to justify its use. Many centers still continue to treat high-count patients with emergent chemotherapy and careful attention to diuresis.

Patients with ALL and white counts higher than 200,000/μl or patients with nonlymphocytic leukemia and counts above 100,000/μl may have signs of leukostasis, including somnolence, dyspnea, and/or priapism. Patients with CLL and CML in chronic phase can tolerate much higher white counts and should not be considered candidates for leukapheresis unless clearly symptomatic.

Patients undergoing leukapheresis for leukostasis should be followed closely by measuring white cell mass with cytocrit and white cell counts. Hematocrit and platelet count should also be followed frequently. Evidence of disseminated intravascular coagulopathy should be monitored with coagulation profiles and fibrin split product screens. Electrolytes should be closely monitored in addition to serum creatinine, calcium phosphate, and uric acid.

In general, large volume exchanges are required to induce significant changes in circulating leukocyte masses. Addition of hydroxyethyl starch during the procedure is usually recommended to facilitate sedimentation and separation of the white cell mass from the red cell mass. In a 3- to 4-hour procedures, 10^{11} to 10^{12} cells can usually be removed with the reduction of the circulating leukocrit by 50 percent.[101–105] Without further treatment, leukostasis rapidly redevelops. Hence leukapheresis should usually be undertaken in close coordination with definitive chemotherapy.

Thrombocytosis and Plateletpheresis

Thrombocytosis (platelet counts in excess of 500,000/μl) is found in association with a variety of diseases, including anemia, infection, splenectomy, and many myeloproliferative disorders. Extremely elevated platelet levels (1,000,000 to 2,000,000/μl) are usually seen only with myeloproliferative disorders. Most patients tolerate thrombocytosis well. However, thrombotic episodes as well as hemorrhagic episodes have been observed in patients with high platelet counts. To date, no investigator has been able to predict which patients are at risk for serious problems.

Patients with platelet counts in excess of 1,000,000/μl and evidence of life-threatening thrombosis or hemorrhage would be considered for plateletpheresis. Care should be taken to ensure that the symptomatology is related to the thrombocytosis and not to premorbid pathology.

Patients usually undergo two to three plasma-volume plateletpheresis procedures. To prevent aggregation of platelets in the cell separator, use of ACD A with a higher citrate concentration is generally recommended. Despite this, microaggregates still occlude the tubing of the pheresis equipment. Plateletpheresis is rarely undertaken as an isolated endeavor. Concomitant therapy with antiplatelet drugs (aspirin, dipyridamole) and definitive suppression of platelets with cytotoxic agents is usually administered.

Erythrocytosis and Erythropheresis

"Blood letting" was performed centuries ago for "plethora." Erythrocytopheresis, the formal term for red cell exchange, has been formalized, as has been its indications. In summary, red cells will cause clinical hyperviscosities with cerebral vascular disease at a threshold of 47 percent hematocrit, with peripheral vascular disease at hematocrits higher than 37 percent and with sickle cell disease at a hematocrit of about 30 percent.

Red cells directly affect blood viscosity and therefore flow rate at concentrations just above normal (45 percent hematocrit) in normal-sized vessels and at lower concentrations in abnormal blood vessels. The effects of relative polycythemia are considered below; the effects of very high red cell concentrations seen in polycythemia vera are obvious.

Cerebral Blood Flow. Cerebral blood flow (CBF) is significantly influenced by concentrations of normal red cells in the hematocrit range just above normal (45 to 50 percent). Transient ischemic attacks (TIAs), strokes, and other thromboic events can be avoided by rapidly reducing red cell concentration by erythrocytapheresis. Traditionally, simple phlebotomy has been the approach as in the following illustrative study in relative erythrocytosis.

Humphrey et al.[106] significantly improved CBF toward normal (68.6 ml per 100 g/min, hematocrit 42) in 52 patients) by lowering hematocrits from 51 to 44 percent. A 33 percent increase in CBF (46 to 60 ml) ($P < .001$) was achieved in the 12 patients' high-normal red cell mass by a hematocrit reduction of 50.4 to 45 percent. In the 11 patients with low plasma volume, CBF increased from 47 to 65 ml, or 47 percent ($P < .001$) after hematocrit reduction from 52 to 43 percent.

This careful study demonstrated significant inverse correlations between CBF and whole blood viscosity ($P < .001$) for both high and low shear rates in the high-normal red cell mass group (not true polycythemia). The CBF-viscosity correlations in the low plasma volume patients were significant ($P < .05$) for both low and high shear rates. Humphrey et al. concluded that patients with hematocrits over 47 percent show a reduction in CBF, which can be significantly improved by lowering the hematocrit below 45. The experience of one of us (R.B.D.) in the hemapheresis center confirms a threshold hematocrit of 47 percent, with TIAs occurring in stable cerebral vascular disease at this level but not at lower hematocrits.

Of Humphrey's 39 patients with hematocrits of 47 to 58 percent, 16 presented with central nervous system signs or symptoms, 7 presented with TIAs, and 5 with mild completed strokes.[106] Three had hypertension, two chest pain, and one peripheral vascular disease. None had red cell mass more than 25 percent above the calculated normal value. Thus, patients with true polycythemia were excluded. it also showed that CBF was reduced from a normal of 70 ml to 56 ml per 100 g per minute in 16 patients with an average hematocrit of 47 percent. Importantly, no patient with hematocrit over 47 percent had a normal CBF.

Peripheral Vascular Disease. Peripheral vascular disease has been demonstrated to be influenced by hematocrit reduction (45 to 35 percent, hemoglobin 15 to 11 gs percent) by measuring leg blood flow in intermittent claudication. This 21 percent average reduction in hematocrit increased resting flow rate by 67 percent (1.8 to 2.7 ml per 100 g), and peak flow rate by 170 percent (2.1 to 6.0 ml per 100g), both significant at $P < .02$. Oxygen-carrying capacity by hemoglobin was increased by 20 percent (0.27 to 0.31) at rest and 50 percent (0.32 to 0.67) at peak flow, the latter being significant at $P < .02$.

In diabetic peripheralvascular disease, hemoglobin concentration was the predictor of healing of distal amputations in all 18 patients with hemoglobin below 12 g percent, whereas all patients with hemoglobin above 13 (hematocrit 39 percent) failed to heal. The threshold hemoglobin value of 12.5 g/dl, below which healing occurred and above which it did not, was significant at $P < .001$ for 59 consecutive amputations, followed for healing at 1 month. Acute normovolemic hemodilution, an operating room procedure often carried out under anesthesia, is an appropriate emergency hemapheresis procedure where available.[107] Manual methods have been routine in many operating rooms for years to conserve blood, as has autotransfusion or reinfusion of shed blood.[108] Many autotransfusion systems involve centrifuges (Haemonetics Cell Saver) or simple filters not requiring a dedicated operator.

Emergency hemodilution by either acute normovolemic hemodilution or autotransfusion systems can benefit surgical or medical patients with red cell flow abnormalities, either primary or secondary to obstructive vascular disease.

Sickle Cell Disease. *Pulmonary Sickling Syndrome.* The most common condition associated with death in the post-Osler Johns Hopkins Hospital sickle cell disease post-mortem study (72 patients and 72 controls) was "crisis," accounting for 20 percent of deaths.[109] What was then called *pulmonary bone embolus* accounted for 7 percent of deaths, with none among controls. Acute respiratory decompression, the major emergency treatment by hemapheresis (now with better management of crisis) seems to be usually a primary sickling event, not secondary to bone infarct and embolus. Importantly, widespread standard usage of supportive measures, especially hydration and oxygen has contributed to this change in presentation of the pulmonary sickling syndrome (PSS).

Raising the inspired oxygen content from the 20 percent

of room air to 100 percent in severe anemia (hematocrit 10) raises oxygen content by 50 percent. This contribution from plasma oxygen varies up to 10 percent at a normal hematocrit of 45 percent.

Red cell exchange with six units of sickle cell-negative red cell units is standard therapy for life- or organ-threatening sickle cell crisis. The goal is to raise hemoglobin A to over 50 percent.[110] Generally the hematocrit is kept below 30 percent to avoid enhancement of "log jamming" blockage by sickled cells. Thus, drawing off a unit of red cells when the hematocrit is around 30 percent is recommended before infusing a unit, even when simultaneous equivalence red cell exchange is carried out. Manual exchange can be lifesaving.

Hepatic Sickling Syndrome. Hepatic sickling syndrome (HSS) is a life-threatening medical emergency that is much less common than pulmonary sickling and sometimes accompanies the latter. Like PSS, it develops over hours to days, allowing ample time for recognition and successful treatment by red cell exchange if hemapheresis is readily available. If HSS develops rapidly, with liver function values worsening over hours, red cell exchange should begin immediately even if it has to be done manually.[110,111] In one series five episodes of HSS as the major component of multiorgan failure developed suddenly in four patients with sickle cell disease on the third or fourth day of treatment with intravenous morphine for painful crises. Four of these patients also developed acute cerebral syndrome and three developed oliguric renal failure, two requiring dialysis. All five episodes involved nonfocal encephalopathy and a rapid rise in creatine kinase, consistent with rhabdomyolysis. Rapid reversal of all abnormalities followed red cell exchange in all five episodes in the two sickle cell anemia patients, who presented with high hemoglobin (9.8 and 12.0 g percent) and high hemoglobin F (29 and 23 percent) and the two patients with sickle cell trait (hemoglobin 13.6 and 14.6 g percent). The high baseline hemoglobin level is suggested as a predisposing factor.[112]

Stroke in Sickle Cell Diseases. In a prospective study, red cell exchange reduced the rate of second strokes from 90 to 10 percent ($P < .001$) over 2 years in young people, which is one of the most dramatic interventions devised in medicine. This study has been followed by acute attempts to limit stroke.[113] In one older patient with sickle cell trait, recovery from a moderately severe hemiparesis was more rapid than predicted after a six-unit red cell exchange.

Priapism and Leg Ulcers. Priapism is an indication for emergency red cell exchange before organ-threatening hypoxia develops. Leg ulcers, a hypoxic disorder in other chronic anemias (e.g., thalassemia) becomes more complicated in sickling disorders. Red cell exchange will not often be an emergency procedure unless acute vascular compromise due to sickling occurs or gangrene sets in. Elective red cell exchange has been used to hasten healing of these ischemic ulcers and preoperatively to promote the success of skin grafting. Low steady-state hemoglobin levels are associated with a higher incidence of ulcer formation ($P < .001$) in sickle cell anemia patients. This suggests that hypoxia may be the primary event in ulcer formation, sickling being a complicating event.

Surgery and Pregnancy. Red cell exchange is appropriate preparation for surgery, especially under general anesthesia or with arterial clamping (as in joint replacements) to reduce the risk of hypoxic-sickling complications. In Baltimore preoperative red cell exchange for major orthopedic procedures in sickle cell disease patients is the practice when available.

Red cell exchange for pregnancy is thought to enhance infant survival, especially when performed in the third trimester. The early experience with red cell exchange at Howard University Medical Center established that a four-unit red cell exchange is sufficient for reducing circulating sickle hemoglobin to under 50 percent and preventing additional sickling (E. Castro, personal communication). This minimal effective red cell exchange has been continued and adopted at the National Institutes of Health.

References

1. Abel JJ, Rowntree LG, Turner BB: Plasma removal with return of corpuscles. J Pharmacol Exp Ther 5:625, 1914
2. Tullis JL, Surgenor DM, Tinch RJ et al: New principle of closed system centrifugation. Science 124:792, 1956
3. Tullis JL, Tinch RJ, Gibson JG II, Baudanza P: A simplified centrifuge for the separation and processing of blood cells. Transfusion 7:232, 1967
4. Freireich EJ, Judson G, Levin R: Separation and collection of leukocytes. Cancer Res 25:1516, 1965
5. McCullough J, Chopek M: Therapeutic plasma exchange. Lab Med 12:745, 1981
6. Guillerin L, Bussel A, Schooneman F et al: Viscosity as the symptom leading to plasma exchange. In Nydegger UE: Therapeutic hemapheresis in the 1990's. Curr Stud Hematol Blood Transfus 57:220, 1990
7. Chopek M, McCullough J: Protein and biochemical changes during plasma exchange. p. 13. In Berkman EM, Umlas J: Therapeutic Hemapheresis. American Association of Blood Banks, Washington, 1980
8. Buffaloe GW, Heineken FG: Plasma volume nomograms for use in therapeutic plasma exchange. Transfusion 23:355, 1983
9. Jandl JH: Autoimmune hemolytic anemia. p. 281. In Jandl JH: Blood: Textbook of Hematology. 1st Ed. Little Brown, Boston, 1987
10. Sprenger KGB, Huber K, Kratz W, Henze E: Nomograms for the prediction of patient's

plasma volume in plasma exchange therapy from height, weight, and hematocrit. J Clin Apheresis 3:185, 1987
11. Alving BM, Hojima V, Pisano JT: Hypotension associated with prekallikrein activator (Hageman-factor fragments) in plasma protein fraction. N Engl J Med 299:66, 1978
12. Dawson RB, Seiguer AS, Edelman BB, et al: Substitution therapy in plasma exchange. p. 65. In Nose Y, Malchesky ES, Smith JW, Krakauer RS: Plasmapheresis. Raven Press, New York, 1983
13. Huestis DW, Thomas SF: Presently available plasmapheresis techniques. p. 1. In Berkman EM, Umlas J: Therapeutic Hemapheresis, a Technical Workshop. American Association of Blood Banks, Washington, 1980
14. Flaun MA, Cuneo RA, Appelbaum FR et al: The hemostatic imbalance of plasma exchange transfusion. Blood 54:694, 1979
15. Thoriacius S, Lefvert AK, Aarli JA et al: Plasma exchange in myasthenia gravis: effect on anti-AChR antibodies and other autoantibodies. Acta Neurol Scand 74:486, 1986
16. Branda RF, Moldow CF, McCullough JJ, Jacob HS: Plasma exchange in the treatment of immune disease. Transfusion 15:570, 1975
17. Bombardieri S, Ferri C, Migliorini P et al: Immune complex behaviour during prolonged plasma exchange in essential mixed cryoglobulinemia and systemic lupus erythematosus. Int J Artif Organs 8:7, 1984
18. Wahlin A, Holm J, Hansson M, Berghem L: Plasma fibronectin levels during daily plasmapheresis. Eur J Haematol 38:39, 1987
19. Lockwood CM, Worlledge S, Path FRC et al: Reversal of impaired splenic function in patients with nephritis or vasculitis (or both) by plasma exchange. N Engl J Med 300:524, 1979
20. Imbach P, d'Apuzzo V, Hirt A et al: High dose intravenous gammaglobulin for idiopathic thrombocytopenia purpura in childhood. Lancet 1:1228, 1981
21. Maharaj D, Fell GS, Boyce BF et al: Aluminium bone disease in patient receiving plasma exchange with contaminated albumin. Br Med J 295:693, 1987
22. Hosokawa S, Oyamaguchi A, Yoshida O: Trace elements and plasmapheresis. The Int J Artif Organs 14:242, 1991
23. Dau PC: Increased proliferation of blood mononuclear cells after plasmapheresis treatment of patients with demyelinating disease. J Neuroimmunol 30:15, 1990
24. Fujishita S, Motomura M, Ohishi K et al: Plasmapheresis changes lymphocyte subsets in myasthenia gravis. p. 297. In Apheresis. Alan R. Liss, New York, 1990
25. Tsokos GC, Balow JE, Huston DP et al: Effect of plasmapheresis on T and B lymphocyte functions in patients with systemic lupus erythematosus: a double blind study. Clin Exp Immunol 48:449, 1982
26. Huestis DW: Mortality in hemapheresis (letter). Lancet 1:1043, 1983
27. Huestis DW: Complications of frequent donor cytapheresis in plasma exchange. Plasma Ther Transfus Technol 6:541, 1985
28. Huestis DW: Risks and safety practices in hemapheresis procedures. Arch Pathol Lab Med 113:273, 1989
29. Sutton DMC, Naire RC, Rock G: Complications of plasma exchange. Transfusion 29:124, 1989
30. Silberstein LE, Naryshkin S, Haddad JJ, Strauss JF III: Calcium homeostasis during therapeutic plasma exchange. Transfusion 26:151, 1986
31. Pearl RG, Rosenthal MH: Metabolic alkalosis due to plasmapheresis. Am J Med 79:391, 1985
32. Tranbaugh RF, Lewis FR: Crystalloid fluid, p. 121. In Dailey RH, Callaham M: Controversies in Trauma Management. Clinics in Emergency Medicine. Vol. 6, Churchill Livingstone, New York, 1985
33. Dawson RB, Cowley RA: Colloid fluid. p. 135. In Dailey RH, Callaham M: Controversies in Trauma management, in Clinics in Emergency Medicine. Vol. 6. Churchill Livingstone, New York, 1985
34. Russell JA, Powles RL: The relationship between serum viscosity, hypervolaemia and clinical manifestations associated with circulating paraprotein. Br J Haematol 39:163, 1978
35. Skoog WA, Adams WS: Plasmapheresis in a case of Waldenstrom's macroglobulinemia. Clin Res 7:96, 1959
36. Schwab PJ, Fahey JL: Treatment of Waldenstrom's macroglobulinemia by plasmapheresis. N Engl J Med 263:574, 1960
37. Solomon A, Fahey JL: Plasmapheresis therapy in macroglobulinemia. Ann Intern Med 58: 789, 1963
38. Beck JR, Quinn BM, Meier FA et al: Hyperviscosity syndrome in paraproteinemia: managed by plasma exchange, monitored by serum tests. Transfusion 22:51, 1982

39. Buskard NA: Blood flow studies in the hyperviscosity syndrome before and after plasma exchange. p. 89. In Borger H, Reuther P (eds): Plasma Exchange Therapy. Thieme-Stratton, New York, 1981
40. Sinico RA, Fornasieri A, Fiorini G et al: Plasma exchange in the treatment of essential mixed cryoglobulinemia nephropathy. Long-term follow up. Int J Artif Organs 8:15, 1984
41. L'Abbate A, Maggiore Q, Caccamo A et al: Long term effects of cryoapheresis and cytostatic treatment in essential mixed cryoglobulinemia. Int J Artif Organs 8:19, 1984
42. Busnach G, Dal Col A, Brando B et al: Efficacy of a combined treatment with plasma exchange and cytostatics in macroglobulinemia. Int J Artif Organs 9:267, 1986
43. Ferri C, Moriconi L, Gremignai G et al: Treatment of the renal involvement in mixed cryoglobulinemia with prolonged plasma exchange. Nephron 43:246, 1986
44. Shaw M, Fenton D, Van de Pette J, McGibbon DH: Mutilating cryoglobulinaemia rapidly improved by plasmapheresis: diagnostic features on blood film. J R Soc Med 78:37, 1985
45. Schifferli JA, Berclaz R, Ryser JE, Blanc E: Neutropenia in a patient with essential cryoglobulinemia type 1: rapid reversal by plasmapheresis. Am J Med 86:139, 1989
46. Moschcowitz E: Hyaline thrombosis of the terminal arterioles and capillaries: a hitherto undescribed disease. Proc N Y Pathol Soc 24:21, 1924
47. Byrnes JJ, Moake JL: Thrombotic thrombocytopenic purpura and the haemolytic-uremic syndrome: evolving concepts of pathogenesis and therapy. Clin Haematol 15:413, 1986
48. Remuzzi G: HUS and TTP: variable expression of a single entity. Kidney Int 32:292, 1987
49. Gasser C, Gautier E, Steck A, Siebenmann RE, Oechslin R: Hamolytisch-uramische syndrome: bilaterale nierenrindennekrosen bei akuten erworbenen hamolytischen anamien. Schweiz Med Wochenschr 85:905, 1955
50. Martin JN, Jr, Files JC, Blake PG et al: Plasma exchange for preeclampsia: I. Postpartum use for persistently severe preeclampsia-eclampsia with HELLP syndrome. Am J Obstet Gynecol 162:126, 1990
51. Bell WR, Braine HG, Ness PM, Kickler TS: Improved survival in thrombotic thrombocytopenic purpura-hemolytic uremic syndrome. N Engl J Med 235:398, 1991
52. Corvetta A, Centurioni R, Danieli G: Plasma exchange in thrombotic thrombocytopenic purpura. Curr Stud Hematol Blood Transf 57:114, 1990
53. Shepard KV, Fishleder A, Lucas FV et al: Thrombotic thrombocytopenic purpura treated with plasma exchange or exchange transfusions. West J Med 154:410, 1991
54. Taft EG: Thrombotic thrombocytopenic purpura and dose of plasma exchange. Blood 54:842, 1979
55. Shulman NR, Aster RH, Leitner A, Hiller MC: Immunoreactions involving platelets. V. Post-transfusion purpura due to a complement-fixing antibody against a genetically controlled platelet antigen: a proposed mechanism for thrombocytopenia and its relevance in "autoimmunity". J Clin Invest 40:1597, 1961
56. Cimo PL, Aster RH: Post-transfusion purpura: successful treatment by exchange transfusion. N Engl J Med 287:290, 1972
57. Deardorff WL: Exchange transfusion vs. post-transfusional purpura. SENN J 2:1, 1972
58. Laursen B, Morling N, Rosenkvist J et al: Post-transfusion purpura treated with plasma exchange by haemonetics cell separator. Acta Med Scand 203:539, 1978
59. Mueller-Eckhardt C: Autoimmune thrombocytopenic purpura: diagnostic and therapeutic actualities. p. 68. Curr Stud Hematol Blood Transf 55:68, 1988
60. Branda RF, Moldow CF, McCullough JJ, Jacob HS: Plasma exchange in the treatment of immune disease. Transfusion 15:570, 1975
61. Williams C, Buskard N, Bussel J: Plasma exchange in idiopathic thrombocytopenic purpura. Curr Stud Hematol Blood Transf 57:131, 1990
62. Bussel JB, Saal S, Gordon B: Combined plasma exchange and intravenous gammaglobulin in the treatment of patients with refractory immune thrombocytopenic purpura. Transfusion 28:38, 1988
63. Guthrie TH, Oral A: Immune thrombocytopenic purpura: a pilot study of staphylococcal protein A immunomodulation in refractory patients. Semin Hematol 26:3, 1989
64. Bensinger WI, Buckner CD, Clift RA et al: Plasma exchange for platelet alloimmunization. Transplantation 41:602, 1986
65. Norris FH, Denys EH, Mielke CH Jr: Plasmapheresis (plasma exchange) in neurologic disorders. Clin Neuropharmacol 5:93, 1982
66. Dau PC, Lindstrom JM, Cassel CK et al: Plasmapheresis and immunosuppressive drug therapy in myasthenia gravis. N Engl J Med 297:1134, 1977

67. Mason PD, Pusey CD: Plasma exchange in nephrological diseases. Curr Stud Hematol Blood Transf 57:152, 1990
68. Antozzi C, Gemma M, Regi B et al: A short plasma exchange protocol is effective in severe myasthenia gravis. J Neurol 238:103, 1991
69. Eaton LM, Lambert EH: Electromyography and electrical stimulation of nerves in disease of motor unit. JAMA 116:1117, 1957
70. Dau PC, Denys EH: Plasmapheresis and immunosuppressive drug therapy in the Eaton-Lambert syndrome. Ann Neurol 11:570, 1982
71. Ropper AH: The Guillain-Barré syndrome. N Engl J Med 326:1130, 1992
72. Van Der Meche FGA, Schmitz PIM, The Dutch Guillain-Barré Study Group: A randomized trial comparing intravenous immune globulin and plasma exchange in Guillain-Barré syndrome. N Engl J Med 326:1123, 1992
73. McKhann GM, Griffin JW, Cornblath DR et al: Plasmapheresis and Guillain-Barré syndrome: analysis of prognostic factors and the effect of plasmapheresis. Ann Neurol 23:347, 1988
74. Osterman PO, Vedeler CA, Rybert B et al: Serum antibodies to peripheral nerve tissue in acute Guillain-Barré syndrome in relation to outcome of plasma exchange. J Neurol 235:285, 1988
75. Vriesendorp FJ, Mayer RF, Koski CL: Kinetics of anti-peripheral nerve myelin antibody in patients with Guillain-Barré syndrome treated and not treated with plasmapheresis. Arch Neurol 48:858, 1991
76. Vedeler C, Nyland H: Plasma exchange in Guillain-Barré syndrome: effect on antiperipheral nerve myelin antibodies. Acta Neurol Scand 82:147, 1990
77. Imawari M, Akatsuka N, Ishibashi M et al: Syndrome of plasma cell dyscrasia, polyneuropathy, and endocrine disturbances: report of a case. Ann Intern Med 81:490, 1974
78. Uldry PA, Steck AJ: Plasma exchange in neurology. Therapeutic hemapheresis in the 1990s. Curr Stud Hematol Blood Transf 57:167, 1990
79. Delauche MC, Clauvel JP, Seligmann M: Peripheral neuropathy and plasma cell neoplasias: a report of 10 cases. Br J Haematol 48:383, 1981
80. Hafler DA, Johnson D, Kelly JJ et al: Monoclonal gammopathy and neuropathy: myelin-associated glycoprotein reactivity and clinical characteristics. Neurology 36:75, 1986
81. Haas C, Tatum AH: Plasmapheresis alleviates neuropathy accompanying IgM anti-myelin-associated glycoprotein paraproteinemia. Ann Neurol 23:394, 1988
82. Zucchelli P, Pasquali S, Cagnoli L, Ferrari G: Controlled plasma exchange trial in acute renal failure due to multiple myeloma. Kidney Int 33:1175, 1988
83. Johnson WJ, Kyle RA, Pineda AA et al: Treatment of renal failure associated with multiple myeloma: plasmapheresis, hemodialysis, and chemotherapy. Arch Intern Med 150:863, 1990
84. Pasquali S, Cagnoli L, Rovinetti C, Rigotti A, Zucchelli P: Plasma exchange therapy in rapidly progressive renal failure due to multiple myeloma. Int J Artif Organs 8:27, 1984
85. Silberstein LE, Abraham J, Shattil SJ: The efficacy of intensive plasma exchange in acquired von Willebrand's disease. Transfusion 27:234, 1987
86. Israel L, Edelstein R, Mannoni P et al: Plasmapheresis in patients with disseminated cancer: clinical results and correlation with changes in serum protein. Cancer 40:3146, 1977
87. Messerschmidt GL, Henry DH, Snyder HW Jr et al: Protein A immunoadsorption in the treatment of malignant disease. J Clin Oncol 6:203, 1988
88. Rock G: Plasma exchange for antibody removal in hemolytic disease of the newborn. p. 100. In MacPherson JL: Therapeutic Hemapheresis, Vol. 2. CRC Press, Boca Raton, FL
89. Dacie JV: Acquired hemolytic anemia with special reference to the antiglobulin (Coombs') reaction. Blood 8:813, 1953
90. Silberstein LE, Berkman EM: Plasma exchange in autoimmune hemolytic anemia, abstracted. Blood: 182a, 1982
91. Dawson RB, Bilenki LA, Wenk RE: Increased albumin levels within two weeks of starting twice-weekly plasma exchange. J Clin Apheresis 2:139, 1984
92. Berkman EM, Orkin JB: Use of plasmapheresis and partial plasma exchange in the management of patients with cryoglobulinemia. Transfusion 20:171, 1980
93. Rachmilemitz EA, Dawson RB, Rachmilemitz B: Serum antibodies against desipramine as a possible cause for thrombocytopenia. Blood 32:524, 1968
94. Dawson RB: Drug induced blood dyscrasias, prevention and diagnosis. Med Times 96:671, 1968
95. Dawson RB, Segal BL: Penicillin-induced immunohemolytic anemia. Arch Intern Med 188: 575, 1966

96. Nordhagen R, Vik H, Wolthius K et al: Immune-immediate hemolysis associated with the administration of radiographic contract medicine. Transfusion 31:843, 1991
97. Morrison FS: Erythrocytapheresis in the management of fulminant falciparum malaria. J Clin Apheresis 2:143, 1984
98. Stuby U, Kaiser W, Biesenbach G, Zazgornik J: Successful treatment of malaria tropica with acute renal failure and cerebral involvement by plasmapheresis and hemodialysis. Infection 16:362, 1988
99. Lichtman MA: Rheology of leukocytes, leukocyte suspensions, and blood in leukemia. J Clin Invest 52:350, 1973
100. Huestis DW, Corrigan JJ, Johnson HV: Leukapheresis of a five-year old girl with chronic granulocytic leukemia. Transfusion 15:489, 1975
101. Carpentieri U, Patten EV, Chamberlin PA et al: Leukapheresis in a 3-year-old child with lymphoma in leukemic transformation. J Pediatr 94:919, 1979
102. Lane TA: Continuous-flow leukapheresis for rapid cytoreduction in leukemia. Transfusion 20:455, 1980
103. Kamen BA, Summers CP, Pearson HA: Exchange transfusion as a treatment for hyperleukocytosis, anemia and metabolic abnormalities in a patient with leukemia. J Pediatr 96:1045, 1980
104. Strauss RA, Gloster ES, McCallister JA et al: Acute cytoreduction techniques in the early treatment of hyperleukocytosis associated with childhood hematologic malignancies. Med Pediatr Oncol 13:346, 1985
105. Bunin NJ, Kunkel K, Callihan TR: Cytoreductive procedures in the early management in cases of leukemia and hyperleukocytosis in children. Med Pediatr Oncol 15:232, 1987
106. Humphrey PRD, Marshall J, Russell R et al: Cerebral blood flow and viscosity in relative polycythemia. Lancet 2:873, 1979
107. Stehling L, Zauder HL: Acute normovolemic hemodilution. Transfusion 31:857, 1991
108. Hauer JM, Thurer RL, Dawson RB (eds): Autotransfusion. The First International Autotransfusion Symposium, Baltimore. Elsevier, New York, 1981, p. 152
109. Haupt HM, Moore GW, Bauer TW et al: The lung in sickle cell disease. Chest 81:332, 1982
110. Klein HG, Garden RJ, Miller DM et al: Automated partial exchange transfusion in sickle cell anemia. Transfusion 20:354, 1980
111. Charache S: Treatment of sickle cell anemia. Annu Rev Med 32:195, 1981
112. Hassel KL, Lane PA: Acute multi-organ failure complicating vaso-occlusive sickle cell pain crises in patients with relatively high baseline hemoglobin levels, abstracted. Blood 78:413a, 1991
113. Russell MO, Goldberg HL, Hodson A et al: Effect of transfusion therapy on arteriographic abnormalities and on recurrence of stroke in sickle cell disease, abstracted. Blood 63:162, 1984
114. Leitman S, Hill EA, Moore RC et al: Efficacy of erythrocytapheresis in the treatment of sickle cell disease. Blood 78:199a, 1991

INDEX

Page numbers followed by t *indicate tables.*

B

C

D

E

G

N

O

P

Q

R

T

W